T0258025

Caring for Patients

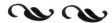

A CRITIQUE OF THE MEDICAL MODEL

Allen B. Barbour

Stanford University Press ⌘ *Stanford, California*

Stanford University Press
Stanford, California
© 1995 by the Board of Trustees of the
Leland Stanford Junior University

Printed in the United States of America

CIP data are at the end of the book

For Joan ↝

Author's Preface

∾ From one-fourth to one-half of the more persistent illnesses we see in medical practice do not respond well to the medical model of diagnosis and treatment we employ. Doctors recognize that these include the common functional disorders with predominantly somatic symptoms as well as the nervous states and depressive reactions with emotional symptoms. Personal distress unrelated to the disease itself can also be a major factor in the intensity and disabling capacity of many organic diseases.

We are well trained to diagnose and treat organic disease. But the illnesses caused mostly by personal distress constitute a far greater problem for medical practice. Diagnosis is sometimes deferred indefinitely. Extended but futile or misleading workups are not uncommon. Or, the illnesses are correctly diagnosed, but the care is restricted to the naming and treatment of symptoms. There may be little attempt to understand the underlying human problem situation. The illness persists or recurs because its source remains unattended.

This book (1) presents a critique of the medical model, its pros and cons, and especially its pitfalls and limitations when applied without perspective; (2) delineates how the faults and inadequacies of the model too strictly applied can be obviated by a better understanding of the relation of the illness to the life of the patient; and (3) outlines the goals, attitudes, concepts, and methods of a more comprehensive, more effective, person-centered care.

This book is not about being kind, thoughtful, or responsive to patients.

These are essential attributes of good care in any circumstance. By *person-centered care* I refer specifically to becoming familiar with the patient's personal situation in its crucial relationship to the source of illness.

Helping patients surmount the impact of chronic organic disease is a traditional concern of medical practice and an important aspect of care. The challenge of rehabilitation, of living as full a life as possible in spite of the disease, is covered in an extensive literature, of which I shall cite here only the major contributions of two Stanford investigators, Moos [1–2] and LeMaistre. [3] But again, these matters are not what this book is about. Here I will focus mainly on the personal distress that *causes* illness rather than the distress that *results from* the disability of chronic disease.

The book is addressed primarily to doctors, medical students, and care providers generally, both in medical and in psychotherapeutic practice. But the medical process, its problems and possibilities, is also of general interest, and the book is intended to provide such broader understanding, as well. Though written in the language of medicine, it is addressed to anyone concerned about the human elements of illness, healing, and health.

My interest in these matters began to take form when I saw my first patients as a medical student. I was an idealist, as are most health-care professionals. I had entered medical school with a scientific background and an insatiable curiosity about human nature. Science was clearly the basis of medicine. I had also read Freud, Jung, Adler, and William James, and although I questioned the validity of certain psychoanalytic postulates, I believed that human behavior and psychological illness could generally be understood. The purpose of medical care, I believed, was to understand the cause of illness and to remove or alter the cause so that healing could begin. The cause might be organic disease, it might be psychological or social, it might involve stress, alcohol or substance abuse, health habits or other problems of human life, or some combination of factors. No matter: I assumed that medical science and/ or psychological understanding could reveal the source of the problem and offer ways to help. I was attracted to general internal medicine as a specialty that combined technical skills with an opportunity to know and work with patients at many levels. So I was interested in all kinds of illness and tried to understand the cause whenever possible.

After six years of residency and fellowship training at the University of California Medical Center in San Francisco, the Massachusetts General Hospital, the Postgraduate Medical School of London, and a tour of duty in the U.S. Navy Medical Corps during World War II, I entered private practice as a general internist with my partner and brother, Donald C. Barbour. I also attended the wards and clinics of the U.C. Medical School as a member of the clinical faculty. After ten years of practice I joined the full-time faculty of the Stanford University School of Medicine as head of the Division of General Internal Medicine. My primary responsibility was the "G.M.C." (General Medicine Clinic) and the Stanford Diagnostic Clinic, its patients, students, and residents.

In medical school I had discovered that medicine was not what I had earlier supposed it to be. I was dismayed by the inordinate split between medicine and psychiatry. In medicine you do not "do psychiatry"; you diagnose and treat disease. In the clinics, however, there were few diseases but many symptoms, and the system of diagnosis and treatment often didn't seem to work very well. Excluding respiratory-tract infections, the most common problem in private practice, I found that organic disease adequately explained the illness in only about one-third of my patients. In fully another third, the illness was strictly functional, with somatic (or "psychiatric") symptoms, i.e., caused by human situations.

Here and throughout the book I use the phrase *human situations*, alternatively *personal situations*, to include all of the stresses, health practices, habits, physical strains, existential dilemmas, personality and behavior patterns, and emotional and social difficulties that can cause illness. These are all personal situations *that can be improved*. In the remaining third of my cases, the patients did indeed have a disease process, but the actual *illness*—that is, *all* of the symptoms and disability—was caused mostly by psychosocial distress not specific to the disease itself. This three-part breakdown is of course approximate, for there are no sharp divisions between these categories, but a similar analysis, with similar categories, appears consistently in published surveys of primary practice (references in Ch. 4).

With perhaps as many as half my patients, I learned that if I didn't know the person I didn't really understand the illness. And if I had no real understanding, it was less likely that the patient would become well, although a diagnosis—tension headache, for example—could be made and something— an analgesic or tranquilizer—could be prescribed to relieve symptoms. That, however, was not satisfying, not why I went into medicine, and usually the symptoms persisted or recurred anyway. I really wanted to understand the source of illness, whatever it was. Not knowing left me intellectually dissatisfied, and seemed unscientific. Care was far more effective when the patient and I came, *together*, to understand the roots of the illness, whether at the physical or the personal level, and better still when something positive could be accomplished at either level.

At the personal level, I found, realistic change in stressful life situations, relationships, attitudes, behaviors, or habits could not always be readily achieved simply because some understanding had been reached about what was most needed. Nevertheless, at that point the patient would have options, paths to health, that had not previously been clear, and that scientific medicine alone had not provided. Most important, the patients became participants in their own health care.

Most patients want to understand their illness. They appreciate the opportunity to share their problems, whether they initially think they can do much about them or not. Some will then make dramatic personal changes and improve immediately. Most feel better from some combination of symptomatic therapy and an understanding of the underlying problems, though real changes can only be made over time. A few patients—surprisingly few, to judge from what I had been led to expect—do not want to share their concerns and feelings and insist on strictly medical interpretations of what are in fact straightforward psychosomatic illnesses.

All in all, if the patient and I—thus you and your patient—collaborate to determine the underlying problem situation and to combine what the patient can do about it with what medicine can do to relieve symptoms, we begin a far more effective patient/doctor relationship. It is also an easier, more satisfying, more straightforward, and more honest relationship. It means fewer visits, tests, drugs, unreasonable demands, and expectations. It is far less costly, and in the long run it takes less time. Gaining an understanding of who, why, and what the patient is all about is obviously most important when the illness itself can be understood in no other way. These points will be demonstrated throughout the text by illustrative case histories.

In contrast, when we try to explain and cure everything solely by the workups, diagnostic labels, and therapies of biomedicine, not only does the patient fail to get well, but serious trouble ensues. Diagnostic stalemates or frank errors, erroneous or misleading workups, ineffective treatments, habituating or hazardous drugs, and even unnecessary surgery are inevitable. Expensive, high-tech diagnostic procedures, often ordered in the search for a disease explanation of what are really unrecognized functional disorders, constitute a major component of the soaring costs of modern medical care.

My patients, and all they have taught me about their lives, illnesses, and medical care, provide the data base for the concepts in this book. The case histories cited are accurately recounted, although I have altered the names and identifying details sufficiently to preserve anonymity. Equally important are the creative perceptions of the students, residents, and colleagues with whom I have shared the unparalleled opportunity medicine offers to know and help patients.

More specifically, I want first to thank the many people who have contributed constructive criticism to the writing of this book: in particular my brother and former partner, Donald Barbour, family members Luzia Krull and Roger Hamilton, and colleagues David Burns, Irvin Yalom, Peter Rosenbaum, Halsted Holman, Daniel Federman, Harold Sox, Jr., Peter Rudd, Robert Glaser, Edward Rubenstein, Barry Rosen, Gustave Freeman, Lincoln Russin, Ami Laws, Dewleen Hayes, Sally Rubenstone, Arnold Gelb, Perrin Cohen, Anne Bergman, Virginia Fowkes, George Hogle, Gene Carragee, David Spiegel, Kelley Skeff, Page Acree, and the late Elinor Kamath.

I am eternally grateful to Richard Blum, who reviewed the entire book, and to my publisher, Stanford University Press, its directors, formerly Grant Barnes and now Norris Pope, and its editors, Muriel Bell, Peter J. Kahn, and William W. Carver.

My deep appreciation goes to Kathy Kirchen, B. J. Kramer, Janice Mason, Mary Kirby, and Nancy Sully, who so uncomplainingly transcribed my many undecipherable drafts to the word processor, and to the Stanford medical librarians who so ably assisted my library research. My thanks also to George Lopatin for his work with literature reviews.

Many thanks go to Stuart Miller and Sara Miller and my colleagues of the Institute for the Study of Humanistic Medicine for the rich experience and early support of the project.

I am grateful for the financial support provided by Bill and Mel Lane, by the Ford Foundation's emeriti faculty development program at Stanford, and by Ted Shortliffe, Chief of the Division of General Internal Medicine at the medical school.

I extend special thanks to Earle Marsh, my mentor during medical-school training.

I was particularly enriched by the close collaboration with my colleagues in the Stanford General Medical Clinics, notably with William Fowkes for the countless hours we spent discussing medical practice, with Mark Perlroth, who directed the clinics during my sabbaticals, with Michael Jacobs, for his ongoing encouragement and wisdom, and with the students and residents, who, in turn, became my teachers.

I have enjoyed the loving support of my family. I thank you all: Sandy, Kent, Grant, Stephanie, Lance, Kim, Kent, and my wife, Joan, who has edited the entire book with me and has been a steadfast inspiration throughout the writing.

A. B.

Portola Valley, Calif.
July 1993

Dr. Allen Barbour died rather suddenly on August 8, 1993, when the manuscript for this book was completed. Allen was a retired professor of clinical medicine at Stanford University School of Medicine. Throughout his forty-year career of clinical experience and teaching, he sought a deeper understanding of the link between the psychosocial aspects of a person's life and the source of illness. His teachings of colleagues, residents, and students in this domain are revered by many.

Through his short illness, the strong advocacy and collaboration of his wife, Joan, and her commitment to the final editing posthumously are a tribute to his memory and this legacy of his life's work.

Virginia Fowkes

Senior Research Scholar
Director, Primary Care Associate Program,
Stanford University School of Medicine

A Note to the Reader

William C. Fowkes, M.D.

∾ I had the privilege of working with Allen Barbour for many years in the Stanford General Medical Clinic and was greatly influenced by his teaching. We spent many hours discussing the kinds of patients described here, and I was an early reader of the drafts of what is now this fascinating book. I have seen some of the patients whose cases are presented in the pages that follow myself, often at times when Allen was not available. I have again and again had the usefulness of the approaches to patients described in this book validated in my own clinical experience, and I believe it is must reading for all physicians who are on the front line of patient care.

In reading the book a final time in proofs, I realized that Allen has presented increasingly difficult scenarios as the book proceeds, and that the relatively "quick cures" in the initial examples may be viewed by some readers as unrealistic. If one stops reading after only a few chapters, the examples may appear atypical, the approaches simplistic, and the conclusions superficial. I particularly want to urge those readers who may react skeptically at the outset to read on. You will see that Allen understands the complexities of the approach he uses, and also recognizes that it will sometimes fail with certain patients—as is the case with all our ministrations.

Whether through modesty or oversight, Allen has not described the precise steps by which he came to classify a patient's illness as being of psychosocial origin. On pp. 183–85, Allen has reported his series of 400 patients seen in the Stanford Diagnostic Clinic and has categorized their illnesses according to organic or psychosocial causation. Again, the skeptical reader may ask, How did Allen finally decide the problem was of psychosocial origin? When we find a specific organic cause whose removal cures the difficulty, we are quite safe in attribution. But how do we decide a problem is psychosocial in origin? In fact, Allen followed an extremely rigorous and meticulous process by which this was done. This involved, first, the complete review of all records available about previous care; second, the interview and physical examination of the patient in the manner described in the text, utilizing many innovative techniques to facilitate discovery; third, the repetition of appropriate previous tests and new testing as needed (though there were certainly times when no further testing was indicated); and fourth, elimination of any organic etiology.

I feel it important to stress that Allen's categorization of illness by organic or psychosocial causation was dependent on the fourth step—elimination of any organic etiology. This determination was based on his clinical judgment, the patient's and/or the patient's referring physician's acceptance of the non-organic etiology, improvement in the course of the illness after intervention, or long-term follow-up either by visits to the clinic or by phone during which time no new organic disease manifested itself. Though we have not established for psychosocial diagnosis the equivalent of Koch's postulates for determining organic disease, the process outlined above—which Allen followed scrupulously—seems the very best possible. I hope you experience, as I did, the excitement of the revelations contained in this work.

Contents

Introduction   1

PART I. The Need for a Person-Centered Perspective

1. *The Limitations of the Medical Model*   9

    *Illnesses as Expressions of Human Predicaments, 12; Splitting
    Patients into Minds and Bodies, 15; Bypassing the Human
    Situation, 23; Knowing What Is Really Wrong, 28*

2. *"What This Patient Needs Is a Doctor"*   31

    *The Doctor's Diagram, 31; Understanding the Personal
    Situation, 38; Two Sides of the Doctor's Diagram: The Emphasis
    Varies, 40; Characterization of Person-Centered Care, 41;
    The Meaning of Care, 43*

3. *The Concept of Disease*   45

    *Disease as Pathological Reality vs. Disease as Conceptual
    Model, 46; Disease as Specific Etiology, Pathogenesis, and
    Treatment, 46; Disease as Disturbance of Structure, 47;
    Disease as a Question of Control over the Pathogenic Forces*

That Lead to the Illness, 52; Disease as Treatability, 54; The
Concept of Disease and the Systems View of the Ill Person, 55

4. **Personal Illness: The Functional Disorders   58**

The Common Functional Disorders with Pain, 59; The Common
Functional Disorders Without Pain, 60; Illness Caused Primarily by
Personal Situations: Prevalence and Recognition, 61

5. **Personal Illness: The Concept of Care Determines
the Outcome   67**

The Concept of Personal Illness, 68; The Patient: Who Is This
Person?, 70; Learning and Growth in Human Illness, 73;
The Medical and Growth Models Compared, 77

6. **Diagnostic Strategies for Unrecognized Personal Illness   81**

Not Making a Diagnosis: Begging the Question, 82; A Diagnosis
Is Established, but Does It Explain the Illness?, 85; Inappropriate
Correlation of the Symptoms with Abnormalities Found in the
Workup, 85; Inappropriate Naming of a Functional Syndrome
as Though It Were a Disease, 92; The Inherent Iatrogenicity of
the Medical Model, 93

7. **Health Practices, Psychosocial Distress, and
Organic Disease   96**

Health Practices and Harmful Habits, 96; Sexual Behavior, Disease,
and Teen Pregnancy, 100; Psychosocial Distress as Precursor to
Disease in General, 100; Psychosomatic Disease, 103; Is Cancer a
Psychosomatic Disease?, 105; Health: Whose Responsibility?, 108

8. **Psychiatric Disorders: The Medical Model in Perspective   112**

The Medical Model of Psychiatry, 113; The Genetic Background of
Psychiatric Disorders, 117; Panic and Anxiety: Emotional Distress
or Brain Disease?, 122; The Psychobiologic Unit, 128

9. **Psychiatric Disorders: Is Feeling Depressed a Disease?   135**

The Spectrum of Feeling Sad, Discouraged, Despondent,
Depressed, 136; The Biology of Major Depression, 138;
The Psychological Basis of Depression, 141; Psychotherapy

*and Depression, 143; "Endogenous" Depression?, 144;
The Continuum of Anxiety and Depression, 145; The
Specificity of Antidepressants, 148*

10. Barriers to Person-Centered Care   151

*The Physician's Point of View, 151; The Patient as Unwitting
Partner in a "Conspiracy," 153; The Organization of Medical
Practice, 155*

PART II. Emotions and Emotional Symptoms

**11. Cognitive/Emotional Dissociation: A Common Cause of
Illness   163**

*Emotional Behavior in Animals, 164; Emotional Behavior in the
Human Species, 166; Cognitive/Emotional Dissociation as the
Cause of Clinical Symptoms, 168; The Major (Cognitive) and
Minor (Intuitive/Emotional) Hemispheres, 170; How Cognitive/
Emotional Dissociation Affects Our Lives, 172; The Dilemma for
Patients and Their Doctors, 173; The Ideal: An Integrated
Personality 176*

12. Emotionally Induced Physical Symptoms   179

*Definitions, 180; Psychophysiologic Reactions, 181; Somatoform
Disorders, 182; The Prevalence of Psychophysiologic Reactions and
Somatoform Disorders, 183; Distinguishing Characteristics of
Psychophysiologic Reactions and Somatoform Disorders, 185;
Somatoform Pain Disorder: Making the Diagnosis, 188; The
Somatoform Disorder: Function and Process, 191; How Emotionally
Induced Symptoms Are Described by Patients, 197; The Spectrum of
Patients with Emotionally Induced Physical Symptoms, 201*

13. Functional Syndromes: Differential Diagnosis   204

*Psychogenic Chest Pain, 205; Chronic Abdominal Pain, 215;
Chronic, Persistent Pelvic Pain, 220; Low Back Pain, 223;
Chronic Fatigue, 228; Aching All Over, 235; Chronic Recurrent
Headaches, 241; Nervous Tension, 244; Problem Drinking, 249;
Pseudoseizures, 251*

PART III. Person-Centered Care

14. *Collaboration Begins: The Medical History 257*

    Listening, 258; Meeting the Patient, 262; Opening the Medical History, 262; The Symptoms: How Does the Patient Feel Sick?, 264; Creative Listening, 265; Emotions and Nonverbal Clues, 269; The Medical History in Perspective, 271; Health-History Questionnaires, 274

15. *Misunderstandings and Hidden Issues   278*

    Common Covert Issues, 279; Secondary Gain, 283; Alternate Belief Systems, 286

16. *Collaboration Continues: First Talks About Personal Illness   287*

    Integrating the Medical and Personal Phases, 288; Opening the Interview, 289; Medical Explanations, 291; Naming the Illness, 291; The Workup, 295; The Patient Parries, 296

17. *The Core of the Collaboration: The Personal Interview   301*

    The Directed Interview, 301; Some Common Problem Areas, 306; The Joint Interview, 324

18. *Engaging the Patient   327*

    Shifting Responsibility, 328; Referrals, 330; Helping Patients Find Their Own Path, 334

    Literature Cited   339

    Index   387

Caring for Patients

Introduction

అ There are many good reasons for our failure to know our patients, particularly the constraints of time and the enormous demands of modern clinical science. We can't do everything. But, pondering this question over the years, I realized more and more that the core problem lay deeper in our thinking: it was the medical or disease model itself, the very process of reducing all patients and all illnesses, regardless of the nature of the illnesses, to the diagnostic names and treatments of disordered parts. We become enmeshed in our own model even when it doesn't work. The model, of course, is absolutely essential for the organic disease to which a scientific approach does apply, and it helps us to understand and relieve some of the symptoms of functional and psychiatric disorders as well, but when it is extended, as a strictly biomedical approach, to the many illnesses caused predominantly by personal situations, the core problem is bypassed in the process of reduction. And that is precisely what we learn to do, except perhaps in a few psychiatry lectures. In the typical medical-school commencement address we are advised to consider the "whole patient," but by then we have been so insidiously locked into the medical model as a solution to *all* clinical problems that we rarely question the process again.

It could be argued, of course, that the problem lies not so much with the model as with the doctors who use it. After all, the patient's history, as taught in medical school, is not just about symptoms and disease. It includes a personal and social survey, and emotional and psychological problems are not excluded. There is no rule against understanding the human situations that cause so much illness, and the medical model in no way prohibits warm, personal, sensitive interactions between doctors and patients. But the medical student soon discovers that the model *actually applied in practice* by most house staff and attending physicians is far more restricted than what was taught in the introduction to clinical medicine. Furthermore, students and residents in training are soon immersed in the management of serious organic disease, mostly on hospital wards where they are overwhelmed by the demands of modern care. There is little time to know their patients as persons. Doctors who try may be viewed as "soft," or as taking too much time away from more important tasks, when they attempt to do so. In my critique of the *medical* model, therefore, I refer to the actual *biomedical* model so commonly applied in practice, rather than to the ideal model taught in the second year of medical school.

Because the physician is mainly trained to think biologically, *medical* comes to mean *biological,* and the *medical* history is rarely pursued in sufficient depth to detect the psychosocial basis of illness, even when that is the main problem. The personal/social history is usually superficial, compartmentalized, and not integrated with the symptoms and other data described in the *present illness* or *review of systems.* Finally, the diagnostic *impression* or *appraisal* is recorded in medical or psychiatric terminology from which the underlying personal situations are almost always excluded, unless a term like *adjustment disorder* (rarely used in primary care) is applied.

The medical model, to be sure, is based on an obvious need for the classification and treatment of disease and illness. But our inordinate focus on this model also results from conventions in clinical thinking that have more to do with our need to find ways to name and treat what we see, to simplify and organize practice, than with understanding our patients or what they need from us. Many axioms of practice, whether effective or ineffective, about how doctors ought to think and act are passed down from one generation of physicians to the next unquestioned. Because so many of these conventions, which define the medical model as inviolable, are such automatic responses, they have taken control of our clinical thinking; we no longer seem capable of evaluating them critically. Instead we think primarily in reductionistic terms. Often we cannot perceive whether this process is appropriate, overly restrictive, or wholly irrelevant.

The problem, then, lies not with doctors personally—with their caring qualities—but with the model in which we have been so indoctrinated. I have known perhaps a thousand doctors in 40 years of private and academic practice, and I know my colleagues, with few exceptions, to be dedicated to the best possible care. But the best care has been defined for us as the biomedical model.

By and large, we were trained for seven straight years, twelve or more hours daily, in medical school and hospital residency, to think disease, diagnosis, and treatment as the sole means of managing illness. The model is embedded in our very bones, and it becomes almost impossible to think clinically in any other way. The illness *is* the disease. That is our problem, and I was no exception. My training led me into every difficulty, every trap, to be described in this book. We focus far more on the "disease" or the "psychopathology" than we do on the person who has it. Even when the illness is caused primarily by human situations, we reduce it to names and nostrums. Or, if we can't make a diagnosis, or the patient fails to improve, we may still believe that we are "doing all that can be done" by ordering more tests and more treatments.

A single-minded biomedical approach is not the only barrier to person-centered care. There are many others (Ch. 10). In this book, however, I will focus on the medical model, because it is not readily perceived how the model, the very foundation of clinical thinking, can be a problem in itself. It is perhaps the least understood and least discussed problem of medical practice.

Since Case Western Reserve University School of Medicine (Ohio) revised its curriculum in the 1950's, the curricula of several other medical schools have been reorganized to emphasize the care of patients as persons in family and social systems as the central focus of medicine. Some curricula are built around community-oriented primary-care programs. [1] Other schools have simply added comprehensive-care courses, beginning in the first year, or comprehensive-care clinics in the third or fourth year, without changing otherwise traditional curricula. Follow-up studies at Case Western Reserve [2] and at the University of Rochester School of Medicine (New York) [3] show an appreciable impact. Nevertheless, most medical schools remain divided into separate basic sciences and clinical departments, with disease the central focus in both. Notwithstanding the innovations introduced at a few schools, [4] and the introduction of better training in interviewing skills and understanding family problems, the reduction of illness to the diseases and treatments of the medical model continues to dominate the mainstream practice of medicine.

The erosion of the patient/doctor relationship engendered by our dominating biomedical focus, and the necessity for greater balance with the needs of patients as persons, have been emphasized in many thoughtful reviews of medical education and practice coming from both within and outside our own profession. [5–17] The elements of a more integrated approach have been described in the writings of our best clinicians, of which I cite but a few. [18–26] Here, with the fundamental goals of medicine in mind, I shall examine the inherent faults and limitations of the medical model. I shall propose some new and more effective ways to view and work with patients. We will see if the illness can be viewed as a signal for understanding, an opportunity for some kind of personal change or growth. As difficult as this may be, it is often the way the healing begins.

Nothing in this book, however, is intended to minimize the fundamental importance of the medical model for all patients. I need not recount here the monumental achievements of medical science. For the many diseases and injuries that respond readily to medical or surgical treatment and are, for the most part, isolated events in the life of the patient, the model is not only necessary, but also sufficient. And for those patients whose illnesses are not so isolated, the medical model is still the foundation of a comprehensive approach. For even with functional disorder, we must first *identify* the illness as one in which personal elements are likely to be important, before we can proceed to explore what those elements may be. Accurate diagnosis is essential. But when the illness includes significant personal causes or consequences, the model itself needs to be incorporated into a more comprehensive framework. The overriding principle must be the need to recognize the human elements in illness, if only to practice good medicine with sound judgment and effective action.

Obviously, a busy practitioner has very little time for each patient, and nonpsychiatric physicians are not always trained for emotional disorders or taught interviewing skills. It will be argued by some that the very concept of person-centered care is unrealistic, that it is simply incompatible with the economic constraints of practice. So it is. Nevertheless, the barriers can be surmounted in many ways (Ch. 10), certainly for those patients whose courses along strictly medical paths are desultory if not disastrous without a deeper understanding. This understanding depends on the physician's motivation to develop a capacity to focus on the central issues, and to move steadily into effective interactions with patients within the time-scale of general examinations and office visits. Alternatively, the necessary understanding might be initiated by a psychosocially oriented colleague, counselor, or therapist, if not by the primary physician personally.

Is understanding possible? Do patients really change? Yes, patients in a medical office are usually aware of the personal situations causing their symptoms or resulting from chronic diseases, and they will tell us about them *if we can learn to listen.* The unconscious conflicts of psychiatry are less common. In the Stanford Diagnostic Clinic, many a student, not yet "well trained" in medical-model practice, has perceived readily what the real problem was—a troubling personal situation—and determined the correct diagnosis of what was really a psychosomatic symptom complex. The referring physician had failed even to consider the correct diagnosis. The student, however, listened!

Patients often remark how a previous physician would not listen, even when they had tried to share the source of their nervous tension. Patients do change and get well.

Untangling the psychosocial dimensions of an illness and turning that diagnostic information into meaningful improvements for the patient can be relatively straightforward, or it can be complex and time-consuming. Many illnesses can be understood and worked out *only* in the context of a stable and caring patient-doctor relationship.

I do not pretend that I can even begin to understand most patients as well as I would like to. I may not find the time. The patient may not respond. And even with the best rapport, understanding can be difficult, or the patient may find no way to make any changes. But unless we keep in mind what might be possible, the healing path is blocked.

Many physicians, I believe, will find a person-centered approach both fulfilling for themselves and crucial for their patients. After all, the repetitious cycle of symptomatic names and remedies that characterizes so much of modern medicine is often not very satisfying. But when the patient is helped to resolve an illness through creative interaction at the personal level, especially when this is found to be the key to understanding the illness, the physician is rewarded by a very special kind of interpersonal relationship and professional satisfaction.

The book is meant to be provocative, and to open options. I do not have answers to as many questions as I will ask, nor have I the only answer to each. If the book serves only to stimulate its readers to question their concepts and modes of practice, and to find their own, better, ways, it will have achieved its objective.

PART I

*The Need for a
Person-Centered Perspective*

The Limitations of the Medical Model

In this chapter, we review the difference between ILLNESS *and* DISEASE, *delineate the essence of the medical model, examine several case histories that illustrate certain inherent problems of the model, and consider how such problems can be surmounted by a more comprehensive view of illness.*

ᕀ Let's begin with what we do so well:

Marjorie L. felt "lightheaded, dizzy." She had noted no vertigo, faintness, disequilibrium, or other symptoms. I knew her from previous checkups to be a sprightly widow of 79 in good health. The past medical history was not noteworthy. On this visit she was found to have atrial fibrillation with a ventricular rate of 150. Digoxin reduced the rate to 70. The symptoms disappeared, and she became well.

Marjorie was indeed the "good patient" we hope to see at every medical encounter. A specific disease with a specific therapy! The medical solution to this problem, as for all clinical problems, is based on the medical or disease model, a concept of illness and a process of resolution so intrinsic to medicine that we rarely pause to consider just what it is, what it does, or what it cannot do. What, then, *is* the model, and how is it applied?

Its core structure is an analysis by which symptoms and physical signs—the complex, mostly subjective phenomena known as *illness*—are reduced to a more specific disordered part, the *disease,* to which science can then be applied. *Illness*—the way in which the person feels sick, functions, hurts, suffers, worries, coughs, throws up, notes something that seems abnormal, etc. refers to a *person,*—whereas *disease*—the pathology, a circumscribed entity identified by predefined objective criteria—refers to a *part.*

The analytic process follows a standard format: examination (history, physical examination, laboratory tests) → diagnosis → treatment. Underlying the model is the implicit assumption that the *illness* (sickness) described by the person, now called a *patient,* indicates a disordered part, or pathology, called the *disease* or *disorder,* which is the cause or basis of the illness. If the disordered part is a structure, it is a *disease* (in Marjorie's case, mitral stenosis). If the disordered part is a functional disturbance of normal structures, it is viewed simply as a *disorder.* When the functional disturbance is physical (tension headache, hyperventilation syndrome, impotence), the illness is known as a *functional disorder.* When the functional disturbance involves mood or emotions (anxiety, depression), thoughts, personality, or behavior, the illness is viewed as a *psychological* or *mental disorder.*

Our purpose is to classify the entity in our nomenclature of disordered parts, called *diagnosis;* to determine the cause, if possible; and to apply a biomedical *treatment* to remove the cause (penicillin), obliterate the pathology (appendectomy), modify its effects (insulin), alter the physiological disturbance (tricyclic antidepressants), or block the symptoms (codeine). The treatment plan includes education of the patient about the condition, with specific instructions regarding related health practices (diet, rest, exercise) or noxious behaviors (smoking, drinking, drugs).

The process is exquisitely designed for its purpose. It works with great precision whenever the disordered part diagnosed fully accounts for the whole illness and its treatment restores the whole system to health. That's how Marjorie got well.

The achievements of scientific medicine result from its remarkable capacity to analyze and alter disordered parts right down to the molecular level. If a patient's illness is due to pneumonia, thyrotoxicosis, cancer, coronary artery disease, myopia, aortic insufficiency, Colles' fracture, phenylketonuria, or any of a host of other diseases and injuries to which medical technology properly applies, the disease model is critical. It is logical and effective. We are fully trained to detect disease and to apply the model to all patients:

Joseph H., 67, also felt "lightheaded, dizzy," beginning 18 months before referral to Stanford. He too noted no specific vertigo, faintness, disequilibrium, or other symptoms, and here again the past medical history was, as we say, "not remarkable."

This time, though the illness appeared similar to that of Marjorie L., the physical exam and routine laboratory tests were negative. Like all physicians in this situation, his doctor pondered: What disease? The differential diagnosis included cerebrovascular insufficiency, cerebellar and demyelinating diseases, a beginning primary degenerative dementia, vestibular disease, acoustic neuroma, and Adams-Stokes syndrome, among others. A workup, completed a step at a time, included EKG, EEG, aortic arch and cerebral arteriography, consultations in neurology and ENT with electronystagmography, audiometry, and other special tests. All studies were negative. Magnetic resonance imaging (MRI) might well be done too today, but this patient was seen prior to the introduction of such techniques.

The working diagnosis then fell into a category of "dizziness of unknown etiology, possibly arteriosclerosis." For three months Joseph failed to respond to therapeutic trials of Hydergine, vasodilators, the "anti-vertigo" antihistamines (although there was no vertigo), and anticoagulants (warfarin). At one point a diagnosis of "depression" was considered, but his illness continued unabated on tricyclic "anti-depressants" for two more months. After all this he was indeed discouraged, as was his doctor. A Stanford consultation was requested.

What went wrong here? Why did the model, which functioned so well for Marjorie, fail Joseph, even though his doctors applied it conscientiously? Was a disease overlooked?

Diagnostic problems are most often solved in my experience, not by more tests, but by a meticulous exploration of the symptoms *just as they are.* Illness is eloquent, and often speaks for itself. So I started by asking Joseph to describe precisely what he meant by "feeling dizzy" and how often he felt that way. To my surprise, the source of his illness was clear from his initial response:

"Doctor, I feel dizzy nearly all the time since my wife died. I don't know what to do with myself. I'm confused. I watch TV, but I'm not interested. I go outside, but there's no place to go." He looked sad indeed as he told of the emptiness of his life. He had moved to California with his wife after retirement. He had no children, no close friends, no special interests.

The crux of the problem here was obvious, though it was revealed more readily than such problems usually are. "Dizzy" was Joseph's way of expressing his confusion. He was a lonely man who had not yet assimilated his grief or learned to develop a new life. His personal situation *was* the clinical problem, and the key to its solution. Biomedical science, attempting to provide answers to the wrong questions, was not a sufficient paradigm through which to view the illness. What Joseph needed was personal understanding rather than biomedical treatment. Only then could a physician begin to outline a plan for health. With the help of our clinical social worker he was slowly guided to accept and surmount his grief and to discover new meanings, friends, and activities. The "dizziness" abated, and over the ensuing five years he remained well. Loneliness is not in the medical nomenclature. Medicalizing it as "depression," and then treating the resulting "psychopathology" with tricyclics, affords neither relief nor change until something is done to relieve the loneliness.

Here we encounter the core problem of medical practice. Unlike Marjorie's illness, caused by specific disease that responded to a specific treatment, Joseph's illness could not be reduced to a disease entity. His symptoms reflected a human situation—the problem of a person rather than the disease of a part. The medical model serves well for illness caused primarily by organic disease—albeit with serious limitations when we know no specific cause or cure. Its limitations are poignantly apparent, however, whenever significant personal problems bring on an illness, or compound an illness associated with organic disease. No matter how hard we try, technology will not help us recognize, understand, or solve human problems in medicine.

Illnesses as Expressions of Human Predicaments

Human situations, problems, and stresses of many kinds are certainly the major cause of the common functional "medical" illnesses that abound in our daily practice: recurrent headaches; chronic weakness and fatigue; various combinations of breathlessness, palpitation, dizziness, and nervousness, or disturbances of normal physiology, especially eating, sleeping, and sexuality; and backache, muscle tension and chronic pain syndromes, nonischemic anterior chest pain, chronic abdominal or pelvic pain, or dyspeptic and irritable-bowel syndromes or other functional GI disorders.

Similarly, failure to cope successfully with the exigencies of the human condition is the main cause of most psychiatric disorders, especially the emotional disturbances of anxiety, panic, and depression so commonly diagnosed and treated in primary care. And personal situations, entwined with the lifestyles of our culture generally, underlie the common clinical problems and diseases associated with tobacco, alcohol, and drug use, abuse, and dependency.

All of these kinds of illness are essentially expressions of human predicaments. Each has biological components, to be sure, as do tears or laughter, but the disordered part that is diagnosed is the *symptom*, not the core problem.

In a patient like Joseph, the doctor's concerns about disease were, of course, entirely appropriate. The symptom of dizziness must be explored to see if it fits a medical category—vestibular dysfunction (vertigo), disequilibrium, presyncope, sensory deficit, dementia, each with its particular differential diagnosis. What wasn't done, however, but could have been, was to listen carefully for the *emotional* aspects of the symptom and the associated human condition. This would seem to be an essential component of the "present illness," for emotional situations are major contributory factors to the dizziness of about 40 percent of the patients with this complaint in primary care. [1] What is rare, for example, is Ménière's disease, [1–2] though this term is sometimes used as a synonym for dizziness and is thereby overdiagnosed. An emotional basis should be seen as a distinct possibility when the dizziness appears not in transient attacks but as a mild, nonspecific, steady state; is not in any way rotational, subjectively or on special testing; fits no special medical category; and yields a general examination that is quite negative, as it did with Joseph.

We are trained to detect disease. To do so, we ask questions. But we are not trained to listen. In one study of 15 physicians, for example, the mean elapsed time from the moment their patients began to express their primary concern to the doctor's first interruption was 18 seconds. [3] From there on the physicians took control of the interview by asking increasingly specific, closed-end questions. The other side of this problem is that we are not well trained to explore or recognize physical symptoms as expressions of emotional distress. Worse still, we labor under an injunction, a medical taboo, as absurd and unwise as it is ancient, that we must rule out every conceivable organic disease *before even considering the possibility* of a psychological disorder. In this frame of mind it is unlikely that the physician will ever get to the source of an illness like Joseph's.

Thus Joseph's doctor did exactly what he was trained to do. Conscientiously seeking to help his patient, he considered every medical diagnosis and tried every test and treatment.

Now suppose this doctor had adopted, from the beginning, a comprehensive approach, and had recognized, from the beginning, the possibility of a psychosomatic symptom. He would still have to decide how much workup to do to rule out possible disease.[1] This calls for careful judgment individualized to each patient. It is true, for example, that "feeling dizzy" without rotation or other symptoms can appear in transient ischemic attacks as the first symptom of cerebrovascular disease (9 percent of a consecutive series of 483 confirmed cases at the Massachusetts General Hospital). [4] The dizziness of these patients was not the vague, constant feeling described by Joseph, however. This study concluded that "feeling dizzy," when an isolated symptom, even in transient attacks, is so rarely vascular that it is best watched carefully rather than approached as a likely vascular problem. Much of the workup, especially the arteriograms, could have been omitted in this case.

In ordering tests, two concerns are paramount. First, an abnormality, if found, should adequately explain the illness; even if Joseph's arteriography had demonstrated occlusive disease, this would not have explained his particular symptoms. Second, the workup, negative or positive, should serve to resolve the diagnosis; if the illness is likely to be emotional, and the workup, sometimes an extensive study, is necessary to be sure, then so be it. When the illness is indeed emotional, however, the investigation must culminate at some point in a definitive judgment in which doctor and patient together understand the illness for what it is. In Joseph's case, however, there was no endpoint. The tests and treatment trials could have gone on indefinitely.

For patients like Joseph the medical model goes awry in several ways. First, when the illness cannot be made to fit some specific category of disease or disorder, it becomes a diagnostic problem, and no resolution is achieved, even at the diagnostic level. Seventy percent of the patients referred to the Stanford Diagnostic Clinic had functional disorders; the referring physicians had failed to make the correct diagnosis because of the extraordinary predilection of many doctors for diagnosing disease, with a corresponding reluctance to recognize functional illness or its personal source. Joseph was such a patient. This can happen to any patient with any symptom not clearly caused by disease, particularly a patient with vague or diffuse symptoms, multiple symptoms indicating no single disease entity, or chronic pain syndromes lacking distinct pathology. Although referred patients are a select group that does not represent the random problems of primary care, there is a useful precept here. In modern medicine there should be few diagnostic problems of undetected organic disease; what still seems enigmatic after an appropriate clinical investigation may well be a functional disorder.

Alternatively, when the illness *does* fit a specific category of functional or psychiatric disorder, then a diagnosis can be established, but how far does that take us? Suppose, for example, that Joseph's reaction to the stress of loneliness had been to develop headaches, to be more depressed than he was, or to drink excessively. Any of these eventualities could occur under similar circumstances, depending on individual proclivities. At the diagnostic level, medical resolution could then be achieved with tension headache, depression, or alcoholism, but at the human level, therapy, though helpful, would result in little resolution. The headaches would recur again and again, no matter what drugs gave temporary relief. Antidepressants are rarely effective in bereavement or adjustment disorders of this kind, and they failed to help Joseph. A patient can terminate alcoholism, of course, by not drinking, usually with the help of an abstinence program, and that is a major achievement in itself. But what cries out for understanding and resolution here is Joseph's lonely predicament.

Any physician encounters a series of problems in cases like this. First are the biomedical problems of differential diagnosis. Nevertheless, the correct diagnosis of a functional illness can be suspected from a careful analysis of the symptoms and the negative workup, even though little is known about the patient personally. Next comes the problem of understanding the underlying difficulty. This can be easy, as it was with Joseph, or it may take some time, even with skillful psychotherapeutic interactions. The third difficulty is convincing the patient. Although Joseph readily furnished the necessary psychosocial data, it took several months for him to accept the fact that this was the whole source of the illness. The final problem is that of effective change. Joseph was reluctant to get involved with a seniors group, and, when finally there, was slow to open up to new relationships. Nevertheless, all this was finally realized.

Joseph illustrates what can be accomplished in person-centered care, as will the other patients with functional disorders whom we shall discuss here. With some patients, however, little or no healing occurs, because there are too many blocks to diagnosis and understanding, or the patient cannot, will not, or for whatever reason does not change in any way, even though the diagnosis, the human situation, and the changes necessary are all clear and obvious. Both the diagnosis and the path to healing may be difficult, but the process does not even begin if the patient founders upon the diagnostic and therapeutic trials of the medical model. All possibilities should be considered from the very beginning.

Splitting Patients into Minds and Bodies

Is the narrow focus of a biomedical model really such a common problem in practice, or was Joseph's condition unusual? The condition, clearly, is not unusual; nonspecific dizziness is a common symptom, as are all manner of functional disorders representing most systems of the body. Was the focus on disease simply the aberrant approach of one doctor with poor clinical judgment? No, not at all; the attempt to solve clinical problems within the medical model is quite conventional, in both primary and specialty practice. Let's shift now to a prestigious medical center where the model evolves even as medical students and residents are being trained.

> *Ruth B., age 21, was a dental assistant, married. Her entire care was administered at one such center by 16 highly trained physicians on 20 outpatient visits (four to the emergency room) and three hospitalizations on the gynecology service.*
>
> *Ruth's main symptom was a persistent pelvic pain unrelated to menstrual*

periods, mostly in the right lower quadrant, with occasional vomiting and constipation, dysuria, irregular menses, and headaches. The illness began two months after a normal delivery and persisted, virtually unchanged, through the 19 months of care. Physical examinations were repeatedly negative except for minimal tenderness in the right lower quadrant of the abdomen and adjoining pelvis on bimanual pelvic exam. The usual screening laboratory tests of blood and urine, cervical and urine cultures, and vaginal secretions were negative.

Culdoscopy, dilatation and curettage (D and C), and a pelvic pneumogram were done on the first two hospitalizations, along with a barium enema and X-rays of the lumbosacral spine. When these studies were negative, a consultation in internal medicine was requested, at which the possibility of porphyria or allergic vasculitis was suggested. Finally, on the third hospitalization, an exploratory laparotomy and appendectomy were performed. The abdomen, pelvis, and appendix were entirely normal. By then, Ruth had lost 15 lbs.

During the 19 months, her 16 doctors had recorded 20 possible diagnoses and tried four drug treatments. The organic diagnoses considered included urinary-tract infection, colon disease, pelvic inflammatory disease, right ovarian cyst (?twist, ?rupture), appendicitis, possible pregnancy (?infected abortion), biliary-tract disease, and hypothyroidism. Psychological diagnoses included anxiety and "psychological reaction," but these were deemed to be "functional overlay," meaning that they were superimposed on some more real underlying disease process. Thus, other sources of anxiety were not explored. Nondescript diagnoses included "lower, or acute, abdominal pain, etiology undetermined," or "due to obscure cause." On some visits the impression was simply "pelvic pains," or no appraisal of any kind was recorded. Ruth had also complained of recurrent headaches and once that "I cannot move my legs," but these symptoms were compartmentalized to their respective body parts and never viewed as parts of the same illness.

Following the negative laparotomy Ruth was referred to the medical clinic. If she were referred to you, what would you do?

In this clinic she encountered a student physician not yet indoctrinated to believe that pain is caused purely by organic disease. He noted the startling correlation of her emotional state with 19 months of continuous pain, and his primary appraisal was that of an emotional illness expressed as pelvic pain. This particular young physician-to-be—kindly, accepting, open-minded—encountered no difficulty in eliciting her material and sexual difficulties. And this particular patient was not at all resistant to the psychosocial interpretation of her illness. She had been ready throughout to share her story with anyone willing to listen.

Actually, she *had* been given one opportunity to share it, with the single psychiatry resident called in consultation during the second hospitalization, six months previously. He not only had listened but had made the correct diagnosis, and recommended a psychological approach. To make a point: none of the physicians attending Ruth then or subsequently had paid any attention to his recommendation, nor had they referred her on to someone who would. It was as though her doctors were not really interested in her personal history; it got in the way of their quest for the elusive disease.

As this case demonstrates, we have evolved a truly appalling practice of splitting our patients into minds and bodies, relegating the former to the "shrinks," the latter to "real" doctors—a schizophrenia of care. The cleavage between medicine and psychiatry inevitably grants the medical doctors a license to disregard what is "psychological," because there is someone else "to do it" if it really becomes necessary. But we don't stop there. We go on to divide bodies into parts, each with its own specialist, every specialist with an advanced technology to rule out that part as the source of disease. Each doctor "rules out" but not "in." There is no one to put Humpty Dumpty back together again. After a negative coronary arteriogram, the cardiologist, for example, diagnoses "nonischemic chest pain" but does not seek to determine if the pain could be emotionally induced, or, if so, to understand the human situation well enough to find out, possibly, what really does cause the pain. Nor does anyone else. Yet that is what the patient needs most of all.

Fortunately for Ruth, the medical student was able to do this in a very few visits by broadening his approach from parts to wholes, to the person and her illness. In this way he was able to understand the personal situation, which was the true "etiology," to make a positive and accurate clinical judgment of psychogenic pain disorder, which represents the diagnosis of an illness rather than of a disease, and, finally, to stimulate the patient to act as a healing force in her own behalf. Most significantly, he did not restrict his responsibility to "disease." He assumed responsibility for the patient as a person, which is the guts of what it means to be a doctor. Our eternal quest for the disease—our process of ruling it in or out—should be the means to an end, not an end in itself. We are supposed to solve problems, not create them.

Ruth's pain abated soon after her first encounter with the student and subsequent joint discussions with Ruth and her husband. With some understanding of the illness and its relation to the underlying tensions in her life and marriage, the couple was able to approach these problems constructively. When seen for a minor illness one year later, Ruth confirmed that she remained well. Note that healing was brought about by a very simple concern and understanding. It required no psychiatric training, no formal psychotherapy.

I do not mean to imply that all patients with this kind of problem do as well as Ruth, any more than that all patients with functional dizziness do as well as Joseph. Healing, nevertheless, often begins with a comprehensive evaluation, clear and honest communication, a concerned physician, and a responsive patient. The outcome cannot be predicted, but it is worth the try.

I chose Ruth's case from a major teaching hospital to illustrate my point about training: it is there that we all learn to detect disease, but not necessarily to understand patients, symptoms, or illness. The 16 physicians who failed to make the correct diagnosis represented as high a standard of practice as there is in the medical community. The residents in gynecology, internal medicine, and surgery would all be certified by their respective specialty boards, and their attendings were already certified. They did exactly what they were trained to do, and they did it well. If Ruth had had an ectopic pregnancy or pyosalpinx, it would have been detected right off.

Note, by the way, the erudite introduction of porphyria and vasculitis in Ruth's differential diagnosis. Like other internists, nothing quickens my academic heart more than the diagnosis of an obscure disease. With regard to abdominal pain I once made a diagnosis of porphyria in a patient who had remained undiagnosed in a major hospital for a year. On another occasion, on a house call, I made a bedside diagnosis of hyperlipoproteinemia type 1 with pancreatitis when I noted the peculiar color of the lipemic serum through the arteriolar walls on ophthalmoscopy. And I have seen two patients with vasculitis causing abdominal pain. That's it: four cases of these three diseases in 40 years of practice! Abdominal pain due to emotional stress must outnumber these three diseases 1,000 to 1. Although it may be well to rule out rare conditions at some point, it is statistically absurd to put them ahead of a functional pain syndrome in the differential diagnosis. In formulating clinical judgments we should never ignore probability altogether, but that is what we often do, because we are taught so little about the prevalence of nondisease or functional illness as the cause of symptoms (Chs. 4, 11–13).

Ruth was fortunate to have had a strictly normal pelvis, anatomically. She eventually recovered with her pelvis intact. But what if she had been found to have a right ovarian cyst? Here we come against still another core problem of the medical model. In our earnest quest for disease to explain symptoms, what happens when we find one? We are very likely to terminate the quest and explain the illness by the disease.

Janet F., 36, married with two sons in their teens, employed part-time in a dress shop, came to Stanford from another state complaining of relentless pain in the right lower quadrant for three years, her complaint no different from Ruth's. In addition to contrast studies of the entire GI tract, gall blad-

der, and urinary tract, one laparoscopy with D and C, and innumerable special tests for rare diseases, she had undergone three laparotomies. At each laparotomy a medical diagnosis was made and treated accordingly. The pain, nevertheless, was severe and continuous, and it recurred shortly after each procedure.

At the first laparotomy, performed two months after the illness began, a right corpus luteum, recently ruptured with a small amount of serous fluid, was noted. A normal appendix, but not the ovary, was removed. At the second, seven months later, a total hysterectomy was performed by another surgeon who noted a "slightly boggy" uterus and two 1-mm red spots on the pelvic floor he thought might be endometrial implants. The pathologist, however, noted only uterine adenomyosis. In spite of the hysterectomy, as well as hormonal suppression for possible residual endometriosis, Janet's continuous pain persisted. One year later she was referred to a major teaching hospital where the gynecologist still considered endometriosis to be the most likely diagnosis and performed the third laparotomy. He released a few adhesions, described the ovaries as adherent to the lateral pelvis wall, and removed both tubes and ovaries. There was no evidence of endometriosis or any other lesion on surgical or pathological examination. I will not describe the many tests, X-rays, diagnosis of "pinched nerve," steroid, Xylocaine, and B_{12} injections, acupuncture, etc., that then ensued in her care by other doctors.

What would your approach have been if Janet had come to you? What would you have done when the pain recurred after the first laparotomy?

Most doctors, I believe, even had they not learned in detail the problems of Janet's marriage, or the divergent personalities of Janet and her husband, would have appreciated the emotional basis of this pain syndrome had they been present when Janet broke out in a tumultuous fit of anger about her marital situation during my second interview, with her husband present.

Emotionally induced pain can be expressed in two ways. It may be physiologically mediated, as in muscle-contraction headache or irritable-bowel syndrome. Or it may be experienced in the absence of a physiological disturbance. This second kind of pain, now known as a *somatoform disorder* (Ch. 12), was formerly described as a *conversion reaction*. Chronic pelvic pain, as with Ruth and Janet, is predominantly somatoform. But whether Ruth's pain was regarded as somatoform, or as mediated through colonic spasm, or both, was beside the point. What mattered was the underlying emotional turmoil. Regardless of the mechanism, the pain is *psychogenic* insofar as this term is used generically to mean emotionally induced. In this sense, any symptom complex, if emotionally induced, is *psychogenic*, whether physiologic, as with the tachycardia and hyperventilation of anxiety, or somatoform, as with Janet. We need to be clear about this, because the term *psychogenic* is often used to distinguish somatoform from physiologically mediated pain, as in descriptions of headaches, but its meaning is not so restricted in this book.

In Janet's case the ruptured corpus luteum could have caused transient pain but not the sustained pain that had already been present for two months. The uterine adenomyosis may have caused some menstrual distress prior to the hysterectomy. But it is unlikely that these lesions, the endometriosis, which was either minimal or nonexistent, or the adhesions, had much of anything to do with the intense, intractable pain that characterized the whole illness. Even a frank ovarian cyst, uterine fibroids, or some endometriosis, if otherwise uncomplicated, would hardly explain the magnitude and continuous quality of this pain. Unfortunately, medical practice abounds with spurious correlations between symptoms and abnormalities found in blood chemistry, X-ray, EKG, surgery, all kinds of special tests—a general problem we will examine in more detail in Chapter 6.

Janet's pain disappeared permanently after a few visits eight years ago, when she was last seen. She later divorced, but then developed other symptoms customarily associated with nervous tension. Eventually, she got into sustained counseling, made other changes in her life, and improved generally. I cannot be sure this illness could have been reversed if the correct diagnosis had been made after the first laparotomy, but that juncture clearly called for a comprehensive clinical judgment rather than a series of medical diagnoses and operations having nothing to do with the illness. At least she might have been saved the next two operations.

Unfortunately, I have seen many, many women like Janet referred for continuing pain after their pelvic organs are gone, removed one at a time in a relentless attempt to cure the pain. Even when the pain recurs after a negative exploration or the removal of a minor lesion, the doctor often fails to consider the possibility of psychogenic pain. The next doctor simply records "status post hysterectomy," etc., without writing for the case history or questioning whether the previous diagnoses were valid explanations of the illness, as was finally done with Janet. With each new diagnosis and treatment, nothing is done about the real illness. Sometimes the patient is blamed for being "surgery prone," even though it is the doctors who recommend and perform the operations, without explaining to the patient that what was found was not sufficient to explain the pain. As the disease model becomes entrenched in this way, it becomes more and more difficult to reverse the process, to understand and heal.

The problem here is compounded by a deeper problem of medical thinking that has to do with the magic of naming. When we can name something we create the illusion that we know what we are doing. Whether the names are right for the findings at the operations but wrong for the illness, as were corpus luteum, adenomyosis, and adhesions in Janet's case, or wrong for both, as was the endometriosis, the names stick, label the patient, and govern our actions. Here, the diagnosis of endometriosis—never demonstrated, merely a conjecture all along—actually resulted in a third operation. Many physicians find it difficult to accept the concept of psychogenic pain of any kind. In patients like Ruth, when no abnormality can be found, the diagnosis switches to physiologic names, such as tension myalgia of the pelvic floor, levator spasm syndrome, pelvic congestion syndrome, pelvic sympathetic syndrome, or the names of neuralgic, arthralgic, or inflammatory conditions used in other countries. The source of the pain must be strictly physical! But the names represent little more than different views of the same condition. Again, however, once the condition is named, that's it! The names fix our thinking. We are diverted into a one-track diagnostic/therapeutic impasse, when what really matters, regardless of the name or the physiology, is to recognize the illness as the emotional expression of a person and not the coincidental disorder of a part. That is the key issue. The name should be the beginning, not the end, of understanding.

Psychogenic pain disorders of the somatoform type are common in both men and women. Sixteen percent of 400 consecutive patients whom I examined in the Stanford General Medicine Clinic had this kind of pain. It tends to focus on sites of previous pain provoked by some disease or injury, or by physical strains or menstrual cramps, especially where the area in question has emotional significance. In men the focus is often on the back or other sites of industrial injury (see Ch. 2), whereas in women this kind of pain often settles in the lower abdomen and pelvis (Chs. 6, 12, 13). I do not refer here to the biologically painful physiological event of dysmenorrhea, or to premenstrual tension syndrome, but rather to a quite different kind of relentless distress all through each month, month after month, as with Ruth and Janet, caused neither by pelvic disease nor by the stressful events of normal reproductive physiology.

Pelvic pain in women is a common symptom, and the ubiquity of psychogenic pain, as a subgroup of patients with pain, was noted long ago by the gynecologists who first studied the question. [5–9] The incidence has been estimated at from 5 to 25 percent of all gynecologic patients, [10] and the syndrome has been elucidated in many careful studies in which there is general agreement about the background and personal difficulties of these women. [11–15] (See also the discussion of other aspects of this problem in Chs. 6 and 13.) If this kind of pain, like dizziness in both sexes, is that common, then all gynecologists should be thoroughly familiar with the differential diagnosis. Unfortunately, many are not. Other gynecologists, oriented to a comprehensive approach, recognize the problem and help their patients to work with its emotional source.

The dominance of the conventional disease-model approach to these patients is obvious from a review of 11 major reference textbooks of gynecology. Psychogenic pain is clearly described in only three. [16–18] In two it is briefly mentioned, but with many reservations, suggesting an organic basis for most cases. [19–20] In six texts, this common condition is omitted altogether. [21–26] Most texts provide no comprehensive approach to the clinical problem of chronic pelvic pain, though the pain of every disease is described, each in its own separate section. If no disease is found, the patient is simply "reassured." The emphasis is strictly on the disease, not the illness or the person in pain. The disease focus also characterized 16 other gynecologic texts surveyed, except for Leonide Martin's *Health Care of Women*, [27] a book by a nurse practitioner for nurse practitioners, and the medical texts of Hale and Krieger [28] and Swartz, [29] which offer excellent descriptions of psychogenic pelvic pain and helpful approaches to the patient.

As with the textbooks, the management of patients varies from doctor to doctor and from one medical center to another. The goal of gynecologists, one might presume, would be the best possible care of the women who consult them. Trained in one institution, gynecologists may indeed view that care broadly as the *health care of women*, their special needs, problems, and illnesses associated with sexuality and the reproductive system, whether physical or emotional. Where gynecologists have been trained in another institution, however, the "care" is restricted to the *detection and treatment of disease*. As emphasized previously, what happens to the patient may be completely different from one situation to the next, depending solely on the physician's concept of care.

The problem of chronic pelvic pain is not an easy one for the doctor. In any somatoform pain disorder the symptom may serve a subtle, unconscious purpose, such as release from a disagreeable job, compensation, avoiding sex, getting sympathy, or expressing hostility (Ch. 12). The patient, unaware of the conversion process at conscious levels of mental activity (though, at dissociated levels of consciousness, knowing very well what is going on), may then deny any problems and appear to be convinced that the pain is caused by a disease the doctor will fix. In this way the emotional aspects of pain, which may be the crux of a chronic pain problem in men or women, are not apparent at first, to either the patient or the doctor. Unless approached judiciously in conjunction with a comprehensive workup, the patient may well resist a psychological interpretation. I have failed to sort this out, sent patients inappropriately for surgery, and other doctors have had to correct my error. This happens to most doctors from time to time, no matter how hard we try to think of everything. In pelvic pain the problem is complicated by the ubiquity of ovarian cysts, fibroids, adhesions, and other lesions, which, though nearly always painless, must be sorted out. Laparoscopy may well be necessary. As for any illness, the cause should be determined by technical procedures, personal interview, or whatever other investigation is appropriate, but the whole process should lead to a realistic appraisal, with the doctor fully aware from the very beginning that some symptoms such as chronic pain can be primarily psychogenic (Chs. 12, 13).

When I encounter a patient with the kind of continuous pain that suggests an emotional source, and a negative physical examination, I have learned to make a special effort to understand the patient's whole situation, explaining that life tensions can aggravate any pain, or even *cause* pain in some patients. If I have discussed this possibility beforehand, then, even though a workup may be necessary, the patient and I are better prepared to use the normal findings as a positive step toward a definitive approach to the real problem, and the surgeon, apprised of the general problem, is less likely to fix the diagnosis on asymptomatic lesions.

Obviously, we need to learn to recognize symptoms for whatever they are: expressions of disease, or personal problems, or both. Any physician, trained to be concerned about all aspects of illness, could have reversed the medical train of events in the three patients cited above, at many points in their care. There were plenty of clues: the symptoms themselves; their unusual course, relentless nature, and emotional tone; and the negative exams and workups, certainly the negative culdoscopy in Ruth and the first negative laparotomy in Janet. The perceptions necessary to understand the nature of the illness begin at any time from the first encounter on through the workup. The physician is indeed responsible for the detection and treatment of disease—no one else can do that. But the greater responsibility is to make an accurate judgment about the whole illness, its nature and its cause, whatever it may be, and to outline whatever needs to be done, by the patient as well as the doctor, to attain health.

Bypassing the Human Situation

It is difficult for those of us trained in medical-model thinking to recognize the extent to which the human situation is invariably bypassed by the reductive process of diagnosis and treatment. The diagnosis of a functional disorder (irritable-bowel syndrome, for example) or an emotional disorder (anxiety or depression) seems to provide an adequate characterization. These terms do indeed describe the functioning of parts—the bowel or mood, respectively. To be sure, these are important parts, distressed and demanding relief, but they are *parts*, nevertheless, not *persons; symptoms*, not *causes*. We still need to know this person in relation to the illness, how this disturbance came to be, what the patient must do to achieve a more positive state of health. No matter how accurate the diagnosis of tension headache, irritable-bowel syndrome, hyperventilation, anxiety, or depression (we have a name for everything) and no matter how helpful the treatment, the aspirin or codeine or Donnatal, the paper bags for rebreathing, the anxiolytics or antidepressants (we have a treatment for nearly everything), true healing will not occur. We have relieved some of the suffering, but health is more than the absence of symptoms.

Even when organic disease is diagnosed, we confront the same problem: the human situation is invariably bypassed by the reductive process of diagnosis and treatment. This makes little difference for patients with readily treatable diseases or injuries to which the medical model applies so effectively. The pneumonia is cured, the fracture is reduced, and that is that. But whenever the human situation is a major contributor to the whole illness associated with organic disease, as it so often is, the medical diagnosis and treatment describe the disease but not the illness. If we focus solely on the disease, we provide very limited care, particularly in certain situations:

1. The disease diagnosed is not the cause of the illness. Robert B., age 40, felt "lightheaded, dizzy," symptoms quite similar to those of Marjorie and Joseph. The examination was negative except for a blood pressure reading of 155/100. A diagnosis of hypertension was established, his doctor's usual workup for hypertension was completed, and treatment was prescribed. A year later his blood pressure had dropped below 140/90, but he felt worse and came in for an opinion. We focused on the illness instead of the disease: Why the dizzy spells? His blood pressure had not really been high enough to cause any symptoms at all. Direct questioning soon revealed that Robert had undergone a stressful two-year period of business pressures and marital discord, during which he had been drinking and smoking more than usual. All this, not the hypertension, was the obvious cause of the illness. When his attention was directed to his personal situation as the source of his symptoms and a major factor in his health and well-being, he set about to make some changes over a period of time. Not only did his symptoms disappear, but his blood pressure remained normal after the therapy was discontinued.

This is a common problem in practice. The presence of a disease diverts our attention from the illness. We get so absorbed in the disease and its treatment that we fail to question whether it explains the symptoms or not. Neither does the patient, who follows our lead and knows too little about medicine to ask about our process. Obviously, the symptoms will persist. Let us look at two other practice situations that illustrate this problem.

A woman at the menopausal stage of life complains of persistent nervous tension, emotional lability, flushing and sweats, difficulty sleeping and concentrating, and feeling breathless and tremulous, or a similar constellation of symptoms. The diagnosis is menopause, and estrogens are prescribed. Just as Robert *did have* hypertension, which was improved with treatment, this patient *is* menopausal, the estrogen deficiency *is* corrected, the flashes and sweats improve somewhat, but most symptoms get steadily worse over the next year or two, even though anxiolytic drugs are also prescribed. Again, the problem is that the disease or disorder diagnosed, menopause, is not the only cause of the illness, nor does the diagnosis of anxiety get to the roots of the problem. It is not that the therapy is inappropriate but that it is the sole focus of the healing plan.

The menopause can indeed be a trying time for the most stable woman in her accommodation to the disturbing, unexpected, and diffuse physical effects of the endocrine realignment, as well as to the import of such a pivotal event. Personal support with an appreciation for the inherent difficulties of this transitional period is important. But this particular patient also needs a more general understanding, because her nervous symptoms are caused mainly by resentments about her marriage and desultory life, not by ovarian failure. The symptoms will persist until something is done about the real cause of her illness. She may or may not find a way to improve the situation, but she cannot begin to act until she becomes more fully aware of the emotional source of the disturbance.

Another patient complains of epigastric distress, severe and frequent, mostly after meals but often persisting for hours. There is no "heartburn." The GI series shows a hiatal hernia. If, then, the diagnosis is hiatal hernia, doctor and patient will focus on the anatomical defect, the possibility of acid reflux, and the usual medical (sometimes surgical) treatment for this condition. The patient responds poorly to H_2 receptor antagonists, antacids, elevation of the head of the bed, and other agents. Because the hernia itself cannot be corrected unless surgery is performed, the patient is led to believe that little more can be done. The patient does, of course, have a hiatal hernia, but is that the cause of the illness? If the situation is explored further, it may be discovered that this man is trying to hold down an extremely stressful job driving a truck 14 hours a day, or that this woman who cooks, shops, and keeps house for her working husband and four children, ages two to eight, also works as a waitress eight hours daily. Neither of these two patients (actual case histories) gets as much as six hours' sleep. The stress and resulting exhaustion are clearly the main cause of what is really a dyspeptic syndrome, and the hiatal hernia is for the most part a coincidental and asymptomatic finding. If the stress can be relieved, the symptoms will improve despite the hernia. These families, struggling to survive, may well find change difficult; the medical regimen may be all that can be done right now, and the patient's distress will persist. But, again, these patients have a right, a need, to understand the source of the illness, so that they can see more clearly where they stand and how they might begin to plan a path toward more effective resolution.

In all these kinds of clinical situations, the wise physician will understand and explain the patient's life situation in relation to the illness, what the disease has to do with it, if anything, what the treatment can and cannot do, and what the patient must do for himself or herself. But that is not what always happens. It is so much easier simply to name a disease and prescribe a treatment. The medical model is seductive, for both doctor and patient. The patient need not assume any responsibility for the illness, and the physician need not take the time or emotional risk of exploring the life situation. Both follow the line of least resistance.

2. The disease itself results entirely or partly from the life situation, but the treatment is purely biomedical. The vital, long-term question in cirrhosis of the liver is not the medical treatment, but how to help the patient stop drinking, or, in chronic obstructive pulmonary disease, to stop smoking. Most physicians will be clear about the key issue underlying these two diseases. In other conditions, however, caused in part by stressful situations, the treatment is all biomedical, and the contributory forces are often bypassed (see Ch. 7, on psychosomatic disease).

A good example is migraine. Because of its unique vascular, electrophysiologic, and neurological aspects, often including cerebral microlesions detectable by MRI, it is appropriately viewed as a disease, although it rarely results in any persistent neurological deficits. Moreover, we have specific drugs to prevent or arrest the headaches or relieve the pain. For all these reasons, the doctor's approach to migraine may be strictly biomedical. If so, what is bypassed are the personal situations that precipitate the attacks in many patients: long hours of mental concentration or physical work, inadequate rest, sleep, or recreation, nervous tension and life stresses, and alcohol. If nothing is done to change the underlying situation, the headaches are likely to recur in spite of the medications, with their serious side effects, and some patients will become habituated to sedatives or narcotics.

Analogous cases abound. An asthmatic patient is a frequent visitor to emergency rooms for intensive bronchodilator or corticosteroid therapy. Though he has been examined many times over the years, no one really knows this person, and it is not perceived how his emotional situations and his ineffective response to them have displaced allergy as the major precipitating factor that most needs attention.

3. Personal distress unrelated to the disease is superimposed. The patient has supraspinatus tendinitis, but the disability that recurs whenever he returns to work is really caused by his resentment of working conditions and his anticipation of disability compensation. Another patient has rheumatoid arthritis, but her wheelchair existence results not from the disease but from a long-standing dependent/manipulative relationship with her husband. A medical student has just recovered from infectious mononucleosis, but his persistent weakness and fatigue are now related in part to his fear of academic failure. Again, the medical model tends to focus on disease and to ignore the human situation. The disability persists, regardless of the therapy, until the personal component of the illness is recognized and dealt with more effectively. The illness, if not the disease itself, is psychosomatic.

4. The disease is caused by multiple factors, but the medical model focuses on one particular cause or treatment. Specificity of cause and treatment are intrinsic goals of the disease model. That is how we prefer to think about all clinical problems. Sore throat is a good example. We identify a specific cause, or *single variable,* as it would be called in experimental models—whether strep, virus, infectious mononucleosis, diphtheria, gonorrhea, syphilis, leukemia, or whatever—and apply a specific treatment, if there is one.

But many diseases or symptom complexes are caused, sustained, or accentuated by multiple factors. An inordinate focus on just one cause or one treatment often yields a poor result. Essential hypertension is a case in point: the specific cause is not yet known, but we do have specific drugs to lower blood pressure, and the doctor's reflex is to zero in on the drugs. Patients are often referred when the hypertension is poorly controlled by two, three, or four drugs, each with its own troublesome side effects. At this point a more comprehensive evaluation may reveal that the patient ingests more than 10, sometimes 20, grams of salt a day (24-hour urine sodium), or that there are other factors that raise the blood pressure, such as alcohol, obesity, stress, nervous tension, or too little rest or recreation. If these factors can be mitigated, the pressure may fall to normal with fewer drugs, perhaps one or none, and, with a healthier lifestyle, the patient may experience a whole new state of well-being.

New patients with moderate hypertension (160/100 ±) can be approached similarly. If they can control the external factors that raise blood pressure before drugs are prescribed, the pressure almost invariably improves and often falls within a normal range where no drugs are indicated. If, however, treatment is necessary, a better baseline has been established, lower doses and fewer drugs are required, and their effects are more accurately evaluated.

Coronary artery disease, hypertension, diabetes, congestive failure, chronic obstructive pulmonary disease, and convulsive states are all conditions that are adversely affected by factors other than the primary pathology. In many cases, the salt or food intake, obesity, physical activities, smoking, alcohol, or emotional tension are more important elements in a comprehensive approach to the whole illness than are the nitroglycerin, diuretics, insulin, or other specific agents.

5. The disease is not the illness, even when the disease, especially chronic disease, fully explains the disability and there are no other contributory factors exacerbating the illness. It is a person, not the paraplegia, the arthritis, or the cancer, who is paralyzed, in pain, or dying, and who needs to surmount the illness with new value and meaning. No disease is disembodied, though we might sometimes wish this were so. To understand the illness we must understand the person. The personal *effects* of chronic disease are just as inseparable from the whole illness as are the personal *causes* of functional illness.

Knowing What Is Really Wrong

Regardless of the limitations of the medical model, we must start with a medical *analysis* of an illness, reducing it to its component parts. When a single cause or very few factors explain the illness, such as the meningococcus or a senile cataract, the analysis itself is sufficient. But when an illness is more complex and includes many elements, either as cause or consequence, especially problems of the human condition, then a *synthesis* or *clinical judgment* about the illness as a whole must follow the analysis of its parts. The diagnosis of adenomyosis in Janet, for example, or of hypertension in Robert, or of menopause, hiatal hernia, asthma, or tendinitis in the other patients, tells us very little about the illness of these patients until we incorporate the diagnosis into a more comprehensive judgment.

The medical analysis precedes the final synthesis, and that is why it is so indispensable to a comprehensive approach. When applied with perspective, with the goal of seeking the truth about an illness, whatever it may be, and evaluating all possible causes of symptoms from the first encounter, the medical model can be the key to the ultimate, definitive judgment. But without perspective it can become a blind alley.

If, for example, the patient is short of breath, we must first determine the kind of dyspnea present. When it is identified as congestive heart failure, we do whatever is necessary to determine the cause. The heart disease may be evident from the physical exam and EKG, or it may require special studies such as arteriography, echocardiography, or cardiolite perfusion scintiscan. If the dyspnea is identified as hyperventilation syndrome, we must also do whatever is necessary to determine the cause, which in this case is usually emotional. This may be evident from a simple query, or may require a special study: an interview in greater depth, the "special procedure" for emotional disorders. We can either do this ourselves or get someone else—marriage and family therapist, clinical social worker, psychologist, or psychiatrist—to do it for us, just as we would get a specialist in nuclear medicine for the scintiscan.

Both patient and doctor must know what is really wrong, or little can be done except to suppress symptoms. The patient rarely gets well when the doctor focuses solely on the symptoms or begs the diagnostic question altogether. Even worse, proceeding strictly within the disease model, narrowly defined, we are likely to do the wrong thing. With pelvic pain the medical route can be particularly destructive.

Think back about Joseph, Ruth, Janet, Robert, and many others you have seen in your own practice, or will see. When we stick too close to the disease model without appreciating the human situation, we often bring to bear:

1. the wrong diagnosis,
2. inappropriate diagnostic procedures,
3. ineffective therapy,
4. unnecessary hospitalization,
5. increased cost,
6. prolonged disability.

Worse yet, the patient is still sick. An iatrogenic illness results from the covert substitution of medical diagnoses and treatments for personal understanding and possible change. The human situation is locked out as medical solutions take over, and the patient cannot get well.

Clearly, the disease model of medicine is critical and life-saving when there *is* a disease, but when an illness is caused primarily by disturbances in the human condition, the results can be disastrous. In this strange dichotomy, the model, depending on the kind of patient and kind of illness, can be medicine's crowning achievement or its core problem.

To avoid this paradox we need to go back over the steps of the medical model—examination → diagnosis → treatment—in terms of our ultimate goal: the relief of illness and the fostering of health. Did we get the information necessary to make the correct diagnosis? Does the part diagnosed fully explain the ill person in all significant aspects of this illness, as it did with Marjorie? Or do we need to understand the person, if only to understand the illness? Whenever we apply a treatment we need to ask ourselves if it is sufficient, as it would be for atrial fibrillation or meningitis, or merely symptomatic, as it so often is with functional and psychiatric disorders.

We cannot solve all problems of human illness with a biomedical model that addresses but one sector of a much broader problem. What is needed is a biopsychosocial model, as outlined by Engel. [30] When we lose our perspective, we inevitably fall into error and cannot recognize our failure even when faced with overwhelming data that the patient is getting nowhere with a strictly biomedical approach. We go on and on, with one test or prescription after another, when we are really foundering in the wrong paradigm altogether. In this way the medical model can undermine the very ideals of care and caring that led us to medical school in the first place.

"What This Patient Needs Is a Doctor"

In this chapter we explore the key features of person-centered care and examine two case histories that illustrate further the difference between responsibility to patients and responsibility for disease.

ᐁ The chapter title here is a quote from one of the most respected clinician/ teachers of our time, E. A. Stead, Jr.: "What this patient needs is a doctor." [1] A strange comment indeed from a chief to his skilled residents on ward rounds!

What did Stead mean? Obviously, the patient needs a doctor to make the correct diagnosis and provide the best treatment, and to do so judiciously, compassionately, and with technical competence.

But Stead meant something more than that, for the skills of his residents were already unsurpassed anywhere. What I believe Stead meant, certainly what is meant in this book, is another dimension of responsibility altogether, not simply for the disease, its diagnosis and treatment, *but for the person who is ill.* This means a commitment to optimal resolution of the illness by whatever means are necessary, and to achieving the best state of health the patient can attain. Often this involves a continuing responsibility until these goals are achieved. In the long run, the correct diagnosis and best treatment may be the least part of what is most needed.

The Doctor's Diagram

In the following diagram, the elements of the doctor's responsibility for the *disease* (the medical model) are noted on the left, those of the doctor's responsibility for the *ill person* on the right:

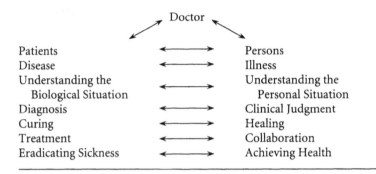

Note that many illnesses can be managed effectively from the left side of the diagram. Others call for a comprehensive approach in which we think clinically from both sides of the diagram simultaneously. The correct diagnosis can be neither firmly established nor acted upon until we understand its relation to the underlying personal situation of the patient, nor can we pursue an interview in any depth for this purpose until we have made the tentative diagnosis of an illness in which psychosocial elements are likely to be significant. Seen this way, the concerns on the right are not restricted to the human side of medicine, nor are those on the left restricted to the biological; they are interdependent, as indicated by the double-ended arrows. Often one side of each pair can be understood clearly only when it is considered in conjunction with its counterpart.

We prefer to think in terms of practice situations in which the *patient* is strictly dependent on the skills of the doctor, working from the left side of the diagram. The *diagnosis* that identifies the *disease* fully explains the illness and provides an ample assessment of its significant features. *Understanding the biological situation* is essential; little or no personal understanding is necessary. The physician has only to apply the medical process with a friendly concern for the needs of the patient while sick. *Cure* lies in the specific intervention—the antibiotic, the surgical procedure, the refraction. *Treatment* comprises all that is done to or for the patient or prescribed under professional direction: the nursing care, fluid balance, symptomatic drugs, diet, physical therapy, etc., as well as the specific intervention. Curing and treatment affect the biological aspects of the healing process. The patient must undergo the treatment as recommended, but recovery may require little other collaboration on the part of the patient. *The sickness is eradicated,* and the previous state of health is restored. The possibility of a more previous state of physical, mental, or social health than existed prior to the onset of symptoms is of little concern in this medical interaction. That is a separate issue altogether.

In contrast, we have seen how little the doctor accomplishes from the left side of the diagram whenever the *illness* results in large part from personal stress, anything that patients have at some level a latent power to understand, modify, surmount in some way. *Understanding the personal situation* is imperative. *Healing* depends on some kind of change, action, insight, or redirection on the part of this *person.* Curing and treatment are not enough. Doctor and patient must work together, but the doctor, who formulates a *clinical judgment* about the whole illness, its source, ramifications, and effects, must assume the responsibility to know this person well enough to point this all out, and to encourage the patient's interaction with the underlying personal situation. *Achieving health* depends on this kind of *collaboration.* The emphasis has shifted from the doctor fixing what has gone wrong to what the patient needs to do for himself or herself.

No matter how straightforward the disease, or how standardized its treatment, the patient is a unique and feeling individual. The back strain, vaginitis, whatever, may be a mundane problem for the doctor who sees hundreds of cases. But it is a very special problem to the person who has it—bringing on the fear of sickness, the role as patient, the examination, the side effects of drugs, the outcome, the surrender to the professional. So, for the doctor, "being there" for the patient is a challenge in every encounter. But we are most concerned in this book with those illnesses that are more intricately intertwined with the human condition. It is then most apparent that "what this patient needs is a doctor," a health professional who can provide medical care embracing both sides of the diagram.

Let us compare the two sides in greater detail. We need to be particularly clear about the differences between disease and illness, diagnosis and clinical judgment, so well delineated by Feinstein. [2]

Example: a 64-year-old male shopkeeper complains of persistent low backache and inordinate fatigue. There are no specific signs or symptoms of a disk syndrome. The examination and workup are negative except for osteoarthritis, or a single disk narrowing, on X-ray of the lumbar spine. A diagnosis of arthritis, or incipient disk disease, is established, and antirheumatic drugs or other medical procedures prescribed, a common approach in this situation but one made here strictly from the left side of the diagram.

Note, first, that the diagnosis is nothing more than the name of a disordered part identified or suspected. It is not, in itself, a clinical judgment. Osteoarthritic spurs noted on X-ray, or the postulated disk condition, may bear no relation whatsoever to the backache, or may be but one of several contributing factors. The diagnosis, in fact, conveys no indication either:

1. That the doctor, after a review of the patient's posture, physical strains, life stresses, and other problems that commonly cause chronic backache, has concluded that none of these factors plays any role in this case and that the arthritis or disk is the sole cause, as implied by the diagnosis, or

2. That no such evaluation has been made and, therefore, the diagnosis is merely an expedient way to avoid understanding and provides no judgment about the cause of the illness.

Now let us suppose that the real cause of this backache is muscle tension from faulty lifting procedures and poor posture at work, combined with the nervous tension and stress of other problems. The diagnosis, though conforming to the X-ray, is an erroneous explanation of the illness. The treatment is no cure; in fact it will provide very little symptomatic relief. The major purpose of the medical model is eradicating sickness, but even that outcome is unlikely here. There will be little or no healing until the real problems are addressed.

What is necessary, then, is a clinical judgment embracing all aspects of the illness. A realistic appraisal in this case would be:

1. Muscle tension backache and fatigue state. Causative factors: faulty lifting, poor posture, and nervous tension.

2. Coincidental, probably asymptomatic, osteoarthritis (and/or single disk narrowing) noted on X-ray.

Patient and doctor can then join in a *collaboration* in which the patient, guided by the doctor, actively *seeks health* by undertaking an exercise program, learning to lift properly and improve his posture, and exploring what can be done about the sources of his nervous tension, while the doctor offers whatever medical treatment seems appropriate for symptom relief.

Whereas *curing* and *treatment* refer primarily to what is done *to the patient, healing* includes, in addition to the treatment, all forces that combine to restore and foster health: the biologic mechanisms of defense and repair; the personal qualities of the doctor, the patient, and their relationship; the overall understanding engendered; the social unit in which the patient lives; and the patient's ultimate propensity, latent in everyone, to restore, strengthen, and enhance physical, emotional, social, and spiritual health. *Collaboration* refers to how doctor and patient work together to activate these forces. Collaboration is the goal of a comprehensive clinical judgment.

Clinical judgment incorporates *diagnosis* but, unlike most diagnoses, explains the whole illness, including (1) its cause and (2) the symptoms, *all* the symptoms. Note that the diagnosis of "arthritis" or "disk" achieved neither of these two objectives. Compounding the problem, it established an erroneous diagnosis for the illness, and, even worse, it blocked further judgment by sealing the diagnosis permanently in the wrong category.

Look back over the diagnoses in the last few pages of Chapter 1. We see that a diagnosis is never a clinical judgment until it explains both the source and the symptoms of the illness. The patient has a right to know both.

Recall also from Chapter 1 how diagnoses of functional syndromes and psychiatric disorders, though medically correct, describe the symptoms but not the cause. The patient has a right to know both.

Clearly, there are many clinical problems in which medical diagnosis and treatment are of little value to the patient until they are integrated into the more comprehensive framework of the right side of the diagram.

> *George B., 42, married, operated machines in a cannery where it was often hot, noisy, and generally disagreeable. He was referred to the Stanford Diagnostic Clinic for persistent disabling pain and weakness in the left leg and foot following a sprained ankle at work two years before. George had been examined by 23 physicians, including his family doctor, several orthopedists, neurologists, and neurosurgeons, and two psychiatrists. The referral jacket was thick with reports, tests, X-rays, and a myelogram. How the illness related to the injury was not clear. The possibility of a disk syndrome with sciatic pain had also been considered, but nothing specific had been found. He was more disabled than ever.*

George B. is introduced here to illustrate further what happens when we get stuck on the left side of the diagram. As we analyze this case, keep in mind Stead's maxim and the diagram above. Note that George cannot begin to get well until the attention of his health-care providers (emphasis on *health*) shifts from the left to the right side of each dyad in the diagram.

The striking feature of all this was that George *himself* had no doctor! The 23 physicians, focused on disease, were trying to take care of *parts* of George—his bones, joints, muscles, nerves, vessels, mind, pain. Some appeared to be taking care of the insurance carrier. But who was taking care of George? Where was the clinical judgment and a plan for getting well?

Once again, find yourself in this picture, perhaps the first consultant (the family doctor), or the 12th, or the 24th. Where would you have focused your responsibility? On the disease or the patient?

Our first response to this illness was that we knew of no "disease" that could explain the whole illness, especially the disability. George had indeed sprained his ankle. Following that, there developed some objective abnormalities. The ankle was still swollen but the edema now seemed due to stasis, not tissue damage. X-rays showed a mild localized osteoporosis probably due to disuse. George had become obese and was "way out of shape." But these disorders did not appear to touch the core of the problem.

The total picture suggested that there might well be psychological elements superimposed on the injury, a sequence known as the *accident process*. [3–5] If so, we had to know George if we were to understand his illness. This part of our judgment was amply borne out as we came to know him and his wife, separately and together; his job stresses, passive personality, and impotence; the litigation; the not-so-subtle advantages of being ill—the whole setting in which this industrial accident occurred.

We explained the illness to them both as a combined expression of the physical and emotional factors we had elicited, superimposed on but no longer due directly to the injury. We were honest but judicious, putting our remarks in a framework of concern for his well-being and recovery. We were encouraging about the latter, but insisted that George agree to participate actively in his own physical and social rehabilitation, and that the litigation be settled.

There are three general ways to approach such an illness. The first is the conventional disease model, destined for failure, but a necessary beginning for obvious reasons. We must start by knowing what disease the patient does or does not have. The second is the deeper personal understanding we have been considering, in which the physician investigates and works with all of the elements that might contribute to the illness. The third is the behavioral-model approach of many pain clinics in which the same illness would be characterized as *pain behavior.* [6–7] Note that in the last two approaches, the physician's responsibility shifts from the disease to the illness, where it belongs when the sick person, not a disease, is the reality. The second, or psychodynamic, approach emphasizes the *source*—the life situation that molded the illness in its present form—and what can be done about that. The third, or behavioral, approach emphasizes the *plan*—a specific program of reeducation to health behavior. In most problems of chronic pain with psychogenic elements, such as with Ruth in Chapter 1, the second approach is most effective. In some chronic-pain problems without demonstrable disease, especially those that are long-standing, complicated by narcotic dependency, and lacking any specific emotional or organic basis, the third approach may be the most effective. We combined both approaches in our healing plan for George. Fortunately, he had not been treated with narcotics, and drug dependency was not an additional problem.

I won't pretend this was all easy. It required seven weeks in a Veterans Hospital, a second myelogram (before the days of CT), and an energetic program of physical therapy and emotional support. George recovered and remained well while working in a small business operated from his home.

At the industrial-accident legal deposition, much to my surprise, my diagnosis of a conversion reaction, as it was then called, superimposed on injury and complicated by disuse effects, seemed to please both sides, and he was awarded a reasonable settlement. Everybody, including the patient, had to know what *it* was, this illness. When the emphasis settled on a clinical judgment about the whole illness, everybody could make progress.

Here again, this case was not unusual. Countless patients have chronic pain in the back, the lower extremities, or both, caused by multiple configurations of physical strain and nervous tension but not by any specific disease process. Very few have a herniated disk, or ankylosing spondylitis, etc. [8]

In terms of the diagram, the problem began with an injury but soon enveloped George, the person, and our attention had to shift from disease to illness. The diagnosis of a conversion reaction (or psychogenic or somatoform pain disorder, or pain behavior, whatever it might be called), rather than of a specific pathology, was then deemed the likely description of the illness itself. The diagnosis was facilitated by *understanding the personal situation.* We were then in a position to formulate a *clinical judgment* that included the etiology, both psychosocial and biological, of the illness, and, thereby, a plan for *healing.* *Eradicating sickness* could not be accomplished simply by curing or treatment, but only by a rehabilitation program directed positively toward *health*, in which George himself had to be the most active participant.

Consider again the usual sequence of events when we allow ourselves to get trapped on the left side of the diagram. The primary physician finds no disease and refers the patient to a specialist—orthopedist, neurosurgeon, neurologist, etc.—who finds no disease either. Neither doctor is prepared to know the patient or willing to explore the stresses and strains, the psychosocial roots of these common problems, which seem too "organic" to merit "psychiatric intervention." The specialist is not happy about the referral of another "functional case," or, to use our most demeaning expression, "crock." The primary physician, who hoped for transfer of a refractory patient, or at least a positive diagnosis, is not happy about the patient's return. Both doctors react with dismay, feeling ill at ease with a patient who has no disease, as though that is not their proper purview. How can a patient complain of a sickness when there is "nothing wrong"?

Even psychiatric consultation may not result in an effective liaison or definitive clinical judgment if the patient is poorly prepared and becomes defensive about the referral. Moreover, psychiatrists, trained primarily for classical mental disorders and psychotherapy, are not invariably familiar with psychosomatic medicine. And the suppressed emotional underpinnings of the symptom may not be touched at all in the verbal interchange of just one or two interviews. Thus in many situations the psychiatrist may be unable or unwilling to commit to a strictly emotional explanation yet finds no evidence of "mental disease." Sometimes the patient is simply reassured about this and returned to the referring doctor.

These desultory interactions culminate when no one can think of another test or treatment to try and the primary physician, if there is one, reassures (!?) the patient that the pain and disability are "not caused by serious disease," without offering any hint about what *does* or *might* cause the symptoms. This remarkable anticlimax, logical as it may seem to those doctors who believe that the presence or absence of disease is the only important decision, is devastating to most patients, who know too little about the ways of medicine to realize that they have been rejected by the medical model, lost in a jurisdictional dispute. They cannot see how the doctor they think they have is not really their doctor. The final comment, "not caused by serious disease," is, of course, a denial that the *illness* is important. The patient is left not knowing even how or when to ask, "What, then, does cause my sickness?"

Understanding the Personal Situation

The next patient illustrates the central role that understanding the personal situation plays in medical care, even when little or nothing can be done about it. Not only was this understanding helpful to the patient, but it also served to facilitate the doctor's role in the patient-doctor relationship. Everyone who practices medicine will recognize this patient.

> *Orvieta T. was a 62-year-old married woman referred by a colleague, a kindly G.P., who found her multiple symptoms quite vexing. He asked me to take over her care if I would. She had asthma, but this was readily controlled by oral bronchodilators alone, and was the least of her problems. For many years she had had persistent abdominal pains, headaches, backaches, and joint and muscle pains. In the previous three years the doctor had seen her 24 times and had obtained several pounds of X-ray films of the chest, spine, and shoulders, and a G.I. series, barium enema, gall-bladder visualization, IV pyelogram, and so forth. His working diagnoses were irritable-bowel syndrome, tension headaches, lumbosacral strain syndrome, bursitis, neuralgia, and asthma, most of which were reasonable descriptions of the various parts of her illness. He eventually had her on eight drugs, one for each symptom, more or less. She got steadily worse.*

The data were reviewed and a complete history and physical exam performed. I found myself in general agreement with the prevailing diagnoses and was tempted to reassure her, change the drugs a bit, and concentrate on a dietary approach. At the same time I knew at another level that there must be a human side to such an illness. The labels here describe only the symptoms. So I asked her to describe the context of this illness in her life.

> *She was quite willing to share. (Had anyone ever listened to her story?) She supported herself, an alcoholic husband, and her delinquent, unemployed, 30-year-old son, by running a boardinghouse with six boarders. She did all the work herself, seven days a week, 5 A.M. to midnight, with just a little time*

for her big vegetable garden in back and her flowers in front, her only appar-
ent satisfactions in life. I won't elaborate on the details, but obviously she was
exhausted—physically, emotionally, spiritually.

I advised her that I thought she had remarkable courage and stamina to support all those people with so little help, that it was amazing she had so few
symptoms, and that what symptoms she did have were clearly due to exhaustion. Orvieta was basically well, but stress like this does indeed cause muscle
tension in the head, neck, back, and bowel, and might even be a factor in her
bronchospasm.

What could I do? I could think of nothing medical that would be truly
effective. What could she do? Very little. Her life was stuck where it was. I
made a few suggestions about regular rest periods, etc.

What happened? Well, she had a latent sense of humor, a wry smile, and
at the end of the interview we were able to laugh a little about the absurdity
of what she expected of herself. I had been honest with her, and she with me.
I understood her process, and she, mine. We respected each other, and the
doctor-patient relationship was off and running.

The surprising outcome: the symptoms virtually disappeared. I took care
of her for the next three years with about two visits per year. Few tests were
necessary. She took only two medications. She remained well. Note that it took
only about half an hour to hear her story. My colleague's 24 15-minute office
visits had taken six hours, but the patient was still sick after three years.

This family doctor was regarded by his patients and the medical community as a model for the art as well as the science of medicine, meaning that he
inspired confidence while applying scientific medicine with skill and compassion. That is precisely how the art of medicine is usually defined: "the skillful
application of [biologic] knowledge to a particular person for the maintenance
of health or the amelioration of disease," [9] or "the translation of the basic
sciences to the immediate problem of the patient ill in bed." [10] These inadequate definitions reflect all too well what usually happens in practice. But an
effective doctor/patient relationship cannot be defined simply as the kindly
application of medical knowledge. That is precisely what Orvieta received—
six correct diagnoses with eight symptomatic drugs, kindly administered. If
that is to be our definition, the art of medicine is little more than bedside
manner. What really counts in such a patient is a deeper understanding of the
meaning of the illness at a personal level. When that kind of understanding
was achieved, the six medical diagnoses were subsumed in a clinical judgment
that included the stress in her life, and the "kindly medical care" was reduced
from eight drugs to two. The patient's improvement was striking. Medical care
from the left side of the diagram, though sympathetic, was ineffective.

I believe that thorough examination, honest communication, and a positive stance about the whole illness were sufficient to resolve Orvieta's concerns about herself. She could then view herself as having but one illness, an illness with a common denominator she could understand and encompass. Without such understanding she was a helpless victim of six seemingly unrelated, mysterious diseases relentlessly getting worse. Most important was the understanding and affirmation, mine of her, hers of herself, that evolved from this simple interview. The illness resolved, even though, unlike Joseph, Ruth, and George, she could make no real change in her life.

Two Sides of the Doctor's Diagram: The Emphasis Varies

If the patient's personal situation is the source of the illness, and this relationship is understood, the whole diagram comes into perspective. The medical diagnoses can then be viewed in the context of clinical judgment, and treatment can be discussed with the patient in the context of a collaborative plan for getting well.

For the patients so far discussed here, note how personal understanding can take the place of treatment. In a sense, it *is* the treatment. The collaborative plan is implicit in the understanding, and without such understanding, we are much too therapeutic. We feel that it is our responsibility to get the patient well. We are bound by a therapeutic imperative. We can only move down the left side of the diagram, fitting patients into diagnostic/therapeutic pigeonholes as well as we can. In this frame of mind we don't like to think across to *clinical judgment* or *collaboration,* because that might get in the way of our medical plan. This leads, of course, to an authoritarian and paternalistic kind of care. We cannot see that our first responsibility is simply to be there, to listen carefully, to understand, to view the illness in perspective, and only then to decide, with the patient, what to do about it.

Personal understanding is not always possible, however, and, even when it is, the patient may not yet be ready or able to make the necessary changes. The physician then seeks a judicious balance between the two sides of the diagram, especially at the juncture of treatment and collaboration. The emphasis varies according to the individual patient: the nature, source, impact, and timing of the illness in the patient's life; the magnitude and frequency of the symptoms; the ease or difficulties of treatment; whether the patient's predilection is toward a dependent or independent relationship; and the patient's responsiveness or resistance to understanding and change.

Ideally, doctor and patient come to understand the underlying situation together. The physician explains the relief, limitations, and hazards expected from symptomatic drugs. The patient considers what can or cannot be done about the basic problem. Medical treatment falls into place as a partial solution to what is really far more than a medical problem. Doctor and patient decide jointly about therapy. When there is mutual understanding, it is surprising how many patients do not want treatment of any kind. They prefer to remain independent of the medical process and to handle the problem in their own way. Or a collaboration is initiated in which the doctor relieves symptoms (for headaches or anxiety, for example) while the patient begins to do something about the underlying stress so that true healing can occur.

I try to achieve as much understanding as I can and to involve patients in their own care as much as possible. Some patients initially reject a suggestion about what they could do to be well, only to advise you weeks or years later that they finally came to the same conclusion and acted upon it. In my practice most patients who could not respond positively from the right side of the diagram, even though they had achieved some understanding about the real personal problem, nevertheless remained my patients. We simply retreated to the medical model, but usually with a better understanding of what it could and could not do, and the resulting care was far safer and less demanding than it would have been had I assumed responsibility for "curing the disease."

In summary, it is our responsibility to understand all aspects of an illness and to be clear about them. Patients should be given every opportunity for whatever change or growth is necessary. They may accept or reject personal responsibility for recovery, but the choice should not be covertly blocked by an exclusively biomedical approach.

Characterization of Person-Centered Care

"What this patient needs is a doctor" has been characterized in various ways: by Engel [11] as *biopsychosocial* in his elegant analysis of the medical model in *Science*, by Miller et al. [12] as *humanistic*, by Tournier [13] as a *medicine of the person*, and by Fox [14] simply as *personal medicine*. Leigh and Reiser also use the term "personal," as I do, to refer generally to the many kinds of human problems that can cause illness and therefore demand our attention. [15]

In the sense that medicine, however practiced, is directed to the health care of both sick and well persons, all medicine is "humanistic" and "personal," but these terms are used here more specifically to indicate a shift in focus from the disease as an isolated entity to the wider problems of the ill person.

Person-centered care may also be viewed as a *change, growth,* or *educational* model. Change and growth are often key features of the plan for healing. The patient whose personal situation is the *cause* of the illness must obviously make some change, in either self or situation, to be well. Similarly, the patient whose life situation is altered *as the result* of severe disease must change in some way to live as full a life as possible in spite of the disability. If an illness such as alcoholic liver disease develops because certain basic personal needs and stresses, as well as the alcohol dependency, have been too long ignored, and these problems can be identified and surmounted, the outcome can be a more positive state of health than was present even before the symptoms first appeared.

Is person-centered care *holistic?* "Holism," from the Greek root *holos,* meaning complete, whole, entire, is used in biology to describe living organisms as unified, organized wholes. In this sense, person-centered care is indeed holistic and shares with *holistic medicine* the common goal of an integrated and individualized approach to each patient as a person who is unique in all aspects of human life—mental, emotional, behavioral, social, and spiritual, as well as physical. [16] Adhering to this goal, many physicians, of whatever persuasion, provide sound medicine with personal understanding, patient education, a view of health as a positive state and not merely the absence of disease, a belief in the capacity of most patients to change and grow, and a shared responsibility for the outcome. Practitioners identified as holistic are likely to add a more concerted program of health promotion, and such approaches as biofeedback, [17] healing imagery, [18] meditation and the relaxation response, [19] and other behavioral, psychological, social, and physical means of stress management, including revision of self-defeating behavior patterns. [20] Such approaches foster self-responsibility, insight, and integration, key goals of person-centered care. The patient's latent healing potentials are activated through personal empowerment, a positive stance toward health, and reduced stress responses. Modalities of this kind should be more widely incorporated into medical practice.

Unfortunately, however, "holistic" is sometimes used to refer, not to wholeness and comprehensive interpersonal understanding, but to a proliferation of "alternative" diagnostic and therapeutic techniques, many of which provide no more understanding of the source of the patient's emotional distress than do the laboratory workups, pharmacology, and other techniques of biomedicine. And if a concept or technique, whether "medical" or "holistic," such as hypoglycemia or clinical ecology, serves to provide a disease explanation for symptoms that are really expressions of emotional distress, then the quest for understanding is blocked altogether.

All healers have techniques, and they use them. Otherwise, patients would not come for care. But any healer, whether a Borneo shaman with a ritual ceremony, [21] a holistic practitioner helping a patient to relax by electromyographic biofeedback, [22] or a conventional doctor prescribing an antispasmodic or benzodiazepine, can rise above the technique and seek to understand the personal problem, if that is the source of the illness, and then work with the person to see what can be done to improve the situation. What Joseph H. needed most was to surmount his grief and establish some new and meaningful relationships. What Ruth B. needed most was to amend the problems in her marriage. What George B. needed most was to adapt more effectively to his personal shortcomings, settle the litigation, and decide on an agreeable job.

If, however, the clinical approach had been restricted to antidepressants, tranquilizers, analgesics, antihistamines, physical therapy, acupuncture, homeopathic remedies, chiropractic, or even a participatory experience such as stress reduction, relaxation training, or biofeedback (if applied as a technique without recognizing or dealing with the core problem), then nothing more than a limited healing response could have been anticipated. It is not that the techniques are not helpful. They may be very helpful. The relationship with a healing person who knows what to do with the procedures at hand is helpful in itself. And if you and the patient are unable to recognize the underlying stressful situation, or the patient can find no way to change the situation realistically, then the techniques for reducing the emotional response may be the most that can be done. But the dizziness, the pelvic pain, the weakness and swelling in the leg, is likely to persist.

Healers of all kinds, once the techniques of each discipline are mastered, tend to attribute the improvement of their patients more and more to the techniques alone, less and less to the inherent healing forces, the relationship with a helping person, and whatever interpersonal understanding may have been engendered. Thus they often come to rely far more on the techniques than on any other aspects of the healer/client relationship. This can happen in holistic medicine just as it does in traditional medical practice. The process goes full circle, from wholes back to bits and pieces again. Because *holistic* is often identified with the techniques rather than the understanding, I use the term carefully, and only to indicate its best connotation of unity and wholeness.

Clearly, the outcome of many illnesses depends not on what the doctor does *to* the patient but on the doctor's capacity to help this person understand and work through the specific personal source of the problem, or the effects of the disease. This in turn depends on the trust, sharing, emotional release, sense of self, confidence, and options for change that the patient has experienced in the relationship with the doctor.

The Meaning of Care

Care can be defined in two ways. It means the performance of necessary services, as for a patient, a child, or a garden. But to care about someone also means showing interest, concern, and understanding. Clearly, all patients need the "necessary services" outlined on the left side of the diagram, where the doctor *takes care of* patients. On the right the doctor *cares for* patients, and some patients need that. "The secret of the care of the patient," in Peabody's celebrated aphorism, "is in caring for the patient." [23] *Taking care of* and *caring for* are not the same, but in medicine they are interdependent.

We usually start by accepting any illness as due to physical or psychosocial forces out of the patient's control, and we do whatever we can to be helpful with medical care. But when these forces include elements the patient *could* change, must change, to be as well as possible, then caring involves a sharing, eventually a shift of responsibility from doctor to patient, as the patient is able to assume the responsibility. It is ultimately the patient who must become aware of self, change, grow, or in some way achieve a more salutary relationship with life situations. Caring means collaboration with respect for, and confidence in, this person. *Taking care of* patients by *taking over* is not necessarily *caring for* them. The patient often needs a doctor who is more guide than therapist.

Comprehensive care, then, means understanding our patients as well as the biology of disease. The Latin origin of the word "doctor," meaning teacher, implies that one of our major functions is to impart understanding. The diagnosis and treatment of disease may be the critical part of that understanding. But often the understanding most needed is our sensitivity to the human condition, our perspective on the relation of the person to the illness, and our confidence in the latent capacity of the patient to surmount the illness in some way. These provide the sparks that fire the healing process.

The Concept of Disease

The concept of DISEASE *dominates our clinical thinking. It seems to represent the ultimate reality of what illness is all about. We apply the concept whenever we think medically as though we know what we mean. The result is that all illnesses appear as objective entities (systemic pathology or psychopathology) for which the medical model suffices.*

Actually, the concept is quite elusive, and is used with different meanings. The purpose of this chapter is, first, to clarify some of these meanings, so that we are not trapped inappropriately in our own model, and second, to indicate how the problem of the concept of disease, as distinct from the concept of illness, can be resolved in a systems analysis of the ill person.

ॐ "Disease" no longer means *dis-ease*, lack of ease, or illness, as it once did; that definition is marked "obsolete" in *Webster's Third New International Dictionary.* "Disease" now refers solely to the disordered part to which the symptoms or dis-ease are attributed. But in the medical model we confound the distinction because, as Magraw put it so succinctly, "In the doctor's view, the patient's illness is not defined and in a sense it has no reality until it can be fitted into a disease frame of reference. Sickness and disease are synonymous. Until the doctor can understand the patient's problem in terms of disease, he does not fully accept the situation as a medical one." [1]

What, then, do we mean by *disease* without the hyphen?

Disease as Pathological Reality vs. Disease as Conceptual Model

An appendiceal abscess is a pathological reality whereas benign positional vertigo, irritable-bowel syndrome, anxiety, and depression are conceptual models, not, as Angrist notes, things that "can be isolated with weight and substance." [2] Such concepts are useful abstractions of medical logic that serve operationally as guides to thinking about what to do, "names for the intellectual locations in which clinicians store the observations of clinical experience," as described by Feinstein, [3] or by Magraw as "a means and not an end." [1]

Note that vertigo, irritable bowel, anxiety, and depression are not things in themselves but rather descriptions of something else—balance, bowel function, or mood, respectively. Even these are not "things," but properties of persons or intestines, as the case may be. Such descriptive diagnostic concepts are "real," to be sure, just as *blue* and *slow* are real, but though used as nouns they are better viewed as adjectives, properties of something else.

The diagnostic categories for functional and psychiatric disorders and many organic diseases are primarily conceptional models of this kind, usually descriptions of symptoms or the functional disturbances by which the symptoms are expressed. Even a term like *tuberculosis*, which represents a pathological reality, namely infection with tubercle bacilli, is used as a broad abstraction to cover a wide range of active or inactive pathologic and clinical events. The same applies to any disease in which the same name is used for both the underlying pathology and the resulting illness.

The problem here is that much of our diagnostic nomenclature is that of pathologic anatomy, and we like to think of all diagnostic categories as similarly substantial. In this way we come to regard migraine, depression, alcoholism, low back pain, and a host of other disorders as "things," "diseases," concrete entities that can be named and treated objectively without understanding the person. But, as Menninger describes, when we think consistently of persons as patients, and of patients as diseases, then the *disease* itself (or the *diagnosis*—we use these terms interchangeably) becomes the ultimate reality. [4] The diagnosis is no longer the *means* but the *end* of the quest for understanding. Magraw's definition has been reversed.

Disease as Specific Etiology, Pathogenesis, and Treatment

Kety describes very well how most doctors like to think of disease: "The medical model of an illness is a process that moves from the recognition and palliation of symptoms to the characterization of a specific disease in which the etiology and pathogenesis are known and the treatment is rational and specific." [5] Seldin goes on to define medicine as a "reductive hierarchy" to "the basic disciplines—physiology, biochemistry, pharmacology and the like"; the disturbance is "illness viewed as deranged biomedical function" and the intervention is the "application of the conceptual framework and tools of biomedical science." [6]

Note that psychology and sociology are excluded from Seldin's definition; *biomedical* presumably means *biophysical.* And the specific etiology, pathogenesis, and treatment of Kety's description cannot be applied to human experience, which involves thousands upon thousands of variables, in contrast to the single variable that is the main cause of an infectious disease, for example. Thus both Seldin's and Kety's definitions break down for that half of all illness that is caused in whole or in part by human situations, for which there is no "specific etiology or treatment." Of the remaining illnesses, which are best explained by organic disease, there may be a specific etiology, but for many there is no specific treatment. These would include acute illnesses, such as viral infections, soft-tissue injury, and muscular pains and strains, as well as the many chronic diseases for which there is no cure. Probably less than 10 percent of all the illnesses we see actually fit all the elements of Kety's ideal model.

If scientific analysis is to include an analysis of *all* the forces that combine to produce natural phenomena, then the science of human illness must include human experience, or it is not scientific. Even a pathologist as eminent as Virchow described medicine as a "social science." [7]

Disease as Disturbance of Structure

This is the basis of the concept of organic disease: disturbance *of structure,* as opposed to the functional and psychiatric disorders, which are, for the most part, disturbances *in the function* of normal structures. All physicians will agree that *disease* properly relates to anatomical abnormality, fault, defect, injury, deficiency, or excess. The spectrum of abnormal structures extends from the atomic level (sickle cell anemia) through cells (leukemia) to tissues (arteriosclerosis) and the whole body (hypothermia). A critical structure may be lacking, such as an ion (hypokalemia), enzyme (phenylalanine hydroxylase), or vitamin (scurvy), or it may be present in excess (endometrial hyperplasia). Sometimes the exact locus of abnormality may be elusive, as when it involves hypertension, asthma, atrial flutter or, epilepsy, but at some level the disturbed function in organic disease rests on disturbed structure.

According to this definition, structural disorders are true diseases, and disorders of the function of normal structures would be viewed as nondisease illnesses. Such functional disturbances may be physical, emotional, cognitive, behavioral, social, or any combination thereof. With concern for this issue the American Psychiatric Association has scrupulously avoided the term *disease* in all three editions of the official *Diagnostic and Statistical Manual of Mental Disorders*, or DSM. [8] Nonetheless, in spite of the A.P.A. disclaimer, we often think of these and all other functional disorders in much the same way that we think of multiple sclerosis or any other disease. But there is a distinct difference:

Mary S. was an 18-year-old woman with attacks of intense discomfort and apprehension, palpitation, tremor, sweating, breathlessness, and numbness, since her marriage three months previously. The past history and physical examination were negative.

The diagnosis was obvious: panic attacks with adrenergic discharge, and hyperventilation with alkalosis. And the treatment? Several choices. Imipramine? Alprazolam? Paper-bag rebreathing?

Mary denied any personal problems when asked general questions about this on the social history. She could not attribute the attacks to any special concern. Directed questions, however, soon revealed that she was virginal at marriage, knew little about sex or birth control, was afraid of pregnancy, and her husband practiced early withdrawal. Though sexually aroused, she had never approached orgasm. Her tears eloquently expressed her frustration. At the same time she was amazed that such a situation could cause so many strange symptoms. The entire syndrome cleared readily in a single interview covering some sexual education, birth-control advice, and reassurance that she was healthy and normal, thereby freeing her natural sexuality to flow unimpeded by fear and inhibition.

In this classical functional syndrome, although a biological psychiatrist might argue the point, there was clearly no fault in Mary's brain, sympathetic nervous system, respiration, or bicarbonate buffers, nor in their functioning, any more than with the lacrimal glands in tears. The usual functional equilibrium was disturbed, but the structures were doing exactly what they have evolved to do in response to emotional distress.

If crying is inhibited, a "lump in the throat" ensues, but the throat muscles, though temporarily tense, are also perfectly normal. Emotional expressions are inherently physical, and they have evolved to unify mind and body in a common purpose. But whenever important needs or emotional expressions are blocked or inhibited, and no action is taken to alter the underlying situation, the frustration aroused is forced into other channels of expression.

Confronted by a child holding back tears, you would deal directly with the human situation and not the pain. Your patient, by contrast, is no longer aware of holding back emotions, or fails to connect the pain with his or her troubled personal situation, and comes to you for help, complaining of pain in the throat. Your attention is drawn to the pain rather than to the emotion, and your training tells you to make a diagnosis and relieve the suffering by treatment. You might diagnose the pain as a psychopathology (anxiety state), a psychophysiological reaction (globus hystericus), or "of unknown etiology." If so, you would probably not notice the sadness, or its intensity, or how the pain in the throat developed only because the tears were denied.

The same holds true for most functional and psychiatric disorders. Here we confront head-on the critical issue of whether we think of these disorders in the disease model or as human events. Our attention as clinicians should be directed to the sadness, not just the pain, for the pain is not the basic "pathology." Similarly, because Mary did not know enough about sexuality to be fully aware of her own situation, and was not even aware of suppressing her own emotional arousal, she developed symptoms she could not understand. She desperately needed a doctor. She suffered a disabling illness, although there was no disease. Mary's hyperventilation was no more abnormal than is the muscular contraction in the child's throat. Mary "ought" to be emotional, in her particular situation. If anything is abnormal here, it is not so much the illness itself as it is our remarkable capacity to inhibit the awareness and expression of our own needs and emotions.

Is there a clear difference between functional illness and structural disease in terms of etiology, that is, between human situations and anatomic pathology? No, there is not. What is "human" and what is "biological" overlap in many ways. The symptoms of a functional disorder such as irritable-bowel syndrome, or a psychiatric disorder such as major depression, for example, are precipitated by stressful personal situations, but the form taken by the symptoms is determined in part by a biological predisposition for the particular response. And in organic disease, though biological determinants predominate, we will see (in Ch. 7) how much the long-term psychosocial substrate of human life determines morbidity and mortality from disease in general. Most important in this regard are the 70 percent of annual deaths in the United States caused by coronary artery disease, stroke, certain preventable cancers, chronic obstructive pulmonary disease, and alcohol-related accidents, disease, violence, and suicide. The prevalence of the first three of these five conditions could be cut in half if their known risk factors, particularly smoking, overweight, and an excess ingestion of total and saturated fats and cholesterol, could be eliminated. Most of the deaths in the two remaining categories could be prevented by not smoking, or by modest, prudent drinking. Thus the major diseases that cause death do indeed develop because of human situations, primarily adverse social situations and health practices, and the settings that lead to smoking and to excessive drinking. In certain conditions, especially hypertension, asthma, and ulcerative colitis, the basic fault is biologic, but the disease itself can be accentuated by ongoing emotional disturbance in some patients.

On the other hand, most diseases of the cardiovascular and respiratory systems (other than those above) and diseases of the eye, ear, nose, and throat, the blood, the genitourinary tract (except for sexually transmitted diseases), the bones and joints, the nervous and endocrine systems, and many cancers develop for the most part independently of human situations. The same can be said for most genetic, degenerative, and immunologic disorders, benign tumors and hyperplasias, and most accidents. Infections are the result of a complex interaction of infectious agents and host resistance.

The conventional distinction between organic disease and functional disorder is useful in many ways, and disease as structural abnormality will be the definition used in this book. At the same time, the human considerations in person-centered care override the differences. As emphasized previously, disease states, especially chronic disease, are "somato → psychic," that is, the disease may be the primary event, but it has significant psychosocial consequences. Certain organic diseases and most functional disorders are "psycho → somatic," caused by strains, stressful life situations, faulty health practices, smoking, drinking excessively, and other behaviors. It is always a "person" who has any illness; what may be most important for healing is the sequence of cause-effect relationships. The turning point for Mary and most patients with functional illnesses, and for many organic diseases such as alcoholic hepatitis/cirrhosis, is when both doctor and patient recognize the personal *source* of the disturbance, and the patient can act upon it. When the sequence is reversed and the disease itself is the primary event, as in paraplegia, the doctor works with the *consequences* of the disease and provides the patient with the guidance necessary for rehabilitation and adaptation.

Obviously, human situations can be directly or indirectly connected with organic disease, as either cause, consequence, or coincidence. The approach in person-centered care varies accordingly. The presenting illness is a vector, and the clinician sorts out the various cause-effect sequences. When we appreciate the interrelationships of person, illness, and disease (if any), we can better balance the diagnosis and biomedical therapy with the person's need for understanding and change.

Think back to the Kety and Seldin definitions and note how disease-model thinking warps our view of functional illness. Because demonstrable specificity of diagnosis and treatment are intrinsic to the goals of the medical model, most doctors feel secure about anatomic disease but uncomfortable about the "nondisease" illnesses or functional syndromes. To circumvent our discomfort, we sometimes simply name illnesses and syndromes and treat them as though they *were* specific entities.

For example, both peptic ulcer and non-ulcer dyspepsia are biologic disturbances of the stomach and duodenum, but only the ulcer can be demonstrated by a GI series or gastroduodenoscopy, and only the ulcer responds readily to standard treatment. [9] Stress is often the major factor in dyspepsia, and stress may also play a significant role in peptic ulcer. Yet other factors now appear more important: Helicobacter pylori infection, [10–12] for example, in conjunction with a baseline hypersecretion; and smoking, anti-inflammatory drugs, and other agents. In the biomedical interaction, the doctor confronting the problem of epigastric pain would rather find an ulcer than not. The crater is impressive. It can be shown to the patient on X-ray. Little explanation is required. The illness is "real" because the disease is real. Dyspepsia, a functional disturbance, is not so "real," even when the pain is far more severe and intractable than that in ulcer. In other words, the *illness* of dyspepsia may be more *real* to the patient, in terms of distress, than the *illness* of ulcer would be, but it seems less so to the doctor, who thinks of illness mainly in terms of structural disease. Even when the disease is demonstrable, however, as Spiro puts it so aptly, "the diagnosis of duodenal ulcer by the physician who is not a mere technician still involves knowing *why* and *who* as much as *where* and *how big*." [13] The *why* and *who* are important for both illnesses, of course, but only the ulcer can be treated effectively without knowing the patient.

The gastroenterologist, who sees many cases, feels secure with either diagnosis. But the primary physician, finding nothing on the GI workup in a patient with epigastric pain, may feel awkward, and unsure of what to say, at the final interview unless the probability of a negative study had been explained beforehand. Meanwhile, the patient, focused on the pain and paying no more attention to the personal situation than the doctor does, "knows" that there must be something really wrong—an "it" like an ulcer, not an "I" like indigestion. At one level the patient, too, would rather have a "real" disease, for similar reasons. An ulcer is not in one's "head"; it seems to indicate less personal responsibility, and the doctor can cure it. So neither doctor nor patient is satisfied with the biomedical interaction in dyspepsia. Sooner or later the patient will drift off to another doctor, another GI series, another treatment regimen.

The same issues apply to most functional syndromes. They can be diagnosed only by clinical judgment, not by physical exam, X-ray, or laboratory tests. They do not respond effectively to strictly medical treatment. It is no wonder, then, that these are the diagnostic and therapeutic enigmas of practice, resulting in so many diagnostic errors, and so little healing from the medical interaction.

Disease as a Question of Control over the Pathogenic Forces That Lead to the Illness

Alcoholism can certainly be viewed as a disease: it is both a medical and a social problem, with a common denominator readily named and categorized, and the dependency or addictive process is the result of biological, psychological, and social forces that are difficult for the patient or anyone else to bring under control. The psychological forces are for the most part unconscious; no one chooses to become alcohol-dependent. Although there is a genetic predisposition of some kind, there is no known primary biologic fault, no marker, that causes the drinking to begin, or to get out of control. The drinking, nevertheless, can eventually cause frank tissue damage and death, and the course is often as relentless as that of amyotrophic lateral sclerosis. The disease concept facilitates the whole process of identification, study, communication, and treatment—meaning outside help and permanent abstinence—for both the subjects and their helpers. An abstinence program that views a person dependent on alcohol as a victim of the inexorable chain of events that characterizes the addictive process, rather than as the cause of the problem, can be both dedicated and compassionate. And the "patient" can accept more gracefully the injunctions of others, whether in Alcoholics Anonymous, professional treatment programs, or both.

Finally, alcoholism fits the Kety definition of disease: it has a specific cause (drinking) and a specific treatment (not drinking). But why the drinking in the first place? Here lies the point at which alcoholism can be viewed more distinctly as a human condition than as a "disease." After all, about two-thirds of all adults in this country drink alcohol, and, depending on how alcoholism is defined, between 3 and 10 percent of all Americans will be alcoholic at some time in their lives. [14] "Normal" drinking shades into problem drinking, with no sharp dividing line. Clearly, there are positive reasons—individual, social, cultural, and many others—for all this, but the most obvious human denominator in persistent drinking is that alcohol helps many people to feel better in one way or another than they would otherwise. This can be described either positively, as more comfortable, secure, relaxed, sociable, spontaneous, powerful, imaginative, or whatever, or negatively, as less uncomfortable, insecure, shy, tense, restricted, anxious, depressed. Many would say that the feeling is "more like myself." However described, no one drinks to feel worse.

I do not intend here to oversimplify an extremely complex problem. Alcohol inhibits certain functions of the brain substrate of human consciousness. But the cognitive, emotional, and behavioral aspects of consciousness are determined by innumerable nonbiological human events, many of them salutary but others detrimental to personal integrity. Problems of the human condition are far too intricate for precise sociopsychological categorization, but it is these aspects of consciousness, nevertheless, that constitute the most likely basis of problem drinking.

At its onset, then, alcoholism develops when a person feels better when drinking than when not, as many of us do, and imperceptibly slips into a state of dependency. It ends when the person assumes responsibility for not drinking, no matter how he or she feels without it. Somewhere between these all too human poles, the alcohol (or narcotic or other psychoactive drug) itself induces a biological and psychological dependency, and that is one but not the main reason for continued use.

The human problem here is most striking in heroin dependency and abuse of drugs other than alcohol. Especially with heroin, there has often been multiple drug use for years, with periods on alcohol, marijuana, barbiturates and other downers, amphetamines, cocaine, or other uppers, and often hallucinogens as well. Because alcohol is legal and socially acceptable, alcoholism may not follow similar patterns of alternative drug use, but it often does. It would appear, then, that the "addiction" of substance abuse is primarily to an altered state of consciousness, rather than to a biological dependency on any one drug at a time. Most telling is that most drug- or alcohol-dependent subjects undergo repeated periods of extended abstinence, for many different reasons, and then return to using, again and again, for the same basic reasons, not because of a primary or acquired biological fault or to get rid of withdrawal symptoms.

Clearly, the biological dependency is but one part of a much broader problem of the human condition. Over and above the physical dependency, a genetic predisposition, and many social pressures to use, the control issue here is that people everywhere drink, or use or abuse drugs, *to feel better or differently than they do otherwise.* That is the principal cause of alcoholism and drug abuse. In the long run, that is the core problem to be solved.

No healing occurs until the subject makes the critical shift from victim of the addictive process to responsibility for abstaining. The paths to this goal are many. They may be negative—avoiding an imminent biological or social disaster. They may be positive—a support system with reaffirmation for one's intrinsic value as a human being; an opportunity to share with others the residual fears, anger, insecurity, and distrust of previous life experience and to move beyond these impoverishing, though often suppressed, negative emotions; a renewed commitment to life, to solving one's own problems, and personal growth and maturation in many ways. Only the person involved can make the final, lonely, existential choice of personal responsibility. That is the ultimate goal of treatment for the disease of alcoholism. But just as patients cannot control cancer by themselves, many alcohol-dependent subjects cannot control their drinking without help; the drinking is simply out of control. That is the key to understanding alcoholism as a disease. The definition of disease has shifted from primarily biologic to one of control and the assumption of responsibility for not drinking.

Does not the same logic apply to *all* illnesses that result in whole or in part from human situations? We do not hold such patients responsible any more than we would a patient with a coincidental organic disease. We accept any illness as it is, caused by forces that have not yet been brought under control, whether the forces are psychosocial, behavioral, or biological. The patient merits our compassion, understanding, concern, medical intervention, and symptomatic relief, when appropriate. But sooner or later, if such patients are to be truly well, we will have to find ways to help them to assume responsibility for the personal components of the illness. One assumes responsibility as one acquires a better understanding and acceptance of self, and learns better ways to approach life's problems. But because individuals can learn, change, and grow does not mean they must be held personally responsible for the way things *were*, that is, for behaviors that evolved in situations over which they had little or no control, at a time when they were not yet in a position to understand, escape from, or handle those predicaments more effectively.

If disease is defined in this way—the loss of control over forces, whatever they may be, that lead to illness—then the disease model could be applied appropriately to any illness, whether functional, psychiatric, or organic. The inertial forces of personal illness are, of course, predominantly psychosocial.

Disease as Treatability

This was one component of Kety's definition. I single it out to emphasize that treatability is often regarded as the "most important criterion [by which] to determine whether a person with the label Disease . . . remains in the medical model," as pointed out by Redlich. [15] This is indeed a common point of view. Unfortunately, it often results in symptom relief but little else.

Benzodiazepines, for example, can block the brain centers that transform psychosocial disturbances into emotional reactions. Propranolol can block the resulting tachycardia. Rebreathing into a paper bag blocks the alkalosis of hyperventilation. But none of this means that anxiety is a "disease."

Similarly, depression is often said to be a disease, because it can be treated by antidepressant drugs. So it can, at least in terms of the biological dysfunctions of major depression, though how much of this is simply the result of feeling depressed, or in part genetically patterned in this way, is not clear (Chs. 8, 9). Most depressions, however, are situational reactions (in DSM terminology, "adjustment disorders") in which no biological fault, either genetic or biochemical, has been demonstrated, either as a predisposing factor or as a resultant factor, and antidepressant drugs are of little or no value. Nevertheless, the disease concept is enticing, and is sometimes invoked, for most depressions. We should, of course, relieve the distress of our patients in any way that we can, but the disease concept tends to lead to drug use not as an *adjunct* but as a *substitute* for the understanding that is often far more important.

The Concept of Disease and the Systems View of the Ill Person

When illness can be reduced to a specific entity with a specific therapy, the disease itself is the appropriate focus of medicine. For many illnesses, however, the reduction provides little more than a fragmentary, if not misleading, view of the illness as a whole. This problem can be resolved in a systems analysis. [16]

In the systems view, an individual is seen as a unitary hierarchy of physical subunits in which subatomic particles are organized into atoms, these into molecules, these into protoplasm and cellular organelles, these into cells, tissues, organs, and organ systems. Each level of organization is but one component of a higher level of organization, culminating in the remarkable integrated unit of the individual person. In turn, each person is but one component of a hierarchical social organization in which individuals are parts of families, which are elements of communities, cultures, nations, and, finally, the human race, which in turn is dependent on a still larger unit, the earth, its physical environment, and the life forms it sustains.

Each level of organization, whether the cells or the families, constitutes a system of subsidiary subsystems that it supersedes or controls in various ways. At the same time, each level is superseded or controlled in various ways by the suprasystems, at higher levels of organization, of which it is a part. The atom limits its protons and electrons to events within the atomic configuration; the molecule limits its atoms to events within the molecular configuration; and so on. At most levels there are interactive forces or feedback loops by which two or more levels can interact with each other. Characteristic forces operate at each level: electromagnetic (subatomic particles), chemical (molecules), physiological (the circulation), child-rearing customs (families), language and traditions (cultures), and so on.

Humankind, with its cognitive, emotional, and spiritual mental functions, a myriad of possible behaviors and social interactions, an awareness of a future as well as a past, and its unique forces of learning, will, choice, and responsibility, is by far the most complex system in nature.

In health, the whole hierarchical system functions harmoniously, but a disruption at any level can initiate the process of illness. Because the levels interlock as they do, the disruption spreads "up" or "down" to involve other levels. The goal of the healer is to analyze any illness in terms of its origins, its ramifications through the system, and its final effects, then to determine which levels can be most effectively modified, through healer/patient collaboration, to restore health.

The disease-oriented reductionist argues that structure and function are opposite sides of the same coin, but in a systems analysis, such a concept is often untenable, especially in functional and psychiatric disorders. Hyperventilation, for example, is not a problem of the lungs; it is a dysfunction superimposed from an emotional disturbance at the higher mental levels of organization.

Consider Sarah T., a teenager with sickle cell anemia. The primary disruption occurred at the moment of conception, when she received two recessive genes, one from each parent, that order the substitution of valine for glutamic acid at position 6 in the beta chains of hemoglobin S. This in turn results in unstable red cells, tissue damage, and pain. Pain is an emotional as well as physical reaction, and the pain experience is accentuated or diminished by the patient's life situation, cultural attitudes, and other factors. In this case, Sarah developed a narcotic dependency, even while the disease was quiescent. Here the disruption had ramified from the molecular level through the cellular and tissue levels to Sarah the person, along with her family and the community. There being no cure for the disease at the molecular or tissue levels, the health-care providers can most effectively interact with Sarah at the personal and family levels. The main problem is to help Sarah restrict narcotics to crises, to continue her education, to develop some confidence and pride in herself, and to surmount her handicaps in any way possible—not an easy path, but Sarah needs such a guide.

Our attention here is directed to the illness as a whole, viewed as a structure of interlocking hierarchical systems. We are no longer focused separately on one entity called the disease and another called the illness. The sickle cells are indeed the root of the problem, the proper focus of biological research, and the clinician must know what is wrong at the cellular level. But the clinician is mainly concerned with the care of a sick person. In the systems view, the disease, however defined, falls naturally into place as but one element, albeit a major one, in a perturbed system.

In the case of Walter G., a married man of 22, the primary disruption began at the political level of the human hierarchy, when his country entered the Vietnam conflict. He was drafted and sent to war. While he was there, his wife took off with another man and sued for divorce. He became despondent, drank excessively, and then got hooked on heroin, a problem indigenous to the soldier subculture in Vietnam. While shooting heroin, he contracted hepatitis B virus from an infected needle, causing hepatic cellular and tissue damage. The liver failure in turn caused jaundice and other systemic effects. Walter, the individual, was then very ill indeed—physically, emotionally, mentally, socially, spiritually. Just as there is no cure for sickle cell anemia, there was no cure for Walter's hepatitis, although both the war and the hepatitis resolved over time. In a systems view, his illness began at the national and family levels, ramified down through the individual to the cellular levels, then back to the individual, as a physical illness. The levels ultimately combined, culminating in a global assault on Walter's personal integrity. What Walter needed most from his health-care team during his recovery was very positive personal support and acceptance as a troubled human being, so that he could regain his self-esteem, stay off drugs, and get his disrupted life moving forward again.

In a conventional medical appraisal we could list here four conditions: hepatitis, alcohol abuse, opioid abuse, and adjustment disorder with depressed mood. As important as these elements may be, the list provides little insight into the guts of this clinical problem. In a systems view we have a map of the entire illness, which shows clearly a continuity of related events, how those known as "disease" connect with those known as "human," and how we might help this person in the healing process.

If we keep in mind the limitations of the concept *disease*, we are more likely to view illness from a comprehensive perspective, and less likely to be subverted by the inherent reductionism of the medical model. A systems view of illness provides a framework in which the disordered parts, or disease, can be perceived in relation to the whole illness, the ultimate clinical problem.

CHAPTER 4

Personal Illness:
The Functional Disorders

The illnesses caused primarily by human situations are designated in this book as PERSONAL *or* HUMAN *illnesses. The personal source of organic disease is discussed in Chapter 7, and of the psychiatric disorders, in Chapters 8 and 9. This chapter summarizes the more common functional disorders with physical symptoms, noting both their prevalence and why we often fail to recognize them for what they are.*

The two main kinds of functional disorders, physiological and somatoform (conversion), are delineated further in Chapter 12, and the differential diagnosis from organic disease, in Chapter 13.

∾ A scientific medicine should address the basic source of illness—infectious, genetic, degenerative, psychosocial, whatever it may be. To identify the cause we direct our investigation along certain lines indicated by the kind of illness present. The laboratory and X-ray procedures for organic disease are well established. But when the source of the illness lies in human situations, the investigation involves a kind of listening or personal interview quite different from that of the medical history. Such a process may be brief or extended, but the physician must make a conscious choice to employ this "procedure," and it must be directed specifically to detect the unique personal problem situation that causes the illness, just as proctocolonoscopy is done to identify the cause of blood in the stools. It is not enough simply to recognize the emotional state of a patient with physical symptoms as one of anxiety, panic, or depression. In some patients, this can be a useful guide to biotherapy, and if the underlying problem situation cannot be recognized or changed, that may be all that can be done. But, as emphasized previously, the disturbance as described in psychiatric terminology is the symptom, not the cause. Stead's dictum: "If one doesn't know what is actually going on, then one doesn't really know how to handle it." [1]

Obviously, a personal interview will not help us solve problems of rectal bleeding any more than proctoscopy will clarify the source of a tension headache. We must have positive interactions for whatever we do. Thus, to proceed judiciously and expeditiously, we must decide, preferably during the initial encounter, which diseases, which functional or psychiatric disorders, are to be identified or excluded, and, overall, whether the illness is most likely caused by an intrinsic pathological process, by human situations, or by both. To pursue the personal side of the investigation we must recognize those illnesses that have their source in problems of the human condition. We begin here with the functional disorders.

The nature of functional illness was illustrated (in Ch. 3) by Mary's panic attacks and hyperventilation. The more common functional disorders expressed as physical illness are noted below. There are of course many others.

The Common Functional Disorders with Pain

Tension and migraine headaches. Ninety-five percent of all patients with chronic recurrent headaches examined in headache clinics have one or both of these two syndromes. [2–3] Migraine, as discussed previously, can be viewed as a disease, but in this book, because the physiological disturbance, so often related to stress, nearly always reverts to normal after each attack, it will be approached as though it were a functional disorder.

Chronic backache. This is caused more often by muscular tension, strain, or sprain, often in concert with other personal problem situations, than by any one specific disease entity such as a herniated disk (Ch. 13).

Chest pain. In studies of chest pain as the main complaint in primary care, a specific disease could be identified as the cause in only one of ten patients in one survey [4] and in four of ten patients in another. [5] Some chest pains prove to be transient, perhaps muscular, the source not clear, but of little significance, physically or emotionally. When, however, the distress is persistent, recurrent, distinctly disturbing to the patient, and characterized medically as "atypical" or "nonischemic" *pain*, not *heartburn*, and there are no esophageal symptoms or other evidence of disease, the pain is often psychogenic, caused by contained emotions. Such pain is less often caused by cardiac, esophageal, pulmonary, or other disease (Chs. 6, 11, 13). Concomitant symptoms of anxiety or panic, if present, are further indications of its emotional source.

Functional GI syndromes. These include certain esophageal-motility disorders, air swallowing, dyspepsia, irritable-bowel syndromes, and "mucous colitis." Symptoms include anorexia, nausea, vomiting, epigastric distress, pain in any or all abdominal quadrants, [6] "gas," "indigestion," diarrhea, and constipation. Functional bowel syndromes comprise 20 to 50 percent [7–8] of gastroenterology practice, and occur in about 30 percent of apparently healthy people. [9] In primary practice, peptic syndromes are found to be more often caused by functional dyspepsia than by peptic ulcer. [10] Most patients with dyspepsia have no histologic signs of gastritis or duodenitis. [11] In one study the cause of diffuse, recurrent or persistent, abdominal pain was considered to be psychogenic in 84 percent of referred adult patients. [12]

Chronic pelvic pain. Pain of this sort, persistent through the entire menstrual cycle, not restricted to dysmenorrhea, ovulation pain, or premenstrual tension syndrome, and not caused by significant pelvic disease, is a common gynecologic problem that is often psychogenic (Chs. 1, 6, 13).

Chronic diffuse pain. Pain throughout the body, either simultaneously or in one area after another, over a period of years, is functional more often than not. A subset of diffuse-pain syndromes is known as fibromyalgia (Ch. 13).

Chronic pain syndromes generally. In pain syndromes lacking clear evidence of disease, underlying adverse personal situations are often important. Disease sufficient in itself to cause the whole illness, but not yet diagnosed by customary procedures, is far less common.

The Common Functional Disorders Without Pain

Anxiety and depression. Emotional distress, viewed in terms of its psychiatric categorization as anxiety or depression, constitutes an immense problem for the physician. First consider its prevalence as disclosed in a national household survey: 27 percent of American adults had experienced "high levels of psychic distress" during the preceding year. [13] Of these, 46 percent reported anxiety with depression; 36 percent, mainly anxiety; 16 percent, mainly depression. Obviously, many of these disturbed people consult physicians. If we turn, then, to another study of new illnesses in primary care, almost half of the patients were found to have adjustment disorders or more conspicuous psychiatric illnesses, predominantly with anxiety and depression, as determined by standardized psychiatric assessment performed separately from the medical visit. [14] About six in ten of the disturbed patients sought medical help for the somatic manifestations of psychiatric illness without presenting any psychological symptoms. This problem of "somatization" has been extensively studied and reviewed. [15–16]

Thus the physician encounters various combinations of adrenergic discharge (pounding of the heart, chest discomfort, sweating), muscular tension and tremor, breathlessness, dizziness, and numbness or tingling sensations— the classic expressions of any disturbing emotion, such as anger or fear. The persistent symptoms that are indicative of nervous tension generally, and of anxiety in particular, are often associated with frank chest pain, functional GI syndromes, headaches, faintness, and/or fatigue states. The patient may or may not be aware of feeling nervous. The physical symptoms can occur singly or in any combination, and they are common. Twenty-one percent of 960 otherwise healthy adults in the Framingham study had been so afflicted. [17] Syndromes of multiple symptoms are rarely caused by disease.

Because feeling depressed is also common, the physician will encounter the corresponding "vegetative" symptoms of apathy, fatigue, or loss of energy; declines in mental clarity, concentration, and memory; waning of sexuality; anorexia and weight loss; insomnia; or, less commonly, increased appetite, weight gain, or hypersomnia. As with anxiety, the depressed patient may not "feel depressed."

Because anxiety and depression are so often conjoint emotional expressions of the same underlying problem situations, the symptoms ascribed to each pole of the disturbance are usually mixed in many ways. The patient may be both "agitated" and "retarded," though either extreme can dominate the total picture. And the symptoms are often associated with any of the functional pain syndromes outlined above, or with chronic pain that appears to be organic, though no definite disease can be demonstrated.

Chronic fatigue and weakness. The dominant complaint is a functional syndrome without any evidence of disease in 80 percent or more of patients so afflicted. This problem and the current controversy about chronic fatigue syndrome are discussed in Chapter 13.

Disturbances of eating, sleeping, and sexuality. The common problems are obesity (though complicated by genetic factors), bulimia, anorexia nervosa, the functional insomnias, and the whole range of inadequate, unsatisfying sexual responses not caused by a specific disease process. Anorexia and weight loss, as isolated symptoms, are often functional.

Illness Caused Primarily by Personal Situations: Prevalence and Recognition

Clearly, functional syndromes are the warp and woof of daily practice. Much less common, for the most part, are the diseases that can cause similar symptoms.

Consider headache, the most ubiquitous of all functional symptoms. Thirty-eight percent of 1,400 random adults (not patients) in a British neighborhood had experienced headache *during the two weeks* preceding the interview! [18] As noted above, most patients seen in headache clinics for chronic, recurrent headaches have migraine or tension headaches, or both. Migraine is not strictly a stress-related phenomenon. Attacks can occur without any previous provocation whatsoever, or they occur only with menstruation and disappear at the menopause. They can also be induced by alcohol, mountain sickness, or dietary tyramines. Yet, on the whole, both migraine and tension headaches are related to the stresses of everyday life. The stress may be desirable (doctor absorbed in work, mother with several children) or undesirable (emotional upset). And both types of headaches are likely to improve if some way can be found to reduce the source of fatigue or tension.

Note, too, how commonly pain is a functional symptom. Of 400 consecutive patients I examined in the Stanford General Medicine Clinics, 170 had pain as the chief complaint. In only 58, or about one-third of these patients, was the pain caused by organic disease. The remaining two-thirds had functional pain syndromes of one kind or another (Ch. 12). A common error in practice is to diagnose each pain episode as though it were an isolated organic disorder: suspected disc syndrome, "arthritis," bursitis, costochondritis, possible pelvic disease, spastic colon, neuritis, thoracic outlet syndrome, etc. Even when many such diagnoses have been made over the years in the same patient, and the patient seems rarely free of pain, we fail to see the emotional thread running through what is really a single long illness with different loci of expression.

If disease were the rule, and psychosocial disorders the exception, the medical model would have far fewer problems. But surveys of practice, mostly in industrial societies, show quite the contrary. Even in times when the infectious diseases dominated practice, functional disorders were next most common: Sydenham noted in 1682 [19] that 17 percent of all illnesses were of this type; and Cabot, in 1904, noted 37 percent. [20] More recently, Stoeckle summarized 68 papers on this question and observed, in the Massachusetts General Hospital Clinic, that significant psychic distress, described by 84 percent of the patients at the time symptoms developed, appeared to precipitate the medical visit in the majority of patients, regardless of diagnosis. [21] Even among patients attending indigenous healers in Taiwan, Kleinman reports a 50 percent incidence of functional disorder. [22] The problem seems universal.

Similarly instructive are the surveys of Bauer in his practice of general internal medicine, [23] Allan and Kaufman at the Lahey Clinic, [24] and Fry in a British general practice. [25] Their data may more closely approximate the experience of most modern practitioners. They report an incidence of

26–33 percent of strictly functional disorders. And when the patient also has an unrelated and relatively asymptomatic disease process, the symptoms may be due mainly to nervous tension. If such patients are included, the incidence of functional disorders rises to about 40 percent. Excluded from this compilation are all patients whose visits are primarily for organic disease, although the disease, for example hypertension, may be in part psychosomatic.

If we exclude respiratory infections and skin disorders, so common in general practice, the incidence of nondisease illness rises in Fry's data to 47 percent. Hodgkin [26], in his textbook, and White, [27] who tabulated the common conditions treated by 171 general practitioners in England and Wales, confirm also that only respiratory-tract infections exceed "nervous" symptoms as a category of illness in primary practice.

My own experience with 400 consecutive patients in the Stanford Clinics, admittedly biased because of the nature of a referral clinic and my known interest in the personal source of medical illness, was a 50–50 split between "nondisease" illness and that caused primarily by organic pathology (see the table given early in Ch. 12). Among the 201 patients with functional disturbances, 174 had primarily physical symptoms (pain, dizziness, etc.) and 27 had primarily emotional symptoms (feeling anxious, etc.).

The data cited above by investigators particularly concerned with the problem of distinguishing functional illness from organic disease are not reflected, however, in such surveys as those of the Virginia study [28] or the diagnostic clusters of the National Ambulatory Medical Care Survey [29–30], which report an incidence of 6.7 percent "behavioral problems," or 3.1 percent "nonpsychotic depression/anxiety/neuroses," respectively. In the surveys virtually no illnesses with physical symptoms were classified in psychological categories. Yet my own experience, cited above, was that 87 percent of all emotionally induced illnesses are expressed as "medical" or physical symptoms, whereas only 13 percent are expressed as straightforward psychiatric disorders. The core problem of medicine—our failure to recognize the human element in illness—can be explained by an analysis of these and similar surveys.

Take backache as an example. Ghormley [31], at the Mayo Clinic, and Dively [32], in private practice, report the cause of backache in 2,000 and 3,587 patients, respectively, all referred for orthopedic consultation. Ghormley makes a strict disease-model analysis that excludes any such thing as muscular tension. Postural or chronic strain of any kind is mentioned reluctantly, and the life situation of the patient is referred to only pejoratively, as "psychoneurosis," in 2 percent of the whole group. Dively's study is also a disease-model analysis, but one that recognizes muscular-ligamentous tension syndromes as a category; again, the life situation of the patients is referred to negatively as "personality problems" or as "compensation," in any case as deterrents to surgery or recovery. The result of their different "knowing," even within the disease model, is that Ghormley finds 70 percent of all backache due to disease and 30 percent due to "indeterminate causes, static disturbances, fibrositis and interspinous ligament syndrome," whereas Dively finds 72 percent due to "strain" syndromes and only 28 percent to specific diseases.

Now let us look beyond the disease model to a more comprehensive analysis. Sarno, [33] analyzing 101 consecutive low-back-pain patients referred to the New York University Department of Rehabilitation Medicine, reports 30 percent due to disease and 70 percent of psychogenic origin (nervous/muscular tension, 42 patients; conversion reactions, 27; psychotic pain delusions, 2).

Obviously, the illness of a patient with muscle tension and a few osteophytes on X-ray would be classified by Ghormley as arthritis, by Dively as lumbosacral strain, or by Sarno as psychogenic if emotional components were paramount. The personal elements contributing to chronic backache are convincingly demonstrated by many investigators. There is no denying the relationship. Whether they are looked for, recognized, or dealt with depends mostly on the clinician's point of view.

There is a critical lesson here. If you "know," like Ghormley, that backache is most likely due to disease, and you then find one, as indicated by an abnormality of the spine on X-ray, you will diagnose what you find and look no further. In this frame of mind you will probably not know that many such abnormalities are to be found in all individuals of the same age, whether they have a backache or not. [34]

Could it be that we diagnose what we "want" to diagnose? Obviously, the best solution to the problem of illness in the medical model is to find a disease that explains the symptoms. So if we order an IV pyelogram for a patient with hematuria, and the radiologist parenthetically notes an abnormality of the lumbar spine, we ignore this altogether. That's not our concern, and it won't even appear on our problem list. But if we order X-rays of the spine for a problem of backache, and the radiologist reports the same finding exactly, we are likely to focus on this as the probable diagnosis. The problem is solved! (Our problem? Or the patient's problem?)

What is important to the patient is the *illness*. What is important to the doctor is the *disease*. This whole problem was succinctly illustrated in a cover cartoon in *Stanford MD* [35]:

Patient, facing doctor in consultation room: "Doctor, I hope you can treat what I've got!"

Doctor, responding: "I hope you've got what I treat!"

We doctors have a remarkable capacity for maneuvering illnesses into medical models. Human situations as the real cause of illness are readily subverted into disease diagnoses that have little to do with the illness. As the saying goes, if all you have is a hammer, you will look for nails to pound. The nails are the disease, and our goal is to find the disease. We don't always stop to question whether the disease has anything to do with the illness or not. What the doctor "sees" and what the doctor does both derive from what the doctor "knows" or how the doctor wants it to be. Atomic physicists know very well that what one observes is determined by the observer as well as by the thing observed. But medicine is a youthful science, and we have not yet achieved such insight.

It is such maneuvering of medical logic that explains the low incidence of emotional disorders reported in practice surveys like the Virginia study. [28] Here, the diagnoses of the 118 family doctors in the study were bound by the USA Modification of the Coded Classification of Disease of the British Royal College of General Practitioners. Imagine yourself in this system, confronted by a tense, hardworking machinist with a backache. You are basically limited to Category 13, *Disease of bone and organs of movement*, from which you may choose *osteoarthritis, back pain alone, muscular rheumatism*, or *sprains and strains*, etc. If you wish to note the nervous tension, you must switch to Category 5, *Mental illness, personality disorders*, and *psychoneurosis*, from which you could choose *anxiety neurosis, physical disorder of presumably psychogenic origin*, or *adult situational reaction*. One category is clearly OK; the other, pejorative, or so it sounds. What would you record?

In a recent study of 12 common symptoms in ambulatory care, namely,

chest pain	back pain	numbness
fatigue	dyspnea	impotence
dizziness	insomnia	weight loss
headaches	abdominal pain	constipation

an organic basis could be established in only 16 percent, but the clinic doctors had considered only 10 percent to be psychologic. [4] What about the other 74 percent? If not classed as "of unknown etiology," they could be described simply by the name of the symptom or diagnosed as disease. If the patients analyzed previously in this book were recorded in the diagnostic system cited above, we would see:

dysmenorrhea	(Ruth)
endometriosis	(Janet)
hypertension	(Robert)
regional osteoporosis	(George)
asthma	(Orvieta)

The human elements vanish into physical categories. Unfortunately, the Virginia survey represents all too well the way we feel, think, and act in medicine, much too often.

A useful rule: common conditions are common; rare diseases are rare! Or, in terms of the adage we all learned in medical school: when you hear hoofbeats, think of horses (unless you're in Africa). We know, for example, that sore throat is more often caused by strep or viral infection than by diphtheria or secondary syphilis. But when it comes to functional syndromes, we sometimes go on looking for zebras indefinitely.

The quality of medical care hinges on accurate, positive diagnosis. The statistics cited in this chapter do not make diagnoses—rare diseases do exist—but the data certainly tell us where to look for the most likely source of certain common symptoms.

Personal Illness: The Concept of Care Determines the Outcome

In Chapter 2 we considered how the resolution of many clinical problems is determined by the physician's concept of care, whether that be restricted to diagnosis and treatment, or driven by a more general concern for clinical judgment, healing, and collaboration. In this chapter we explore more specifically how our views about psychosomatic and psychiatric disorders determine the outcome in this whole sector of clinical care.

ᢙ The power of physicians is enormous. We have seen that what we actually do in practice is often determined more by our medical philosophy, conception of purpose, and attitudes toward patients, illness, and care, than it is by our scientific knowledge. Our goals govern the information obtained, the kind of appraisal and how it is explained to the patient, the plan for getting well, and, therefore, the ultimate resolution or nonresolution of the illness. We have virtually total control over the entire medical process. This means that we have an awesome power to influence the attitudes of our patients toward their own illnesses, especially in psychosomatic medicine and with depression and the anxiety disorders. If we focus predominantly on diagnosis and treatment—that is, on what has gone wrong and how to fix it pharmacologically—the persons who consult us will soon regard themselves as patients, sick, and dependent on the care provided. If, on the other hand, we focus on their needs as individuals, their strengths as well as difficulties, and their latent potential for whatever change is necessary or possible, we may be able to turn the illness into a positive learning experience.

The Concept of Personal Illness

I have introduced the term *personal illness* here to distinguish those illnesses caused primarily by human situations from illnesses caused primarily by an organic pathology, or what in that case could be called a *disease illness.* No firm line can be drawn between the two sources of illness, which interact and combine in many ways. Nevertheless, I find the terms *personal illness* and *disease illness* useful ways to indicate the relative importance or sequence of the major causal events.

I prefer to think in terms of *personal* illness, problems, or conditions (instead of *psychogenic, psychosomatic, psychophysiological, psychiatric, psychological, psychosocial, mental,* or *neurotic disorders*) for three reasons:

First, I seek a positive view of my patients, as people who strive, albeit with difficulty, to fill the basic needs that we all have.

Second, I want to avoid the negative, pejorative connotations inherent in the terminology used in medicine. To most people, doctors and patients alike, the prefix *psych-*, as used in the italicized terms above in conjunction with *disorder*, means mental disorder, an abnormality of the mind or psyche. If *mental disorder* "is conceptualized as a clinically significant behavioral or psychological syndrome . . . that is associated with present distress (a painful symptom) or disability (impairment in one or more important areas of functioning) or with a significantly increased risk of suffering, death, pain, disability, or an important loss of freedom," as defined in DSM-III-R, [1] then many of the patients whose cases are discussed in this book do indeed have mental disorders. But following the definition quoted, the manual makes this important point: "A common misconception is that a classification of mental disorders classifies people, when actually what are being classified are disorders that people have."

Here lies the rub. Most people identify *mind* with *self.* Thus it is difficult to avoid the misconception noted above. Furthermore, psychiatric diagnoses are classifications of "behavioral signs or symptoms," not of minds. The common misconception is that the mind itself is abnormal. In general medicine, our patients with personal illness have human problems, to be sure, but are they or their minds "abnormal"? They have not yet learned how to solve a problem, or to live more effectively, harmoniously. They may have suppressed their emotions since childhood, as most of us were trained to do, and they need more fully to experience their feelings. They may be under inordinate stress, and may not yet have learned to cope with it effectively, or to change it. Symptoms develop in countless ways, but if our patients or their minds are all "abnormal," then all of us are abnormal at one time or another.

Third, the prefix *psych-* ties us into an either/or dichotomy, *organic* or *psychological*, whereas the nondisease illnesses are really caused by combinations of psychological, social, physical, and other factors. As emphasized previously, *personal illness* is a more encompassing term that can be used to view those illnesses caused predominantly by problems of the human condition, in any of its manifold ramifications: outmoded and unproductive behaviors, cognitive constructs, values, purpose, and meaning, as well as emotions, relationships, occupation, sexuality, a difficult childhood, poverty, racial prejudice, physical strains, the stress of modern life, faulty nutrition, smoking, alcohol or drug abuse, and many others.

The medical terms are clear and useful, and I use them as all doctors do. Though I think conceptually in terms of *personal illness*, I record more conventional terms in institutional charts. Even there, however, I prefer simple phrases such as *nervous* or *stress reaction* to more formal psychiatric nomenclature. Most important is that my relationship to patients is quite different when I view their problems in a person-centered framework. When I think in terms of psycho*pathology*, as indeed I do in the medical model, I see mostly what has gone wrong, what symptoms to suppress, rather than what is right, and what is needed for health. Every person with a personal illness is a person in need. I am far more effective when I ask myself not "What is wrong?" but "Who is this person?" and "What is the need?" I do not like to label. I want to understand.

In the same vein I think first in terms of *understanding*, and defer *psychotherapy* for later consideration. That is the approach emphasized in this book. Doctors rightfully regard *psychotherapy* as a special skill for which they are not trained. Therefore, they do not do "it," that is, "psychiatry." But in medicine, unfortunately, basic *understanding*, one person for another, as occurs naturally with one's family or friends, is too often relegated to the realm of psychiatry, to be "done" only in the formal matrix of "psychotherapy." Consequently, many doctors do not seek to understand the source of the very illnesses for which they assume responsibility.

This is a sad situation, for several reasons. Most of the problems causing the common personal illnesses of daily practice can be recognized by anyone with a reasonable interest in human nature. No harm is done by listening. Many patients can handle their personal situation effectively on their own once the situation is identified and connected to the illness. You don't have to *do* something, but you and the patient *do* need to understand what the core problem is. "Psychotherapy" is often unnecessary; if indicated, it may simply be unacceptable to the patient, or out of reach financially. When it is necessary, patients cannot begin to consider referral until they become more aware of the problem to be solved. Until that happens, nothing else happens, one way or the other.

The Patient: Who Is This Person?

When I approach a patient with a personal illness by asking "Who is this person?" and "What is the need?" I do so aware of certain basic needs most people must confront sooner or later—the universal challenge to be fully human. Most of us travel only partway along that path.

"To be human is to be a problem," notes the theologian Abraham J. Heschel. [2] In medical practice we lose this perspective. We divide the world into those who are patients and those who are not. The patients get the diagnostic labels and lose their "personhood"; it is they who are abnormal. The others are OK, or ostensibly so.

> *Ann F. was a 50-year-old married homemaker who was obviously nervous, tense, and shaky. She complained of pains throughout her body, pounding of her heart, shortness of breath, and dizziness. There was no evidence of disease. Medically, she would be classified as having a hyperventilation and muscle-tension syndrome and/or an anxiety or panic disorder.*
>
> *She impressed us as a "nice" person, well-meaning, anxious to please, physically attractive. She had raised a family and worked hard to make something of her life. She communicated courteously. We asked many questions about possible sources of nervous tension, but little was revealed.*
>
> *Her husband, Seymour, was invited to join the final discussion in our attempt to understand her problem. Throughout the interview he appeared overbearing and arrogant. He ignored his wife, showed no feelings or concern for her or her illness, had nothing to offer about it, and made it clear in many ways that it was his life that was important, not hers. I sought to limit the alienation disclosed in this exchange by asking him to describe the two or three best things about his wife and marriage. There ensued a long silence embarrassing to everyone but him.*

Who is sick here? The label is fixed upon the one who reacts (the "identified patient"), in this case Ann, who tries the hardest and cares the most. Those who are cruel, selfish, egotistical, inconsiderate, intolerant, rigid, abusive, etc., feel no need for doctors. They have a human "pathology," but medically they are normal; that is, they fit no DSM category of mental disorder. It is their children or spouses, who know not how to escape, nor how to change the situation, whom we label as "abnormal." In such situations, do we not blame the victim?

Here we see the futility of trying to understand Ann, or any personal illness, no matter how "abnormal" it may seem, solely in terms of individual "psychopathology." The illness makes sense only in the context of her needs vis-à-vis her life experience and relationships. To understand Ann (or anyone else, for that matter, including ourselves), we must view her in the mainstream of human needs and aspirations. She is not a "case" apart.

What are these human needs? We need, of course, family, food, home, health, education, work, and economic security, and doctors see many patients who must struggle just to hold to these basics. But at deeper levels, with those who are closest to us, we need to share our humanity comfortably, to love and to be loved, to trust, to give and to receive gracefully. We need to feel good about ourselves, and to feel appreciated by other people for those special qualities that distinguish each of us as unique human beings. Other people, of course, need the same from us. We need to feel free, to experience and embody our innate vitality, exuberance, spontaneity, and joy of life, to be involved in the process of realizing our own potential for personal growth, creativity, and fulfillment.

Relationships, too, are critical to personal fulfillment, and we must achieve an optimal balance between individuation and mutuality in our more intimate relationships. We need to be able to communicate easily, clearly, effectively, to share our ideas and feelings with those of other people. We need to be aware of our needs, fears, anger, and other difficulties, so that we can express our concerns when appropriate, so that we can act upon these barriers to our well-being, or in some way move beyond them. We need to express and share our sexuality in caring relationships, and to feel adequate and right about our sexual roles. We need to form meaningful relationships with friends and associates at school, at work, and in social and other activities. We need to feel good about what we do, both at work and in other activities, and to realize a pride of accomplishment. We need, in short, to feel worthwhile, both to ourselves and to others.

We need to develop meanings, value, and purpose with spiritual as well as personal, material, and social goals. We need to feel secure and confident, to know how to be responsible, and to have the strength, the resourcefulness, to make wise choices and decisions and to act on them effectively as we reach toward realistic goals and our higher aspirations. We need to be able to handle stress, to accommodate to and grow from the inevitable losses, sicknesses, and eventual reality of death that mark our lives. Though the balance of forces is often disturbed in many ways, we need to maintain an inner harmony as well as we can: our spiritual, cognitive, emotional, and physical selves integrated, no one of these contributors to the human comedy so deprived or accentuated that it adversely affects the function of the others. Work, play, and rest, too, must find their proper balance.

Most of all, we need compassion, both for ourselves and for others, for the path toward being fully human is fraught with difficulties, detours, and absurdities.

Inherent in all this is a brief introduction to mental health. But what happens? Life is an exciting adventure, but personal growth is not easy. There is much to learn and few teachers. Many people start life in families that nourish few if any of these needs. Worse, the parents may be absent, rigid, neglectful, or abusive. Then schools train minds, not persons. Personal growth depends on enriching life experiences, but these may be infrequent and fortuitous, and many experiences block growth. Our worlds can be competitive, unjust, impersonal, and threatening. We look out primarily for ourselves. Often we overemphasize the importance of success, wealth, social norms, or an image, if not the reality, of happiness. If we allow these goals to dominate, we may fail to grow in ways more important for other vital needs.

Intimacy may be frightening. On the basis of previous negative experiences, we fear being exposed, vulnerable, hurt, rejected, misplacing our trust. We may not know how to receive from another person, to express our anger or disappointment, to state our needs, or ask for help, to communicate honestly, to work together. We are not fully aware of our own feelings and emotions. We may not feel secure about ourselves, or our relations with others, yet we try to appear as though we are. Our concerns are focused on past events and future expectations, and we are not fully attentive to the present. We are so involved with the immediate demands of life that we do not seek higher goals. Change can be threatening, and we settle for stability in the status quo. Often we dwell on our limitations, our failures, our isolation, as deficiencies derived from arbitrary standards of how we believe we ought to be, and we do not feel right about ourselves or our path through life. Many of us simply do not know how to be self-responsible, and so we become victims of what appear to be the whims of fate.

As fine as life can be, the problem of becoming more of what we could be can be overwhelming—for some people, most of the time; for others, some of the time. Unresolved problems gnaw at the core of one's being. Childhood behavior patterns, which evolved when basic needs were denied, circumvented, or only partially satisfied, may be deeply entrenched, difficult to change. But unfilled needs demand expression. No wonder, then, that they result in the multitude of physical, mental, mood, emotional, and behavioral disturbances that physicians see as clinical problems.

I introduce this fragmentary sketch of needs and problems, drawn from many sources, of which I cite just a few, [3–15] and from my experience with patients and my own life, to remind us of the common humanity that is the real basis for so many of the problems we see. There are, of course, many other psychosocial [16–17] and religious [18] ways to view human needs, problems, and their resolution.

Viewing life from the perspective of human needs, we can readily understand Ann's problem and feel compassion for her predicament. We can even begin to wonder about Seymour—what has driven him to his self-centered ways? Though this kind of understanding provides no immediate solution to the problem, it is a beginning. Ann cannot begin to act on her needs or her problems until she sees what they are. In the long run, she needs understanding and compassion more than she needs a label and a treatment.

If Ann is viewed as a psychosomatic or psychiatric "case," the diagnosis, whatever it is, shifts our attention away from her problem as a person to the dysfunctional "part." From this perspective, emotions are deemed undesirable mental phenomena that should remain contained in the head, where they belong. Those who cry or get angry have poor control; those who hold back the tears or suppress the anger and develop symptoms have a psychopathology. In short, there seems to be something about the emotion itself that is not right. Ann and other patients with similar disorders ought to be able to recognize and deal with their problems rationally, or adjust to them with constraint. If emotions cannot be dispelled and spill over into an outburst or into clinical symptoms, should not the disturbance be suppressed? Especially if we regard the patient who feels anxious or depressed as having an essentially biological disorder?

But this is not just a problem of the way physicians view symptoms. Patients view themselves the same way. The patient seeks relief. The physician seeks to provide it. One or the other or both may be reluctant to accept or to explore the underlying human anguish. We all get caught up in the idea, more or less, that emotions are not OK, and, therefore, that to be fully human (emotions and all) is not OK. We try to suppress our feelings, but we can't. In medicine, the result is a focus on the dysfunctional part. The "disorder" is labeled and treated.

It is our emotions, nevertheless, that express the intensity of our needs as well as our values, our highest aspirations, and our peak experiences. Our emotions tell us who and where we really are. When they express needs, they are a call for action, a signal for change. They are eloquent, and they demand an audience. Who listens?

Learning and Growth in Human Illness

Jean G. was a married woman of 55 whose intermittent headaches during her adult life had become more intense, almost continuous, for three years. She was taking codeine, 240 mgm daily, an unusually high dose, and visiting an emergency room about twice a month for Demerol injections. Jean's headaches had earlier been characteristic of migraine, but often more like tension headaches. Now they fell into no specific pattern but had become incorpo-

rated into the daily fabric of her life. Neurological and other consultations and many tests were negative. The usual treatments for both kinds of headaches had provided but temporary relief. Her physician referred her to the diagnostic clinic, seeking a more effective management.

So far Jean's headaches have been managed strictly in a model of disease, as though they were inevitable faults of nature having little to do with her patterns of life. Migraine attacks, however, are often precipitated by human situations, though the form of the physiological disturbance is determined by a specific biological substrate. Jean's medical examination was, again, normal. Nothing suggested a brain tumor or other organic disease. I decided to shift from the medical to a psychiatric model. If not organic disease, there must be an antecedent psychosocial cause, some stress or conflict. But what? When we shift from physical to psychological causes, note that we are still looking for past causes of present effects. This is the classical format of psychoanalysis. We remain in the basic cause-and-effect linear model of science.

In an extended interview with Jean alone, and then again with her husband, we found no stress or conflict. She had done well in school, had a happy marriage, had raised three children with love and affection. In the past she had held a satisfying job as a salesperson. Her husband was clearly loving, thoughtful, communicative, and open with his feelings, as she was. They enjoyed each other. They had a nice home, no economic problem or other stresses, and no concerns about their sexual relationship. Their children were married and successful, and visited often. Jean and her husband were cooperative, even enthusiastic, about our psychosocial exploration of their lives, displaying no detectable evasion or resistance. So what was the problem?

Such a patient is sometimes said to have a masked depression, "endogenous" or "involutional." Should I switch from the biology of headaches to that of depression and prescribe antidepressant drugs? Or would traditional psychoanalysis provide a better insight into the background of this illness?

I decided to view Jean in terms of her human situation. If she is a person in need, what is the need? Could Jean have needs for purposiveness, for new meanings?

I asked, "What do you do?" "Housework." "Then what?" Long silence. So I asked, "What else?" "More housework." A few more exchanges like this, and it was apparent that Jean had run out of purpose. With the children gone, no need for a job, her husband employed and helpful around the house, she had moved beyond her previous identities as daughter, student, mother, and employee. Little remained but homemaking and a nice husband. During the years of devotion to the major concerns of her life she had not developed any meaningful social, athletic, recreational, intellectual, artistic, or other special interests of personal significance for her. Life was barren. Her husband confirmed that he had regarded this as her main problem for some time.

Her illness could then be explained by (1) her dependence on medical solutions to what she had been led to believe was a biomedical problem, (2) the resulting drug dependency, and (3) the real problem, her need for personal development. After a discussion with Jean and her husband about the probable nature of the whole problem, she agreed to discontinue the narcotics. No psychoactive drugs were substituted. She was assured that this could be done, and that it was an essential step in her recovery. We stressed her apparent need for meaningful activity and enlisted her husband as an ally. She was able to withdraw from the codeine, and the headaches improved steadily. In the next few months she managed to develop several new interests and activities, including the development of a previously minor hobby into an active business, making and selling greeting cards. In the ensuing eight years she remained well, with only occasional minor headaches, controlled with over-the-counter analgesics.

Jean's predicament was not at all unusual. Many people do not consider personal growth their responsibility. They have not learned to do this from their parents, schools, or other influences. Nor have they been taught not to. They are unaware that they have options. It is simply not a principle embedded in their being, and they go through life doing more or less what is expected of them. When the need for change or growth becomes a problem, as it did with Jean, they cannot act toward filling a need of which they are not aware. Meaning and purpose, nevertheless, are vital for most people, and such needs may surface at any time, from adolescence on. This realization can become acutely poignant after a heart attack, or when cancer is diagnosed. Many patients then discover how they have failed to realize, or even to think about, the most significant values in their lives. If the need becomes a problem but finds no way to awareness or action, it may be expressed emotionally, either as tears or frustration, physical symptoms, anxiety, or depression. The need to assume personal responsibility for one's own interests, growth, and meaning can be a difficult concept to get across. In working with patients toward this kind of responsibility, I fail more often than I succeed, but Jean cast no blame, viewed herself positively, and had the full support of her husband and family.

Note that there was no *cause* for the human side of Jean's illness, so long as cause is seen as antecedent events. The cause, her need to learn something new and important for her own personal expansion, was something that had not yet emerged. In this sense Jean's problem cannot be made to fit the cause-and-effect model of science, unless cause is redefined to include a person's destiny as well as past experience! Fulfillment is more important than where one has been.

Learning thus adds a new dimension to the healing process. Most patients do not have specifically existential problems like Jean's, but most patients with personal illnesses do need to learn something new about how to move forward from their present predicament.

The diagnoses and treatments of the medical model, by contrast, focus on what has gone wrong. The psychopathology is the result of what has already happened. This being the sole focus, the purpose of therapy would be to discover and detach the causal events from their present effects, or, that failing, to control or suppress the symptoms. The past, however, is not readily uncovered or eradicated like tubercle bacilli, even in psychoanalysis. And when locked into a model of psychopathology, most physicians fall readily into a discouraged view of patients with psychosomatic or psychiatric disorders.

In the inorganic world the present is indeed determined by the past, if we choose to deal in the cause-and-effect model of science. So are human predicaments, but these can also be viewed in an alternative frame of reference. Though *shaped* by previous events, they are also determined by what one has *not yet learned* about more effective ways to be, more effective ways to solve a problem. With some patients, especially those with deep-seated unconscious conflicts, the past is most important. The patient must first reexperience the source of the problem. Only then can subsequent growth begin. The release of repressed emotions can sometimes effect a "cure" without new learning. For most patients, however, undoing the past is primarily a process of becoming more fully aware *of the present problem,* then learning better ways to proceed along future paths. In medical as opposed to psychiatric practice, the kinds of situations causing the common functional illnesses can usually be appreciated without an extensive understanding of past influences. What the patient can do to improve the situation is often clear, and several of the patients we have seen in this book illustrate this point. Orvieta's condition (Ch. 2) improved simply with a new and positive view of herself. If these patients had been seen in formal psychotherapy, it would have been helpful to them perhaps to explore the roots of their attitudes and behaviors, but this was not essential for healing to proceed. Jean's inherent vitality and individuation were presumably displaced, for example, in the course of being brought up to be an obedient child, a "good girl," to do as she was told and little else. For the present illness, however, Jean was quite able to learn what she needed to learn so as to change her attitude about herself and to fill some of her needs without such an anamnesis. Ideally, many patients could benefit from psychotherapy or from other, more extensive, counseling than can be provided by physicians in regular medical practice, but for many reasons referral is usually difficult, as we all know. By offering a comprehensive clinical judgment and a beginning understanding of the patient's current problems, the primary physician provides an indispensable service.

Thus the *therapy* of *psychotherapy* has a dual meaning. Undoing the present effects of past causes is the classical meaning of *therapy* in the medical or scientific model, and the legacy of Freud in psychiatry. Learning and growth, on the other hand, evoke the uniquely human attributes of choice, freedom, responsibility, values, meaning, and purpose, all of which fall beyond the realm of science.

Unlike other natural systems, human beings are not simply determined by inexorable extrinsic or internally biologic or instinctual forces. A person is a force her/himself, both creator and reactor, stimulus and response, cause and effect, responsible choice-maker as well as "victim." As emphasized by William James, [19] Carl Jung, Alfred Adler, and others at the turn of the century, and continuing through to the more recent humanistic and existential emphasis in psychiatry, learning and growth, values and meaning are now essential components of psychotherapy generally. A growth model is the necessary complement of the medical model. Healing is a problem of learning as much as it is one of treatment. The same holds true in many ways for surmounting the illnesses of chronic organic disease.

The human dimensions lead us to a positive view of human life and a correspondingly positive stance toward personal illness. A patient who needs an opportunity to learn or experience what has not yet taken place can be viewed more constructively than one with a "psychopathology." Learning and growth are the key issues serving to switch our attitudes from what is wrong to what is needed. If we regard our patients as inherently healthy, their emotions as valid and understandable, and their symptoms as expressing a need to reengage in the process of life in new ways, then we are more accepting, more sensitive, even enthusiastic about the possibilities for change. Regardless of the medical interactions, the true feelings of a physician toward the patient as a person are invariably communicated, overtly or covertly, and the patient tends to respond accordingly.

The Medical and Growth Models Compared

Let us now consider more systematically the differences between what is called here a growth model for psychosomatic and psychiatric illness and what I take to be the conventional medical model in such cases.

By no means can the growth model be applied to all patients. Some cannot seem to make a move, and remain dependent indefinitely on medical care. Some patients need, and many expect, prescription drugs to relieve distress, at least at the beginning of care. Others accept a psychological approach, but it never seems to move much beyond understanding past causes and present conflicts, self-validation, support, and reassurance; the patient finds it difficult to be responsible for real change or to act on it effectively. It is important, then, to accept and work with patients at whatever level is possible between dependency and independent responsibility for change, but if the growth model is kept in mind we are more likely to understand patients wherever they are, and less likely to overlook interactions that may lead to real change.

In the following table the differences between the two models are accentuated, to clarify each point, but in actual practice the two sides are integrated according to each patient's situation, as discussed in Chapter 2.

Approaches to psychosomatic and psychological disorders

The medical model	The growth model
1. The emphasis is on the physical or the psychopathological, and elimination (treatment) of the disordered part. The patient is sick. "Neurosis" is a kind of disease. The doctor focuses on the sickness.	The emphasis is on the change(s) necessary to achieve a harmonious whole. The patient is potentially well but stuck on, and struggling with, a problem of living, a need for personal growth. The doctor focuses on the wellness of the patient. [20]
2. Physical symptoms are abnormal reactions of the body. Emotions should remain confined to the mind.	There is a pervading mind-body unity; all emotions are physical. If appropriate action or emotional expression is not possible, symptoms are inevitable.
3. A diagnosis of psychogenic disorder should be considered only after organic disease is ruled out.	Psychogenic disorders are sufficiently characteristic that a tentative early diagnosis can be made and the source explored beginning with the first visit.
4. The medical or psychiatric diagnosis is the essential description of the patient's problem. The anxiety or hyperventilation or whatever *is* the illness. The patient's feeling of depression or anxiety is caused mainly by the biological disturbance.	Diagnostic categorization of a personal illness is useful, but the underlying life situation is the core of the problem. The anxiety or hyperventilation—or whatever—is the *symptom*. The biological disturbance is mainly the result, not the cause, of the emotionally disturbing personal situation, though the situation and its somatic emotional expression combine to produce the ultimate clinical picture.

The medical model	The growth model
5. It is the patient who has the pathology, and receives the treatment, and who should adjust better to his or her life situation. Examination of the individual patient is sufficient.	The identified patient often expresses a marital or family problem, or a social problem of the wider community. Patients cannot be understood apart from these relationships. Family interviews are often helpful.
6. The crux of the interaction is the treatment. That is why patients come for care. The symptoms should be modified by medication. There are specific therapies to counteract most psychosomatic disturbances, anxiety, and depressive reactions.	The crux of the interaction is the understanding. That is why patients come for care. They expect relief of suffering, but in conjunction with an understanding of the illness, what causes it, and what they themselves can do about it. Psychoactive drugs are helpful but less specific than is suggested by their "anxiolytic," "antidepressant," designations. Their effects are often marginal or negligible if no change occurs in the underlying personal situation.
7. Implicit in the "contract" between patient and doctor is the doctor's responsibility to get the patient well. There is little discussion of the patient's responsibility for change. Even in psychiatry this may not be emphasized.	What the doctor can and cannot do, and what the patient can and cannot do should be made explicit. The doctor seeks to activate the latent capacity of the patient to be more aware of his or her own choices, and to be increasingly responsible for his or her own welfare, change, and growth.
8. The emphasis is on cause and effect. Current difficulties are bound to past events. Growth is expected to occur when these links are released. Therapy, as with organic disease, means to correct what has gone wrong.	The emphasis is on growth as a process that should go on continuously. It builds on the past but need not be bound by it. The path to health is not so much a *therapy*, or undoing of the past, as it is a *learning opportunity* for the discovery of better ways.
9. The interaction remains mostly at the verbal-cognitive level. Emotional breakthroughs are disturbing and best avoided.	The interview is informative, but if the symptom converts to an actual expression of the suppressed emotion, the core of the problem will be clarified. Healing can flow from this experience. The doctor is not afraid to allow patients to experience their own emotions.

The medical model	The growth model
10. Both understanding and change are difficult. The doctor is not optimistic.	The patient already knows at some level what the real problem is, and change is possible. The doctor is affirmative, and holds to a vision of the patient's potential.
11. Patients with psychosocial disorders should go to psychiatrists.	This is not always possible, even when indicated, and it may not be necessary. "What this person needs is a doctor." (Chapter 2)

Diagnostic Strategies for Unrecognized Personal Illness

The detection and treatment of organic disease is the clear responsibility of every doctor. This dominates our training and practice. Functional disorders—the realm of "nondisease"—may consequently become viewed as a distinctly secondary concern. When a physician has an over-ridingly organic focus, what is really a functional disorder may be unrec-ognized, and perceived instead as a "diagnostic problem." Alternatively, if physical abnormality is disclosed in the workup, it may be wrongly diagnosed as though it were the cause of the illness. In either case, the diagnostic quest for disease serves as a "strategy" (though not recognized as such by an organically focused physician) that effectively bypasses the correct diagnosis and its source: the underlying personal problem situ-ation of the patient. This chapter delineates these strategies, particularly with respect to those diseases which, though often diagnosed, may have little or nothing to do with the patient's illness.

The "organic" approach, when applied inappropriately to personal ill-nesses, is inherently iatrogenic, for two reasons: the psychosocial cause of the illness is neither recognized nor dealt with in any way, and the whole problem is compounded by the diversion of attention to a disease that is not really the cause of the symptoms.

ᴄᴧ Doctors and patients share the same goal: to find out what is wrong and what can be done about it. When diagnosis and treatment are specific, the problem is relatively simple; when either is uncertain, the problem is difficult.

Illnesses caused directly by problems of the human condition, with its bound-less variables and ambiguous pathways for change and growth, are especially difficult. Our time with patients is limited, as is our capacity to fathom the human condition. Obviously we prefer to work with problems that are far more specific. Patients, too, hope that something simple and straightforward can be done to make them well, strongly preferring that their attending doc-tors—or other kinds of healers, for that matter—not tell them that a major change in their pattern of life is necessary.

For these and many other reasons, our reluctance to face, explore, and deal with the personal aspects of illness is understandable. We saw in Chap-ter 4 that the emotional basis of functional disorders with predominantly physical symptoms often remains unrecognized. What happens instead is that we bring into play a variety of practices that serve to maneuver these illnesses into organic categories. By these means the complexities of psycho-somatic medicine are reduced to presumably manageable guidelines, prefer-ably a specific diagnostic/therapeutic dyad that provides a positive biomedical approach.

The practices described here, sanctified by years of use, are acquired "by osmosis" if not by actual instruction, and they are readily incorporated into the ethos of an organically focused model of care. From this perspective, such practices appear to be logical and helpful. It then becomes difficult to realize how such practices, as ways of thinking, are really subtle expedients for by-passing human complexities. By becoming more aware of this problem, we will be in a better position to view illness from a more useful perspective. That is the purpose of this chapter.

Not Making a Diagnosis: Begging the Question

In this situation, as with Joseph or Ruth (Ch. 1) or George (Ch. 2), the doctor cannot establish a diagnosis of organic disease but is also unwilling to consider a functional illness, especially a psychogenic pain disorder. The doctor persists in the assumption that the illness is caused by a primary or-ganic disease not yet detected, and continues the workup with more tests and X-rays. This is not perceived as a strategy to beg the question because the exclusion of clinical judgment is not noticed in the erudite and conscientious search for the elusive disease.

The search often begins by formulating a problem list with a differential diagnosis for each group of symptoms (Ch. 14). This would constitute an ap-propriate means to an end if it incorporated a realistic judgment about the probability of a functional disorder, as opposed to organic disease, but often it does not. The "differential" here is merely a list of diseases to be ruled out, but there is no plan for resolution when X, Y, and Z *are* ruled out. Sometimes at the end of the list one finds the enigmatic phrase, "rule out psychoneurosis," but there is no indication *how* this is to be ruled "out" or "in," which means, in effect, that a functional disorder is not likely to be considered seriously even when it is the correct diagnosis. Usually a problem list so devised never gets resolved, because its very format indicates an unwillingness to make a judgment. Further tests and therapeutic trials may divert the clinician and, therefore, the patient's cure for years.

Unknown etiology. The problem of nondiagnosis can be couched in the vernacular of medicine: *idiopathic,* or pain of *unknown etiology,* or *cause not yet determined.* These terms invariably refer to undiagnosed organic disease. Clinicians would rarely if ever describe an illness in this way if their intentions were to explore its psychosocial basis. When applied to an undiagnosed symptom complex, therefore, these terms usually block such a quest.

Meador's whimsical solution to this problem in his paper, "The Art and Science of Non-Disease," was simply to label certain syndromes as "non-Cushing's disease," "non-anemia," etc. [1]

Status/post-. This is a legitimate term used in the appraisal to refer to the patient's status following a medical event such as pulmonary resection for carcinoma of the lung. As pointed out in Chapters 1 and 14, however, such terms as "*status/post* hysterectomy, 1982; *status/post* oophorectomy, 1984," often abbreviated to the familiar "S/P," may serve conveniently, perhaps unconsciously, as an evasive strategy for avoiding a judgment about whether the previous diagnoses were appropriate, the operations were necessary, the pathology is sufficient to explain the pain or other symptoms, the present pain is really a continuation of the former pain (or is perhaps psychogenic), and so forth.

Another way of avoiding judgment is to say that the patient "carries" or "is said to have" a diagnosis of diverticulitis, schizophrenia, or whatever, where, by so doing, the physician makes no ongoing commitment to agree or disagree with the previous diagnosis. The patient may then continue to carry an ambiguous diagnostic label.

Functional overlay. Where the psychological aspects of an illness are too obvious to overlook, but the doctor is still unwilling to consider a functional or psychiatric disorder, a common strategy is to record a "functional overlay." This implies that the symptoms, though viewed as caused by a "real" problem of organic disease, are accentuated because of superimposed nervous tension. Virtually every time I have seen this phrase utilized, however, a functional "underlay" seemed more to the point; that is, the illness was mainly emotional, and bore little or no relationship to the relatively asymptomatic disease in question.

Similarly, the term *endogenous* is often appended to a diagnosis of depression to suggest that the condition is predominantly physical (Ch. 9). As with "functional overlay," however, the phrase is used frequently with little or no effort to understand the patient's situation. Again, a premature use of such terminology blocks the quest for understanding.

Referral. Consultation is often important, either for the care of a disease or simply to convince both patient and doctor that no disease is present. But the consultation should be but one part of a specific overall plan. In particular, when the specialist has ruled out disease, the referring physician must be prepared to resume responsibility for the patient and the illness, which in this situation is often a functional disorder. Too often, however, as with George (Ch. 2), there is no such plan. Instead, the referring physician had hoped to escape the dilemma by transferring responsibility, [2] often a futile pursuit. Though many specialists provide excellent care for their patients with the functional disorders that fall within their field (headaches in neurology, backaches in orthopedics, etc.), most medical specialists are not prepared to assume responsibility for nondisease. In short, the consultation request is sometimes used as still another strategy for evading the problems of human illness. When both the referring doctor and the consulting doctor believe that the other should be responsible, the patient is caught in the crossfire. Unfortunately, this may happen even in tertiary-care centers, which are divided by disease and specialty, therefore affording less clear responsibility for the patient than is typical in private practice. Balint refers to all this as the "dilution of responsibility" by the "collusion of anonymity." [3]

Shifting the focus from diagnosis to therapy. When a workup is completed and found to be negative, physicians are usually satisfied that major disease— their main concern—has been ruled out. The actual diagnosis, whatever it is, no longer seems so important. Perhaps the problem is an ill-defined "rheumatic" or "neuralgic" condition, muscle tension or spasm, etc. In any event, we need to provide relief and get on with therapy. Suppose, for example, the problem is chest pain, and the coronary arteriograms are negative. Still, regardless of the etiology, calcium channel blockers, alprazolam, or nitrates might relieve this nonischemic pain. The emphasis then shifts from diagnosis to therapy. Again, in our earnest desire to help our patients, we may not perceive that the treatment itself constitutes still another strategy for begging the question about the nondiagnosis. A two-line note is recorded in the medical record at each visit. The first line describes the symptoms, the second, the treatment, visit after visit, sometimes for years, without an established diagnosis or reevaluation. Even the patient may not be curious. I frequently ask, "What is your idea of the nature of your illness?" Even after years of care, including psychoactive drugs, many patients seem bewildered by the question. Then I ask, "What do you think your doctor thinks about it?" "I'm not sure." "Did you ever ask?" "No."

A Diagnosis Is Established, but Does It Explain the Illness?

A not-uncommon custom of practice is to rule out every possible organic disease before considering the diagnosis of a functional disorder. In the preceding discussion, no disease was found, and the illness became a diagnostic problem. If, however, an abnormality is found, is it the cause of the illness? Though most clinicians are quite aware of inappropriate correlations, the organically focused physician may well establish the abnormality as the diagnosis. If so, the corresponding focus of attention soon shifts from the illness to the disease, with the implication that the disease is the cause.

In some of the spurious correlations between symptoms and diagnosis to be described in what follows, the physician may or may not believe that the symptoms are fully explained by the disease diagnosed, but such doubts are often not discussed with the patient. The doctors who performed Janet's hysterectomy or treated Roger's hypertension (Ch. 1) may have realized that the conditions diagnosed were too minor to explain Janet's intense continuous pain or Robert's dizziness, but they did not say so. They may have thought that Janet had a "low pain threshold" or that Robert was an exception to the rule that moderate hypertension is not a cause of dizziness. Or they may simply regard the disease, not the illness, as the proper focus of care. In any event, the customary mindset in this situation is to give the patient the "benefit of the doubt" and do what can be done about the physical condition.

In this way, as the focus shifts from the illness to the disease, neither doctor nor patient perceives how the illness itself has been bypassed. The correct diagnosis of the functional disorder is not made, nor is its source explored. The shift in focus is so embedded in medical thinking that it cannot be recognized as a strategy for evading the key issues. The physician is relieved that an organic diagnosis can be established. If, on the other hand, nothing had been found, the doctor would have had to deal in some other way with the symptoms, or perhaps even with the underlying personal situation!

Sometimes the disease that is discovered, though recognized as asymptomatic, should be treated anyway. But whether treated or not, the patient needs to know what does cause the symptoms, if not the disease. Otherwise, patients are hooked inappropriately into the disease model, as were Janet and Robert. They can only assume that the disease was the cause of the symptoms.

Inappropriate Correlation of the Symptoms with Abnormalities Found in the Workup

The abnormalities I list here are common and usually asymptomatic. When found on a physical, laboratory, X-ray, or surgical examination, they rarely explain the symptoms for which the exam was done, unless there are other, more specific, data to demonstrate the relationship. The correlations indicated are for the most part inappropriate:

Chronic Low Backache: Abnormalities of the Lumbosacral Spine on Standard X-Ray

Roentgenographic comparisons of patients with and without backache show virtually the same incidence of osteoarthritis, single disk narrowing, transitional vertebra, spina bifida occulta, and mild to moderate scoliosis. [4] Other studies have demonstrated similarly significant abnormalities in about 50 percent of young, asymptomatic, male work applicants who gave no history of backache. [5–6] For the most part, there is no way to know that these conditions cause backache in individual patients, though such abnormalities may cause some patients to be more vulnerable to the effects of physical trauma. Regardless of the findings on plane radiographs, the clinician must still consider the usual stresses and strains and psychosocial issues that often result in chronic backache (Chs. 1, 2, 4, and 13). Conditions like disk rupture and spinal stenosis that more clearly cause back pain and sciatica are demonstrated by special studies. [7]

Headache, Tinnitus, Epistaxis, and Dizziness: Hypertension

A survey of 6,672 subjects showed no relation of these symptoms to either systolic or diastolic blood pressure, with the sole exception of dizziness, which was somewhat more common in patients whose diastolic pressure exceeded 110 mm/Hg. [8]

Fatty Food Intolerance, and/or Dyspepsia (Epigastric Distress, "Indigestion," "Gas," Belching, "Fullness") in the Absence of Biliary Colic Type Pain: Gallstones

These ubiquitous symptoms occur in subjects with gallstones no more often than in those without stones. [9–10] Pain, not dyspepsia or food dyscrasia, is the hallmark of cholelithiasis; cholecystectomy cannot be expected to relieve such nonspecific symptoms. The decision for surgery must be based on other grounds.

Dyspepsia, Epigastric Pain, Heartburn: Hiatus Hernia

Thirty-three percent of asymptomatic volunteers had a hiatus hernia on barium swallow [11], compared to 30 percent of patients studied for peptic disease by the same technique. [12] Heartburn is caused by esophageal reflux, which occurs independently of hiatus hernia; the latter usually has little or no effect on gastroesophageal sphincter competence, except perhaps for an occasional sliding hernia. [13] For the most part, hiatus hernia is an asymptomatic anatomic variant. [14]

Dyspepsia is a common functional disorder in which all kinds of stress or nervous tension, eating too much or too fast, excessive ingestion of fats or coffee, smoking, drinking, inadequate rest or sleep or recreation, and other factors can play a role. These issues need to be explored with the patient, whether or not gallstones or a hiatus hernia are found.

Chronic Lower Abdominal Pain: Diverticulosis

In one study, the incidence of diverticulosis in 70 asymptomatic volunteers over 40 was 35 percent, increasing from 19 to 42 percent according to age. [15] When diverticulosis is found in patients studied for symptoms indistinguishable from irritable-bowel syndrome, experienced observers regard the diverticuli as silent except in attacks of diverticulitis, as indicated by localized pain and tenderness, fever, leukocytosis. Such inflammatory episodes are generally transient, infrequent, and readily managed medically. [16] Severe attacks and complications are uncommon. In one series of 294 referred patients found to have diverticulosis and followed for an average of 15 years, 86 percent of the 73 patients who had at least one attack had only one to three attacks in all this time. [17] Diverticuli are rarely the source of chronic or frequent recurrent abdominal pain.

Dyspepsia and chronic abdominal pain syndromes are discussed in greater detail in Chapter 13.

Anxiety States

Depending on the particular cluster, symptoms are sometimes correlated inappropriately with the following conditions:

1. Reactive hypoglycemia. Episodes of frank hypoglycemia, usually with a blood sugar less than 40 mg %, occur in patients with insulin reactions, insulinomas, and several other disease states. Each episode causes cognitive impairment or confusion and a compensatory adrenergic discharge, but the patients rarely if ever complain of chronic nervous tension. The persistent or frequently recurrent symptoms that characterize nervous states, as described previously, and occur in otherwise healthy individuals, are not caused by hypoglycemia. Such symptoms cannot be so ascribed unless (1) a comparably low blood sugar is demonstrated whenever symptoms are present and (2) the symptoms are consistently, immediately, and completely relieved by the ingestion of sugars. [18–20] This is rarely the case, and the attribution of persistent anxiety symptoms to reactive hypoglycemia is nearly always spurious.

Advocates of the syndrome suggest that the diagnosis should be considered if the blood sugar falls below 59 mg % on the glucose-tolerance test.

Surveys of glucose tolerance in healthy subjects, however, show how commonly (and how far) the blood sugar normally falls below this level: in 17 percent of adult women [21] and 24 percent of young male adults. [22] Carefully controlled studies of the five-hour oral glucose-tolerance test, correlated with symptoms, demonstrate clearly that there is no way this test can be used as the sole means of establishing a diagnosis of reactive hypoglycemia. [23]

2. *Mitral-valve prolapse.* Because cardiologists have noticed that many patients with mitral-valve prolapse (MVP) complain of chest pain, dyspnea, palpitation, lightheadedness, and other symptoms of anxiety, [24] a link has been suggested between these symptoms and MVP. [25] The association, however, except for palpitation due in some patients to arrhythmias, is spurious, and a clear case of ascertainment bias. [26] Patients attend their family doctors for symptoms of anxiety. Those with the systolic click or murmur of MVP are referred to cardiologists; symptomatic patients without a click, and asymptomatic patients in which a click is noted on routine physical exam, are not referred. The cardiologist, therefore, sees a highly selected group of patients. Prospective studies (screening for MVP) of presumably healthy subjects, [27–30] or of the relatives and spouses of previously identified patients, [31] show no difference in the frequency of these common symptoms, or of anxiety or panic attacks, between those who have MVP and those who do not. Other studies show both groups to be asymptomatic. [29, 30] If patients with long-standing panic disorder are found to have a higher incidence of MVP than do control subjects, as suggested by one study, [32] it would seem more likely that the emotional disturbance with persistent adrenergic discharge, or some other factor such as low body weight, [30] underlies the MVP, rather than the other way around. There is no reason to believe that symptoms of anxiety are caused by the relatively common anatomic-physiologic variant of MVP, any more than such symptoms are caused by frank mitral stenosis or insufficiency.

3. *Nonischemic chest pain, a disease of unknown etiology.* Psychogenic chest pain is a common symptom. It occurs in about three-fourths of all patients with anxiety states. [33, 34] Some of these patients have the discrete attacks of panic disorder, [35] but in most the persistent pain and other symptoms are better classified in the current *DSM* terminology of generalized anxiety or adjustment disorder with anxious mood. [36] As with all the other physical expressions of anxiety, however, the chest pain often appears as the predominant or only symptom. In this case, it must be distinguished from cardiac or esophageal pain, and in the absence of other symptoms its emotional source is less obvious, thus a problem for the physician.

With the advent of coronary arteriography, such pain began to be described simply as the *anginal syndrome associated with normal coronary arte-*

riograms. [37] Similar names have been used in a host of papers, many of which imply that the chest pain is caused by an organic disease of unknown etiology and is, therefore, "unexplained." [38] Actually, most emotionally induced chest pain differs from that of true angina, and its psychogenic basis has been demonstrated in many recent studies. Nevertheless, the extensive literature about "unexplained nonischemic" pain has distracted a generation of physicians from seeking to understand its emotional source in many patients. The current emphasis on panic disorder and on microvascular angina as predominantly biological entities has the same effect. These problems are discussed in greater detail in Chapter 13.

Chronic Fatigue

Feeling tired and feeling a lack of energy are common features of anxiety, depression, or simply feeling discouraged about one's life situation. As with chest pain, there may be no other symptomatic expression of the underlying personal problem. Inappropriate correlations with various disease states, particularly hypothyroidism and chronic fatigue syndrome, are not uncommon.

1. *Hypothyroidism.* In the past, owing in part to inaccurate tests for thyroid function, or to the tendency to prescribe thyroid for low-normal test results in the quest to find something positive to do for tired patients, chronic fatigue was often diagnosed as hypothyroidism. Among my own patients checked years later with the more accurate T4 and TSH determinations, after withdrawing thyroid medication for four weeks I found that many such patients had normal function. This should no longer be a problem, because all common endocrine diseases can now be known or ruled out by precise techniques.

In studies of patients with fatigue as the major complaint, the prevalence of hypothyroidism varies from 0 to 4 percent. [39–43] Many patients with frank hypothyroidism (TSH >20 mU/L) have no symptoms at all; the disease is discovered on routine laboratory testing. Those who do have symptoms, even with myxedema, rarely complain primarily of fatigue or weakness; the diagnosis is suggested by other signs or symptoms. And when mild hypothyroidism is found in the study of a "tired" patient, the fatigue may be psychogenic, and may persist after the TSH reverts to normal with thyroxine therapy. [43] On the other hand, some euthyroid patients with functional fatigue become psychologically dependent on prescribed thyroid and soon complain of a symptomatic rebound if thyroid is discontinued, though withdrawal would cause little or no distress in a myxedema patient for several weeks.

2. *Chronic fatigue syndrome.* This controversial issue is discussed in Chapter 13.

Identification of Symptoms with Age or Sex

The vasomotor instability (flushes and sweats) and urogenital atrophy of the menopause are strictly biological effects that respond to treatment with estrogens and progestin; the diagnosis is appropriate for the symptoms. When estrogens first became available, "menopause" was at times the main categorization of any or all psychologic, physiologic, or psychosomatic symptoms in women between 40 and 60. The symptoms persisted because this inappropriate correlation diverted attention from the life situation, which was often the real cause of the symptoms. [44] This usage is far less common today.

Similarly, many mental symptoms in the elderly (the lightheadedness of Joseph, Ch. 1), attributed to "arteriosclerosis," "old age," or "senility" are really due to the social deprivation, loss of purpose, and other psychological problems of declining years.

Continuous Pelvic Pain in Women: Uncomplicated Ovarian Cysts, Uterine Fibroids, and Certain Other Lesions of the Reproductive Tract

Intense protracted pelvic distress that is present most of the time, throughout the month, is often psychogenic. It is well known that most uncomplicated ovarian cysts and tumors or uterine fibroids cause little or no pain. Nevertheless, when these same lesions are found at laparoscopy or laparotomy in a search for the cause of chronic pain, there is a tendency to apply the "benefit of the doubt" hypothesis. The involved organ is removed as though it were the cause of the pain, especially by surgeons who are not familiar with the syndrome of psychogenic pain or are resistant to the concept. The inappropriate correlation of the pain with the pathology results in an often unnecessary operation, sets the stage for a second operation when the pain recurs, and blocks the possibility of dealing with the issues that really cause the pain (recall Ruth, in Ch. 1).

A more controversial problem is *endometriosis.* It can cause premenstrual or menstrual pain in some patients and acute episodes of pain if an endometrial cyst ruptures, but many patients experience no pain at all. In a recent series of 1,000 consecutive celiotomies performed for any gynecological indication, endometriosis was found in 50 percent of the patients; of those with the disease, only 15 percent had complained of dysmenorrhea, and fewer still of any other kind of pelvic pain. [45] Endometriosis is often found at laparoscopy performed only for the investigation of infertility in women free of pain. [46]

Thus endometriosis is usually an asymptomatic disease, except for dysmenorrhea in some patients. Nevertheless, when the disease is found during the investigation of a patient complaining not of dysmenorrhea but of unremitting, long-term pain, it is usually regarded as the cause. But is it? Probably not, and the rare exceptions certainly do not include the minor lesions alleged to have caused Janet's intractable pain (Ch. 1). The most telling evidence against endometriosis as the cause of chronic pain is to be found in the reports of laparoscopy performed for the investigation of chronic pain, and for infertility in pain-free patients, by the same gynecologist. The incidences of endometriosis and of adhesions were the same in both groups. [47–49] Thus no correlation between chronic pain and these two conditions is demonstrated. The only exception was found in one series that included patients with dysmenorrhea as well as chronic pain. [50]

Textbook descriptions of the symptoms of endometriosis commonly note how patients with the extensive lesions of advanced endometriosis are often free of pain, whereas those found to have minimal lesions may have disabling pain! [46, 51, 52] This apparent enigma is better explained as another form of ascertainment bias: the surgeon obviously hopes to cure the "disease" of chronic pain; asymptomatic endometriosis is a common condition; psychogenic pelvic pain is a common symptom; and the two often coexist. The disease-minded physician, however, cannot dissociate the two. Thus the same doctor who operates on a pain-free patient with a prominent pelvic mass and expresses surprise when the pelvis is found studded with "chocolate cysts," continues to attribute intractable pain in other patients to minor lesions.

In most patients, unremitting pain of three to six months' duration is probably psychogenic, regardless of the presence of minor to moderate, uncomplicated endometriosis, though the psychogenic-pain syndrome may have been superimposed on the previous physical pain of primary or secondary dysmenorrhea. Old, inactive pelvic inflammatory disease, uterine adenomyosis, and the various syndromes involving incompetence of the supporting structures of the pelvic floor are also unlikely causes of unremitting long-term pain. To understand the pain, the physician will have to know the patient at a level other than the anatomic. And as with any other disease, one must combine a knowledge of its usual symptoms with an understanding of the patient as a person in order to make a tentative judgment of whether the disease is responsible for all, some, or none of the symptoms.

Adhesions rarely, if ever, cause pain. If the disease causing the adhesions is still active, such as a pelvic abscess, then the disease itself is the cause of the pain, not the adhesions. In the comparative studies cited above, [47–49] adhesions were found in a third of all pain-free patients studied by laparoscopy for infertility, *less often* than in patients with chronic pain. And patients with acute bowel obstruction caused by entrapment by adhesive bands give no history of chronic pain prior to the moment of obstruction, no matter how thick or tense the adhesions. I have seen patients with the entire bowel matted by adhesions caused by the retroperitoneal fibrosis of methysergide therapy, or by metastatic carcinoma of the colon, without any pain whatsoever. The most desultory correlation of all occurs in patients with long-standing psychogenic-pain syndromes when the pain, no different than it has been all along, recurs after the last remaining pelvic organs have been removed, and is then ascribed to adhesions! As Thompson puts it, attributing chronic-pain syndromes to adhesions is the "cry of the diagnostically destitute." [53]

In this discussion of pelvic pain, I do not mean to oversimplify an extremely complex issue. Depending on the condition found, surgical treatment may well be appropriate even though the disease is not the cause of the pain. The question of surgery is especially complex in regard to the uterus. For some women, hysterectomy represents a physical and symbolic dissolution or loss of femininity. [54] The operation is often followed by depression, most commonly in young or middle-aged women who have symptoms of pelvic pain or menorrhagia in the absence of significant pelvic disease, and previous or concurrent nervous disorders and/or marital discord. [55, 56] These correlations, along with a higher incidence of sexual and menstrual difficulties, are similar to those that characterize patients with psychogenic pelvic-pain syndromes. [57] On the other hand, for many women who have had all the children they want, hysterectomy brings welcome relief from menstruation, fertility, and concerns about uterine disease. It also allows replacement hormonal therapy toward prevention of osteoporosis, without periodic bleeding or the hazard of endometrial carcinoma. Thus hysterectomy may provide pain relief for some women even though the pain has been psychogenic [58], yet 41 percent of the patients in another study who had had pelvic surgery for chronic pain still had pain four years later, even though the pathology in question had been excised. [59]

Obviously, gynecologic surgery carries many connotations over and above the medical indications. Persistent pelvic pain, unlike other functional disorders, most of which are not approached surgically, constitutes a unique problem. The surgery, after all, is irreversible, if not curative. As in few other fields of medicine, the physician must know the patient well, explore all possibilities, arrange psychologic consultation if necessary, discuss with the patient all aspects of this sometimes complex problem, and actively, knowledgeably, involve her in the choices to be made. [60]

Inappropriate Naming of a Functional Syndrome as Though It Were a Disease

Here the name of a disease is substituted for the name of the functional syndrome, mostly by patients, sometimes by doctors, not by inappropriate correlation with an abnormality in the workup, but simply by inference, without any clear evidence that the disease is actually present.

Some terms are colloquial, such as "flu" or "virus" for feeling weak and achy, "arthritis" or "neuritis" for muscular aches and pains, "sinus" for headache, "allergy" for many kinds of symptoms that are rarely found in truly allergic patients.

Some terms are medical misnomers, such as fibrositis for the functional syndrome now known as fibromyalgia, or costochondritis, a term often applied to nonischemic chest pain (Ch. 13). An inflammatory disease has not been demonstrated in these conditions. [61–63]

In other situations, disease terminology is simply stretched to fit the illness. Examples would include labyrinthitis or Ménière's disease for nonspecific dizziness, ulcer syndrome for dyspepsia, colitis for irritable-bowel syndrome, radiculitis for trunk pain.

In some situations a major medical diagnosis must be seriously considered even in the absence of confirmatory data. For example, since the interval electroencephalogram may be borderline or negative in a patient with grand mal seizures, and since it may be difficult to obtain a tracing during an attack, "fits" resembling seizures are often diagnosed as epilepsy. I have seen several patients with pseudoseizures ("hysterical fits") diagnosed in this way and treated uselessly for years with anticonvulsant drugs. When an illness could well be functional, the physician must be especially circumspect in establishing a diagnosis of organic disease in the absence of objective data.

Hypotheses for diffuse symptoms change like fashions. "Colitis" was a favorite in nineteenth-century France. [64] "Autointoxication," "foci of infection," and "brucellosis" faded in the 1940's. "Reactive hypoglycemia" dominated the mid-twentieth century until recently, when a series of critical evaluations and controlled studies demonstrated it to be an unlikely source of symptoms. Mitral-valve prolapse is only now beginning to fade as a correlate of anxiety symptoms. The "yeast connection," [65] and "clinical ecology" [66, 67] are current favorites.

The Inherent Iatrogenicity of the Medical Model

Note that the patients whose functional illnesses are inappropriately diagnosed as organic disease, as discussed in this chapter, start with one illness and end with two. The patient's primary illness, for example, is psychogenic pelvic pain, but this is not recognized by either the patient or the doctor, because its emotional basis is not obvious, and no effort is made to understand it. When the appendix and right ovary, the latter with a 4-cm cyst, are removed, the pain usually abates, for several reasons. Because the pain is now attributed to the cyst, and the cyst is gone, an emotional component to the illness is no longer suspected by anyone, whether family or physician. The diagnosis of the disease has actually served to confirm the conversion process

(Ch. 12). The patient is exonerated from having played any role in the illness. For a while the post-op disability takes the place of the pain as the covert way in which the underlying personal problem situation is concealed and managed. Both doctor and patient are gratified that the clinical problem has been solved. A short-term gain has been achieved. The patient now "knows" that the cyst was the cause of the pain. A second illness, ovarian cyst, was thereby added to the first illness, psychogenic pain. The latter, however, remains unattended and will recur sooner or later. If you are the doctor, what will you do six months later when the pain recurs in the mid or left pelvis? If you and the patient both remain convinced by the disease concept, the next series of steps is inevitable. If you had had misgivings about the original surgery but didn't say so at the time, what would you say or do now? If you are now convinced about the possibility of psychogenic pain after all, will the patient believe you?

Sadly, the patient has lost an opportunity to deal with the real personal problem that not only caused the pain but continues to have a profound effect on her whole life. On top of all this, she must now contend with a second problem, the "disease" in her pelvis and all that that entails. The inherent iatrogenicity of the medical model when inappropriately applied is obvious.

If this patient has three operations in ten years, and we add to the hospitalizations all the doctor's visits, tests, and treatments that such a case involves, the total cost is enormous. If the doctor had recognized the possibility of psychogenic pain early in the care and, in addition to laparoscopy, had arranged for what might turn out to be only three 50-minute psychological interviews at $100 each, which would usually be enough to confirm the pain's emotional basis, the total cost would be far less! If we are going to remove a major source of the skyrocketing cost of medical care, we should start by teaching medical students and residents to make positive primary diagnoses of psychosomatic symptoms from the beginning of an encounter, and to direct the workup and treatment accordingly. But the monetary loss is nothing compared to the human distress caused by the inappropriate biomedical focus.

The iatrogenic element is obvious when the diagnosis is wrong for the illness, even though it does describe an abnormality detected on the workup (the second major section of this chapter). If, however, the patient is trapped in a diagnostic quandary (the first section), the patient is locked into the disease model just as securely as if an error had been committed. Finally, as emphasized previously, even when the functional or psychiatric diagnosis is correct and the biotherapy helpful in relieving symptoms, but patients are not made aware of other options, an iatrogenic element is superimposed as the patients are drawn into a system in which they are led to hope, expect, or believe that the treatment will accomplish what it will not, that is, the need to effect some change in the underlying stressful situation. The important principle here is that *many patients with personal illnesses will remain ill indefinitely until the doctor has provided insight into the true nature of the problem.*

In all of these situations, iatrogenicity is reinforced by the doctor's authority, the sanctity of the names by which the illnesses are known, the avoidance of discussion of the personal source of the illness, and the shared illusion that all is being done that can be done. There need be no hemostat left in the abdomen, no drug toxicity, no specific malpractice of any kind. The iatrogenesis results from medicine doing exactly what many believe it is supposed to: classify and treat disease.

CHAPTER 7

Health Practices, Psychosocial Distress, and Organic Disease

Adverse health practices, harmful habits, and psychosocial distress are major precursors of organic disease. About 40 percent of the diseases that cause premature death could be prevented by eliminating such factors. Data that document the personal antecedents of preventable disease, and the effects of changes for health, are reviewed in this chapter.

Care providers play an important role in converting disease-provoking behaviors to health-promoting practices in individual patients. The health of the nation, however, is primarily a problem of family and individual responsibility.

Health Practices and Harmful Habits

A prospective neighborhood survey in Alameda County, California, showed clearly how health practices affect overall mortality rates. [1–2] The seven salutary practices surveyed were basic and simple: no smoking, regular physical activity, modest alcohol use, adequate sleep, normal weight (from 5 percent under ideal to 15 percent over), routinely eating breakfast, and not eating between meals. Life expectancy varied with the number of these health practices maintained, as follows:

Years of life expectancy, at age 45, per number of health practices maintained

	0 to 3	4 or 5	6 or 7
Men	22	28	33
Women	29	34	36

In short, a male of 45 with the most good health practices can expect to live 11 years longer than a male with the fewest!

If the kinds of food eaten had been examined in this study, rather than the regularity of meals, the results would have been even more striking. Of the four major risk factors for coronary artery disease and stroke, [3] only smoking and obesity were examined in the Alameda County study; hypercholesterolemia and hypertension were not included. Yet cholesterol levels, hypertension, and obesity are interrelated in various ways to what and how much we consume. Obesity is a risk factor in itself but may exert its main effects through the almost linear relationship of weight to serum cholesterol and blood pressure. [4] Elevated cholesterol levels are almost inevitably related to an excess of total calories but more specifically to total and saturated fats and cholesterol per se. [5] Hypertension, in addition to its relation to obesity, can also be induced or accentuated by excessive use of alcohol, or of salt in salt-sensitive subjects. [6]

The probability of coronary artery disease bears a linear relationship to each of the four major risk factors. Slender individuals with low cholesterol levels and low blood pressure have a longer life expectancy than those with average, "normal" levels. Furthermore, as first demonstrated in the Framingham Study [7–8] and later summarized for general use in Farquhar's *The American Way of Life Need Not Be Hazardous to Your Health,* [9] the risk factors for coronary disease, which also include stress and lack of exercise, are additive. Individuals with several inimical risk factors can have a probability of premature heart attack or stroke of well over ten times the probability of those with the fewest.

Let us next examine the question of health practices in relation to the five conditions that cause 81 percent of the annual deaths in the United States. [10] Cardiovascular disease (mostly coronary heart disease and stroke) accounts for 49 percent, and cancer, 22 percent. The remaining 10 percent are caused by accidents, chronic obstructive pulmonary disease, and suicide/homicide, in that order.

In many ways, these conditions don't "just happen." If the known risk factors for coronary disease, stroke, and certain cancers, particularly smoking, dietary factors, and overweight, could be eliminated, the deaths from these three conditions could be cut in half. [11, 12] Cessation of smoking, alone, would prevent 80 percent of the deaths from chronic obstructive pulmonary disease, as well as from cancer of the lung, larynx, and oral cavity. [13] If we consider as a group all conditions related directly to excessive drinking (motor vehicle and other accidents, suicide, homicide, drug overdose, and medical disease such as cirrhosis of the liver), alcohol overuse would constitute the next most common cause of death in the United States after heart disease, stroke, and cancer! [14]

In summary, about 40 percent of the conditions causing premature death could be prevented. Mortality statistics, dramatic though they may be, disclose only the final result of a vast morbidity caused by behaviors that lead to disease. Alcohol-related death figures, for example, do not measure the personal and social devastation of the 10 million or more people in the U.S. who are alcohol-dependent without specific medical complications.

What can we expect if the risk factors described above, once established in a person's lifestyle, were to be turned back toward normal?

Overweight. The excess mortality rates noted by life insurance companies for subjects who were overweight when insured, compared to all persons insured as standard risks, over the period limited to the first 20 years or less from the onset of the policies, [15] are striking:

Excess mortality rates (percent) for overweight subjects, by percent overweight at time insured

	10%	20%	30%
Men	13	25	42
Women	9	21	30

The same actuarial source shows that those who succeed in reducing their body weight reduce their mortality rates correspondingly, owing to a reduced incidence of vascular as well as other diseases. [16] In maturity-onset diabetes in obese patients, for example, blood sugars often return to normal if weight reduction can be accomplished.

Smoking. Similarly, for smokers who stop smoking, the mortality rates for coronary disease and lung cancer, which increase steadily with age and the amount and duration of smoking, drop steadily toward normal (depending on the amount smoked previously) during the years after cessation. [17] The relationship of smoking to chronic obstructive pulmonary disease is also well known; when smoking ceases, the bronchospasm and bronchitis, if not the alveolar damage of emphysema, subside.

Reducing serum cholesterol. When distinctly elevated levels of cholesterol, particularly of low-density lipoprotein (LDL) cholesterol, are reduced in high-risk men by diet [18] or pharmacologically, [19, 20] *before the advent of coronary disease*, the incidence of ensuing disease is clearly reduced. Dropping cholesterol levels in conjunction with weight reduction in overweight subjects is especially effective. From many other epidemiologic studies it can be inferred that lowering mild to moderate elevations of cholesterol by dietary control in nonobese subjects will also reduce the incidence of disease, though this has not yet been demonstrated in prospective clinical trials. Finally, even the progression of *established disease* has been demonstrably retarded by lowering serum cholesterol with drug regimes in major clinical trials. [21–23]

Hypertension. About 60 million American adults have an elevated blood pressure, 140/90 or greater. [24] Long-term actuarial studies of blood pressure show clearly the inverse relationship of blood pressure to longevity. The value of reducing blood pressure by antihypertensive drugs when diastolic levels exceed 100 mm/Hg is well established, but because the end-organ complications of mild hypertension—with diastolics between 90 and 100—do not appear for many years, it is difficult to demonstrate the value of therapy at those levels in short-term clinical trials. Nevertheless, a modest benefit, especially in terms of stroke reduction, has been noted. [25] From the long-term actuarial correlations, however, one infers that reducing mildly elevated pressures to normal would be found beneficial if long-term studies were to be undertaken. Even so, the gains of drug therapy have to be weighed against costs, risks, and inherent side effects. Although hypertension can occur in the absence of any extrinsic provocative factors, such as nervous tension, blood pressure in most subjects with mild to moderate elevations can be lowered significantly by weight reduction in the obese, restriction of excessive salt intake, regular exercise, limitation of alcohol, stress reduction, and/or adequate rest, sleep, and relaxation. [26] In mild hypertension, changing what can be changed readily and safely should be the first consideration.

The problem in perspective. The good news is the 36-percent decline in the U.S. death rate nationwide for cardiovascular disease during the 20 years prior to 1983. [27] The decline is due in part to improved medical care for coronary disease, hypertension, and stroke, but perhaps most important has been a healthier lifestyle generally, particularly the control of specific risk factors noted in the countries with reduced rates. [27–29] Enough individuals have stopped smoking, consumed less fat and calories, and obtained better control of their blood pressure, to make the difference.

The bad news is that about one-third of all U.S. adults still smoke, [13] one-third are more than 15 percent overweight, [30] and some surveys suggest a trend toward a decline in certain other health practices, such as more drinking and less sleep. [31] For many people, health is not a concern—until they become sick.

Sexual Behavior, Disease, and Teen Pregnancy

The health problems related to sexual behavior are now an international concern. The increasing incidence of AIDS (172,000 deaths in the U.S. as of 1992) [32a] dominates our attention, yet the incidence of gonorrhea and syphilis in recent years still exceeds that of AIDS by about 20 to 1. [32b] The ongoing epidemic of teenage pregnancy is an overwhelming problem. Though the means of prevention are relatively effective and available, the problems of sexually transmitted disease and unwanted or socially costly pregnancy are likely to persist. Individual responsibility is obviously essential, but a solution to these problems, especially in sexually active youth, will require a broad foundation of family and societal understanding, realism, education, and self-discipline. Sex itself is a "health practice" with the most far-reaching consequences.

Psychosocial Distress as Precursor to Disease in General

There are those, like Mary Baker Eddy, who believe the ultimate cause of all human illness, even organic disease, to be mental. [33] And there are those who believe the ultimate cause of illness, even psychological disorders, to be physical. Pauling: "I believe that mental disease is for the most part caused by abnormal [chemical] reaction rates, as determined by genetic constitution and diet, and by abnormal molecular concentrations of essential substances." [34] Gellhorn: "If it were possible, it would be best to omit the term 'psychological.' Many modern psychologists are in agreement with this proposal. They study behavior by objective methods and believe that it is an overt expression of activity of the brain. It seems safe to assume that disturbances of the mind are due to a faulty physiology of the central nervous system." [35]

Most physicians and psychologists would categorically deny Gellhorn's extreme position. Nevertheless, when our approach, even to functional and psychiatric disorders, is exclusively biomedical, we are acting as if biophysical disturbances were indeed the core of the problem.

The truth lies somewhere between. Concepts of psychosomatic disease have always been integral to general medical theory. From Plato's "Timaeus": "We should not move the body without the soul or the soul without the body, and thus they will aid one another, and be healthy and well balanced." [36] In the first half of the present century, psychosomatic relationships were elaborated by Dunbar, [37] Alexander, [38] and others who focused on emotional disturbances and personality types in relation to disease. Meanwhile, Selye proposed the concept of stress and the diseases of adaptation on the basis of his study of external physical stresses on animals. [39] The early clinical studies of psychosomatic disease were mostly retrospective anecdotal accounts or psychoanalytic evaluations of patients with disease. Most of the studies were neither "blind," nor controlled, nor prospective.

Since then, however, many careful epidemiologic studies have demonstrated a clear relationship of untoward preexisting psychosocial situations and certain aspects of personality to a premature increase in morbidity and mortality rates from disease in general, when the troubled subjects are compared with others in more favorable circumstances. The diseases studied are those that cause most of the deaths in the industrial world—cancer, coronary and cerebrovascular disease, diabetes, hypertension, emphysema, etc. The studies cited here are mostly prospective; those that are cross-sectional or retrospective are objective.

The personal situations that correlate with increased morbidity and mortality rates from physical disease include the following:

Parental deprivation and quality of childhood experience [40, 41]
Quality of social support [42–45]
Marital status (divorced, single, or widowed, as opposed to married)
[46, 47]
Stressful life events [48]
Bereavement and grief [49]
"Type A personality," particularly hostility and related aspects of nervous
tension [50–52]
Socioeconomic status [53, 54]
Race and ethnic group [55]
Overall quality of mental health [56, 57]

The consistent correlations of these personal situations to subsequent disease in many studies is impressive. In the Berkman and Syme prospective study of almost 7,000 adults, [42] for example, the mortality rate over a nine-year period for men aged 50–59 with the best social networks was 10 percent compared to 31 percent for those with the fewest interpersonal connections.

The relation of stressful life events to illness has been well documented, but poses many problems of interpretation. [58] Does the stress cause an individual to adopt a sick role and complain of symptoms, or does it actually cause illness?

The problem of impaired socioeconomic status and opportunity is illustrated by the U.S. infant mortality rates of black babies, which are almost twice that of whites, [59] and the life expectancy of black adults aged 25, which is about five years less than that of whites. [60] Access to medical care, health practices, genetic/biological differences in regard to certain diseases (hypertension, for example), and other factors are also pertinent.

In Vaillant's study of psychologic health, 185 men were evaluated in college and thereafter. Followed for 32 years, only 2 of the 59 men (4 percent) with the best mental health had become chronically ill or died, compared to 18 of the 48 men (38 percent) with the worst mental health. [56] Palmore followed 268 volunteers aged 60 and over for 15 years and found that work satisfaction and overall happiness were the best predictors of longevity. [57] Other studies of specific aspects of mental health, such as stress responses [61] and temperament [62] in medical students, or coping styles, [63] have found similar correlations.

Vaillant concludes "that stress does not kill us so much as ingenious adaptation to stress (call it good mental health or mature coping mechanisms) facilitates our survival." [56]

It is clear that many kinds of adverse personal and social circumstances lead to far more than functional and psychiatric disorders, alcoholism, substance abuse, and suicide. The ultimate consequence is an increased incidence of major disease. How does this happen? An individual in distress may well smoke, drink excessively, or neglect health generally. Such factors could explain the correlations in some patients. In the Vaillant study, however, the relation between previous mental health and subsequent physical health remained statistically significant when the effects of alcohol, tobacco use, and obesity were excluded by multiple regression analysis. [56] So there is a more distinct relationship. This does not mean, of course, that the personal situations directly *cause* organic disease, as they do functional illness—recall Joseph's loneliness, which caused him to feel dizzy (Ch. 1), or Mary's sexual frustration, which caused her to hyperventilate (Ch. 3). Subjects with the most favorable personal situations develop the same diseases as do those with the worst situations, but they do so later in life. The correlations show only that host resistance to many disease states is somehow compromised, presumably through complex biological interactions that are poorly understood at present [64] and vary from one person, or one disease, to another. Interactions of temperament, childhood experience, personality, life situations, personal strengths and weaknesses, nervous tension, and health habits, both good and bad, are difficult enough to sort out. What is stress to one person is a welcome challenge to another. How all this relates to the possible roles of the hypothalamus, [65] neuroendocrine, immune, [66] and other biological systems in the evolution of disease remains to be determined. [67]

The link between stress and vulnerability to disease has been imputed by many investigators to impaired immunocompetence—the field of *psychoneu-roimmunology*. [68] But for the two most important diseases of the modern world, coronary disease and cancer, it has no explanatory value. Arteriosclerosis is not immunologically related. Nor can it be proposed that psychoimmunological mechanisms activated by psychosocial disturbances might lead to cancer. After all, patients with AIDS and immunosuppressed patients with renal transplants, all of whom have grossly impaired immunocompetence, are not more susceptible to most cancers (except for Kaposi's sarcoma, tumors of lumphorecticular origin, and perhaps squamous cell carcinomas). [69] The extensive investigations of psychoneuroimmunology are indeed provocative, but we do not yet know that stress-induced impairment of immunocompetence plays a significant role in the pathogenesis of disease, or, if it does, how much so. [70]

Psychosomatic Disease

Certain diseases, particularly duodenal ulcer, [71] essential hypertension, [72] asthma, [73, 74] and ulcerative colitis, [75] have been viewed as psychosomatic, in that stress can be one significant factor that directly initiates or exacerbates the disease process, at least *in some patients*. These four diseases are caused by primary organic pathophysiology independent of emotional stimuli. Helicobacter pylori infection now appears to be the major factor in ulcer recurrence and perhaps also in its inception (Ch. 3). Nevertheless, the gastric-acid hypersecretion in ulcer, the arteriolar vasoconstriction of hypertension, and the bronchial constriction of asthma are all mediated through neuroendocrine and autonomic nervous system mechanisms that are also activated by emotions. In this way, personal distress can sometimes directly accentuate the physiological basis of the disease. The final common pathway in ulcerative colitis is unknown, but the association between emotional distress and bleeding occurs repeatedly in some patients. [75]

Whereas the pathways connecting emotional and social adversity to the ultimate development of the major diseases here discussed are extremely indirect, the pathways connecting personal distress with the so-called psychosomatic diseases are direct and immediate. There is considerable overlap, however; for example, the peak increase in mortality risk from any major disease for a young adult bereaved by death of spouse occurs within the first year of the loss. [49]

Thus emotional distress, if indeed it does accentuate a disease process, acts on the constitutional basis of or predisposition to the disease, usually emerging in conjunction with other factors. Blood pressure, for example, can be elevated by obesity, salt, alcohol, [76] and/or nervous tension, but severe hypertension can develop in the absence of all these factors. In many patients, nervous tension plays a negligible role, and even under stress the blood pressure does not rise. In other patients, stress can be a major factor. If the patient can resolve the problem, the effect can be dramatic. In my residency, for example, before antihypertensive drugs were available, I followed the course of a woman of 28 in a turbulent marriage. She had a persistent pressure of 220/120. After her divorce the pressure dropped to 140/90, where it remained without treatment for years. Another patient in a comparable marital situation had chronic ulcerative colitis. She was admitted to the hospital before the advent of steroids with the toxic megacolon, pseudopolyposis, and other complications of advanced disease. On discharge she too separated from her husband and later was divorced. She remained well for two years without treatment; a barium enema was negative except for scarring.

It may be that healing in these anecdotal accounts was simply the result of supportive medical care. In view of the usual course of each disease without treatment, however, it seemed likely that a total change in the life situation, which each patient was able to achieve, was essential to the healing process.

In many patients with "psychosomatic" disease, no underlying stress can be identified, or, if it can, the patient may be unable to do much about it. For these reasons, and because the biotherapies for the four diseases listed above are so effective, a common practice is to focus exclusively on the biomedical approach. Many patients would do far better, however, if they could recognize and resolve the personal distress that may accentuate the disease process.

Many studies have suggested that Graves' disease and rheumatoid arthritis are "psychosomatic." [77] The evidence for this and the clinical experience of most doctors, however, is far less convincing than that for the other four diseases. Though emotional distress may well intensify the symptoms and the disability, as in any disease, I do not believe that a direct effect on thyroid function or joint inflammation has been clearly demonstrated.

Anorexia nervosa and bulimia begin as functional eating disorders but often develop into frank disease states with serious inanition, endocrine and other metabolic abnormalities, and death. The psychosomatic basis for these conditions is expressed through the patient's compulsive eating behaviors.

Cirrhosis of the liver and carcinoma of the lung are not generally regarded as psychosomatic diseases. If, however, alcohol and smoking are their major causes, respectively, and if drinking and smoking have psychosocial antecedents responsible for the later physical consequence, then these two diseases are also psychosomatic. From this point of view, the same could be said for all diseases to which alcohol, smoking, substance abuse, or other behaviors contribute.

Is Cancer a Psychosomatic Disease?

The question in turn raises several others, related in the main to the antecedents of the disease and its course and treatment.

The antecedents of cancer. We have seen that different kinds of psychosocial adversity can be correlated with the premature appearance of many diseases, cancer included. Is that all that can be said about the psychosocial background of cancer? Or is there a constellation of personality traits and disturbing events that more specifically predisposes some individuals to cancer?

Affirmative answers to the last question began with Galen in the second century A.D. Many recent studies provide data suggesting that several interrelated psychosocial characteristics do play a specific role in the inception and course of cancer. [78–82] Animal studies, "notwithstanding the experimental difficulties and conflicting results, . . . demonstrate that stress is capable of influencing various disease processes, including some neoplastic disease." [83]

In the human studies cited, it is proposed that cancer-prone individuals, when faced with the difficulties of life or disease, tend to respond with a stoic acceptance or, at the extreme, a giving up or "helplessness and hopelessness," as opposed to a fighting spirit. It is further proposed that they tend to be conforming, appeasing, unassertive persons who deny, repress, and fail to express negative emotions. And they fail to rebound from significant losses or to take charge of their own lives. Critical reviews of this question, [84–89] however, point out the methodological difficulties of these observations and conclude that a clear relationship of personality to cancer has not been established.

All in all, I find the cancer-prone personality hypothesis unconvincing. First of all, unlike such conditions as hypertension or asthma, in which emotional effects can be transmitted through known physiological pathways to the disease process, there is no obvious way that such effects could be transmitted to the evolution of cancer cells. The only process postulated is suppression of immune surveillance, but this has not been demonstrated in otherwise healthy individuals as a significant factor in the cause of cancer, and it is not likely to be.

Second, I am impressed by the many patients I have seen who had quite the opposite of a "cancer-prone personality," yet were hit by cancer at the peak of productive lives. And in contrast, every doctor sees countless patients who give up on life early, appear "helpless and hopeless," cannot express their repressed emotions, and go on to suffer years and years of nervous symptoms but never develop cancer. The "helpless and hopeless" aspects of the "cancer-prone personality" in its most eloquent form would be characterized as frank depression, but a clear correlation of depressive symptoms to cancer morbidity or mortality has not been demonstrated. [90]

The question of a cancer-prone personality will be settled only by more definitive, longer-term, prospective studies with greater numbers of patients than those reported to date. It will probably turn out that the relation of personality and stress to cancer is not more unique or specific than has been demonstrated in other ways for major disease in general. [40–57]

The course of cancer. There are other ways to approach the same question. Two are of particular interest. First, if cancer is in part psychosomatic, is the progress of the disease, once established, influenced by the same variables? Second, conversely, can the course of cancer be improved by reversing the psychological sets that are thought to act as adjuncts to the disease process? Or, even if the biology of cancer is not in any way psychosomatic, can survival times be extended if the patient's psychosocial well-being can be improved in various ways?

Concerning the first of these two approaches, many studies, well controlled, do demonstrate a positive correlation of personality characteristics and coping style with survival time. The long-term survivors have qualities opposite to those that are thought to comprise the cancer-prone personality. They are said to have a fighting, even feisty, spirit. They tend to participate actively in their own care and to be responsible for their lives and health. They express their needs and feelings readily; they do not suppress their emotions. In general, they respond to crisis with flexibility and self-sufficiency. These observations are summarized in recent reviews of this question, both supportive of the correlations [81] and critical. [91]

Again, we encounter a controversial literature. Cassileth et al., in a meticulous prospective study of 359 patients with specifically defined and comparable cancers, found that those with the most favorable psychosocial attributes had the same survival or relapse times as those with the worst. Their conclusion: "Although these factors may contribute to the initiation of morbidity, the biology of the disease appears to predominate and to override the potential influence of lifestyle and psychosocial variables once the disease process is established." [92] Jamison et al. had the same findings in a similar study and reached the same conclusion. [91] The editorial, [93] subsequent correspondence, [94] and other rebuttals [95] in response to the Cassileth study and editorial show the strong feelings held by health professionals on both sides of the controversy.

As for the second of the two approaches, the studies cited above simply correlate personality variables with outcome. There was no intervention. The significance of such variables could be better demonstrated by controlled studies designed to change the outlook and behaviors of patients while undergoing medical therapy.

The most widely known advocates of such intervention on behalf of survival are Matthews-Simonton, Simonton, and Creighton [96] and Siegel. [97, 98] They provide eloquent accounts of improved quality of life as well as unusually extended remissions. Unfortunately, they provide little or no controlled data about survival.

The favorable preliminary reports of Simonton et al. were of a highly select group of about 200 patients with metastatic cancer of many types and no concurrent controls. [99, 100] Few details were provided, and comparisons were extracted from the general literature. Similarly, Siegel's remarkable recoveries, attributed to his Exceptional Cancer Patient program, are also anecdotal. The only published controlled account of his patients did not demonstrate a clear extension of survival time. [101]

Nevertheless, their contentions about survival may be valid. The recent controlled study of Spiegel et al. [102] does indeed show that psychosocial intervention lengthens survival. This study is particularly convincing in that the group was organized merely to determine the emotional value of such support for patients with metastatic breast cancer; the extended survival of the support group for an average of three years, compared to one and one-half years for the controls, was the unexpected result.

The outcome is not surprising. Though the value of support groups has been debated in various ways, [103–106] the medical, psychological, and social benefits have been clearly demonstrated in a variety of institutional studies. [107–114] Combined sometimes with other therapeutic modalities, such as self-hypnosis or imagery, support systems can reduce the intensity of pain, the sense of suffering, the fatigue, and the anorexia, nausea, and vomiting of many patients, concurrent with a reduction in their anxiety, depression, and generally discouraged state. [108, 115, 116] The value of a support system is further substantiated by the data in references [42–45]. If patients suffer less pain, need fewer narcotics or other psychoactive drugs, are more active, eat and sleep better, and hold weight, they *are* likely to live longer. I suggest that positive results, when they do occur, as in Spiegel's study, [102] are nonspecific and do not rest in any way on a psychosomatic theory of the disease.

I believe that similar results could be achieved in the Simonton and Siegel programs, not through reversal of a cancer-prone personality as postulated, but because of their very positive support systems. I make this point because the psychosomatic concept has so captured the attention of the public that people often ask: what did he do, or I do, to bring the cancer? Simonton et al. did indeed base their approach in part on the concept that personality factors combined with disturbing events, though not postulated as the basic cause of cancer, "permit" the disease to develop. In this way patients unknowingly "participate" in getting the disease, though they are not, so it is said, "to blame," because they have not yet learned to replace outworn patterns of behavior with more positive attitudes toward self and life. "By acknowledging your own participation in the onset of the disease, you acknowledge your power to participate in regaining your health and you have also taken the first step toward getting well again." [117] That *is* blame, after all, and I believe wrongly attributed.

I offer the following comments. First, though there may be psychosocial precursors that play a role in cancer, their effect is far outweighed by more important organic causes, and the disease is not *psychosomatic* in the usual meaning of the term. The concept lays an unnecessary and unwarranted burden on cancer patients. Second, though some patients accept this concept as the stimulus for change, many others are beset with a sense of guilt, especially when the disease recurs after treatment. There is a fine line here between participation, responsibility, and guilt—an inherent problem for the psychosomatic hypothesis, valid or not, depending on how it is put to the patient. Third, the changes necessary to achieve a positive philosophy of life, loving relationships with a resolution of conflicts and discharge of negative emotions, and a state of peace with a sense of personal dignity and responsibility for self—the positive attributes of the Simonton and Siegel programs—are important in their own right. Many patients discover this for themselves when faced with any serious disease. Said one busy surgeon after a massive myocardial infarction: "Just give me three months so I can be with my family the way I should have been the past 20 years." In short, a new approach to life and self need not rest on a psychosomatic basis for the disease. If the changes achieved affect cancer biology favorably, well and good, but that is not the main issue.

Siegel puts it well: "We are asking people to play an active role in their health care, not demanding of them that they get well. Exceptional patients don't try not to die. They try to *live* until they die. Then they are successes, no matter what the outcome of their disease, because they have healed their lives, even if they have not cured their diseases." [118] Suitable support programs can provide patients and their families an opportunity to do this in a constructive environment if they are unable to do so with their own resources and the guidance of their doctors. The enhanced quality, meaning, and excitement of life, perhaps even length of life, that many patients experience is striking.

Health: Whose Responsibility?

The World Health Organization defines health as "a state of complete physical, mental, and social well-being and not merely the absence of disease or infirmity." [119] Two principles in this definition are important here. First of all, the three aspects of well-being, each a desirable goal in itself, are intricately interrelated. Second, health and disease are often opposite sides of the same coin. True healing results only when health-promoting practices replace the contrary situations that caused the condition in the first place. Both principles are evident from the data in this chapter and throughout the book.

The pursuit of health as a complement to the treatment of disease has been an essential constituent of medical practice since Hippocrates. [120] Disease prevention and health promotion are, or should be, a major thrust of pediatric and obstetrical care. They should be more prominent features in the general medical supervision of adults, as well. [121, 122]

Physicians usually encounter patients only after sickness occurs. We find ourselves at the far end (fix-it-if-you-can) of an overwhelming problem of preventable disease. Nevertheless, in spite of our late involvement, any illness that results from unfavorable psychosocial situations or health practices provides a signal for change, an opportunity for what might be viewed as preventive medicine in reverse. There is no healing in alcoholic liver disease without sobriety, no healing for tension or migraine headaches until the underlying stress is replaced by more salutary life situations. The health-promotion aspect of the doctor-patient encounter can be its most important aspect.

In spite of the critical functions of health providers in patient care and education, however, health is a problem at many other levels. The personal antecedents of disease involve far more than can be approached by doctors.

A problem of family life. The foundation for health is built largely in infancy, childhood, and adolescence. The script for the drama of life is written then. An appreciation of oneself as a unique, worthwhile, lovable human being is established. A sense of self-worth or self-esteem is critical. [123, 124] On that basis, security, trust, independence, strength, responsibility, joy, caring, all have their beginnings. The family is where our basic needs, as suggested in Chapter 5, are fostered, blocked, or thwarted. The family is also where health and health practices are respected and modeled, or ignored altogether.

Yet parents have no special training for this critical process, apart from their own families and whatever other influences may have been acquired along the way. Children from nurturing families, when adults, tend to nurture their own children similarly. Children from troubled families, unfortunately, may not learn to do better for their own children. These problems are compounded by the enormous pressures facing single mothers and families experiencing poverty, unemployment, impaired nutrition, parental abandonment, deficient education, racial and sexual discrimination, sexual and physical abuse, crowding, and homelessness. Socioeconomic deprivation is a formidable barrier to personal dignity, opportunity, and social responsibility.

Most of us discover sooner or later how difficult it is to change our attitudes about ourselves, our lives, and other people, as well as the diets and other health patterns we acquired in childhood. It is no wonder, then, that we have so many individuals dependent on alcohol, and widespread substance abuse, so many functional and psychiatric illnesses, and so much preventable organic disease, to say nothing of crime and a host of other social problems. The whole problem is of such magnitude that it led the State Legislature of California to establish the California Task Force to Promote Self-esteem and Personal and Social Responsibility, a program introduced by Assemblyman John Vasconcellos. [125] The family is where the health of nations begins, as Leonard Sagan eloquently argues. [126]

A national problem. The overwhelming national problem of preventable disease has been made explicit by the Minister of National Health and Welfare for Canada, [127] and by the Surgeon General of the U.S. in a series of reports from that on smoking in 1964 [128] to the 1988 report on nutrition and health. [129]

Smoking, the nation's most significant source of preventable disease, illustrates the enormity of the problem. The annual death toll that can be attributed thereto is about 350,000. [130] The total direct health-care costs associated with smoking alone exceed $16 billion annually, and the indirect costs from lost productivity and earnings due to disability and premature death run to $37 billion annually. [131] This means an annual per capita social cost of about $200. The economic burden on each nonsmoker for providing medical care for smoking-induced illness exceeds $100, paid mostly through taxes and health insurance premiums! [132]

A problem of individual responsibility. Health education begins in families and continues through schools, the work place, the media, books about health, medical centers, and national institutions, both governmental and private. All of this has some effect. The Surgeon General's report on smoking, for example, may have been instrumental in reducing the proportion of U.S. adult male smokers from 52 to 35 percent, though for women only from 34 to 29 percent. [13]

In the last analysis, however, health is primarily a matter of individual responsibility. [133] The positive forces of health education outlined above are not so effective. The antagonistic forces of peer pressure and the general social acceptance of habits adverse to health, the prevalence of high calories, fats, and salt in our diets, the immediate pleasures and availability of abuse-potential drugs, alcohol, and tobacco, and many other toxic influences, are strong. Before disease appears, it is clearly each person's responsibility, with whatever support may be helpful, to prevail over such contrary pressures.

Finally, in the medical encounter, when an illness is manifest, the doctor can treat and advise, but it is up to the patient to make the necessary changes. An inherent problem of medical care, unfortunately, is the patient's covert transfer of responsibility for getting or staying well to the doctor, the psychotherapist, the program for weight control or smoking cessation, etc., which can sometimes subtly undermine the patient's own assumption of responsibility. Physicians have a remarkable opportunity to help patients stop smoking, [134] for example, but the vast majority of smokers who have achieved long-term abstinence quit on their own. [135] Similarly, successful weight control is more common among self-initiated dieters than it is among clinical populations. [30, 136] Is it not the emphasis on individual responsibility for not drinking, albeit with the support of the group and surrender to a "higher power," that makes Alcoholics Anonymous so effective? It is by no means easy to establish a commitment to personal responsibility for health in our patients, or, for that matter, in ourselves, but that is a goal toward which we all can strive.

Psychiatric Disorders:
The Medical Model in Perspective

In response to complaints of physical or emotional distress that can be classified as a psychiatric disorder, the doctor's attention readily shifts from the main cause, which lies in the LIFE SITUATION OF A PERSON, *to its effects, the* SYMPTOMS OF A PATIENT. *This is an inevitable result of the medical model of psychiatry in which the symptoms (feeling depressed or anxious, for example), not the cause, are identified as the diagnosis. This is the reverse of the medical model for organic disease in which the cause (appendicitis) is the diagnosis, not the symptoms (pain, vomiting). This chapter provides a perspective on this transformation. It points out the inherent difficulties and contradictions of a descriptive-phenomenologic diagnostic system based on symptoms. The purpose is to expand our focus—which is often restricted to the symptoms, their genetics, physiology, diagnosis, and treatment, as important as that may be— to include the personal problems that constitute the basic difficulty in most patients.*

ॐ Disturbing symptoms of emotional distress afflict 80 percent of all U.S. adults at some time in any one year. In household surveys, most of these people describe the distress as mild to moderate, but about one in four are seriously "impaired" [1] or experience "high levels of psychic distress." [2] In terms of DSM categories [3] at least one in six would be diagnosed as having a mental "disorder," [4, 5] and one in three as having had such disorders at some time in their lives. [6]

These astounding figures demonstrate a virtually universal predicament of the human condition. Emotional distress is often intense and intolerable. It is not surprising that so many people seek relief, as they have done for 5,000 years, with opium or alcohol. [7]

The Medical Model of Psychiatry

When individuals become aware of intrapsychic or interpersonal difficulties, feel generally troubled or dissatisfied with life, or experience symptoms of emotional distress, they may seek the advice of a psychotherapist (marriage, family, and child therapist, clinical social worker, psychologist, psychiatrist), pastoral counselor, or others. In most situations there is little need for a medical or psychiatric diagnosis. The therapist focuses on the client's personal problem and proceeds directly with counseling or psychotherapy. Other than "therapy," there are, of course, any number of ways to personal, social, and spiritual growth, by which many people, troubled or not, find what they need to change or enhance their lives.

Many troubled persons, however, are but dimly aware of the source of their distress, or, if they know the cause, are overwhelmed by it. The tension mounts until they experience emotionally induced physical symptoms, feel intolerably anxious or depressed, or otherwise have symptoms fitting a psychiatric diagnostic category. Focused on their symptoms instead of the personal situation, or defining themselves as sick instead of troubled, they seek relief from doctors. The complaint of symptoms, instead of a request for counseling, evokes the medical model. The focus shifts, at least at the beginning of the encounter, sometimes indefinitely, from the *life situation of a person* to the *symptoms of a patient*, as such persons are then known.

Medical interactions are based on diagnosis. There is no way, however, to classify the thousand and one variables of the human condition that constitute the real cause of the distress in most patients. Nor is there a way to classify the genetic or biological components, poorly understood at present, that contribute to the kind of distress experienced by patients with schizophrenia, major affective and panic disorders, alcoholism, and certain other psychiatric conditions. Instead, the resulting symptoms or clinical syndromes are diagnosed. Unlike the medical model of organic disease, in which the cause of the illness, not the symptoms, is identified as the diagnosis, the procedure is reversed in psychiatry. The symptoms, not the cause, are used for the diagnosis and thereby come to be regarded as the basic pathology. Feeling depressed ("depression"), for example, is the pathology, not the life situation, the personality factors, or the biological reactions that cause the person to feel that way. Delusional thinking or hallucinatory perceptions combined with mood and

other disturbances ("schizophrenia") is the pathology, not the brain disturbances or psychological forces that cause the illness.

The next question in a medical interaction is treatment. For true healing
to take place, most troubled patients need to bring about some major personal
changes, but (from the doctor's point of view) listening carefully, striving with
the patient to understand the underlying problems, providing appropriate
guidance, and encouraging change can be difficult. Furthermore, individuals
who seek medical attention usually expect the doctor to do something. The
distress of anxiety, the major affective disorders, and psychosis can usually be
relieved pharmacologically to some extent. The biomedical model provides a
remarkable shortcut to relief—often, for those with the more intractable psychiatric disorders, the only effective relief. Thus the physician, prepared as
always to relieve suffering, and dismayed by the difficulty of being effective
in other ways in the limited time available, prescribes psychoactive or other
symptomatic drugs. If the cause of the illness is regarded as a dysfunctional
biological system—the symptoms the key to diagnosis, biomedical relief the
essence of therapy—there may be little or no attempt to help the patient understand, or work through, the underlying personal distress.

In this way the *patients* of doctors often undergo a process quite different
from that experienced by the *clients* who opt for counseling or psychotherapy,
*even when the symptoms of the patients are caused by the same kinds of personal
problems.*

The diagnostic model of psychiatry, like that for the functional syndromes
of medical practice, based as it is on a description of symptoms, provides a
restricted view of the whole illness. But in spite of the limitations, the symptomatic model is indispensable. Both doctor and patient need to know what is
wrong, at least at some level of classification. Certainly at the beginning of any
encounter, the patient is focused on feeling depressed or paranoid, for example, not on the psychodynamics. Such symptoms are devastating and
demand relief. The DSM is a thoughtful, useful compendium of those very
symptoms. If the symptoms have significant biological components, or can be
treated biomedically, categorization provides a guide to this aspect of psychiatry. In any event, patients need to be assured that the doctor's goal is symptom
relief, whether the therapy is psychological, pharmacological, helping them to
learn better ways to handle life's problems, or whatever.

The biomedical model is uniquely relevant when the symptoms of distress are those of schizophrenia, bipolar (manic-depressive) disorder, major
depression, or the more florid panic and general-anxiety disorders of psychiatry. Such disorders often evolve when adverse psychosocial situations trigger
genetically patterned psychobiological reactions that modify the resulting
emotional expressions of distress along the lines of one disorder more than

another. At this level of the most extreme and refractory psychiatric disorders, even though the cause includes prominent psychogenic components, psychotherapy often fails to reverse the cognitive, perceptive, or affective reactive sets that have been established, whereas psychopharmacology may relieve the symptoms effectively. Thus such patients are often in greater need of the biomedical than the psychosocial aspects of a biopsychosocial approach.

Most troubled patients in medical practice, however, do not have such intractable disorders, nor do they have intermediate syndromes such as cyclothymia [8] or dysthymia (depressive neurosis). [9] In current psychiatric nomenclature, they would be classified as "adjustment disorder" with anxious mood, with depressed mood, with mixed emotional features, with withdrawal, or with physical complaints, etc., [10] "psychological factors affecting physical condition," [11] conversion or somatoform disorders, [12] or in other clearly psychogenic categories. Healing will depend, sooner or later, on a redirection of focus from the symptoms of distress (the "illness") to the needs of a person.

If 80 percent of the adult population experience emotional distress annually, then obviously most symptoms are caused by problems of living, not by coincidental "disease" or biological faults. Even in the major disorders of psychiatry in which a genetic diathesis plays a role, psychosocial factors are often most important, especially in depression and anxiety. The diagnosis of any psychiatric disorder should serve as a signal for the need for personal understanding. But what happens? Constant usage of psychiatric terminology hallows the diagnostic names as descriptive of truly basic entities such as sickle cell anemia or tuberculosis. We no longer perceive that the terminology refers only to symptoms like jaundice or hemoptysis. The quest for understanding often ends when the diagnosis is established. Most physicians rarely use such informative phrases as "adjustment disorder" or "psychological factors affecting physical condition." The diagnosis is simply anxiety or depression, as it may be migraine or fibromyalgia. This process readily diverts our attention from the needs of a troubled person to the diagnosis and treatment of an illness. Psychoactive drugs, though quite specific for certain symptoms, appear to be more generally specific than they really are. The long-term strategic goals of personal change and growth are readily eroded by biochemical theories of etiology and the short-term tactical goals of psychoactive drug relief. The psychosocial aspects of a biopsychosocial model tend to be excluded as the biological predominates. [13] This happens, even in psychiatry. [14–16] And psychiatric care tends to be limited to biotherapy, at the expense of psychotherapy, as more and more restrictions are imposed by medical insurance.

Psychosocial distress is the major source of one-fourth to one-half of all illnesses seen in primary practice (Ch. 4). Of these patients, physical symptoms are far more common than complaints of psychic distress per se. Most disturbed patients, therefore, are diagnosed by the medical names of the common functional syndromes (Chs. 4, 12, 13) and treated accordingly, usually with symptomatic drugs. When emotional distress so dominates the illness that the medical model must be shunted along psychiatric lines, there is a tendency to stick close to two diagnoses, anxiety or depression, not so much to indicate a need to understand the underlying personal situations, but because the diagnosis leads directly to a medical response with "anxiolytic" or "antidepressant" drugs.

It is not surprising, then, parallel to the self-medicating use of alcohol and opium, that psychotherapeutic drug prescriptions, received each year by one American in five, account for 17 percent of all prescriptions filled in drug stores; and 85 percent of the recipients have never seen a psychiatrist. [17] The problem is similar to most western industrialized nations. Benzodiazepines, sedatives, and hypnotics account for 60 percent of all psychotropic drugs dispensed; antidepressants, 26 percent. [18] In office practice, primary-care providers prescribe most of these drugs mainly for emotionally charged physical symptoms; they also attend 60 percent of all patients with frank mental disorders. [19]

Clearly, these agents fill an important need of patients and their doctors. *If* the doctor has

1. explained the symptoms and their probable emotional basis,
2. explored with the patient the likely psychosocial source of the problem, and what the patient may be able to do about it, with or without the help of a therapist,
3. described the pros and cons of psychopharmacology, explaining what it does to relieve symptoms as well as what it does not do in regard to the basic source of the symptoms, and
4. decided, with the patient an informed participant, that a psychoactive drug would be helpful at this stage of their collaboration,

then the biomedical model as an integral component of a comprehensive approach is invaluable.

Unfortunately, (1) the benzodiazepines, though they do suppress feelings of anxiety, can result in undesirable side effects and drug dependency, and the antidepressants, though often effective in major depression and panic disorder, are usually ineffective in the kinds of depressions and anxiety most common in medical practice; (2) the drugs are often prescribed not as adjuncts to understanding but as substitutes for it; and (3) the patient may become bound to the biomedical model as the only path to healing.

The Genetic Background of Psychiatric Disorders

At the most disruptive end of the spectrum of emotional distress are the major psychiatric disorders in which, for several reasons, the medical model is particularly appropriate: a genetic/biologic predisposition for certain types of symptom formation, the availability of effective psychoactive drugs, and the difficulties of understanding or changing the psychologic components of the illness in many patients. Although very few "nervous" patients in medical or psychotherapeutic practice have such conditions, the biology of the major disorders has had a profound influence on the attitude of many physicians toward all "psychopathology." Are most symptoms of nervous tension primarily problems of deranged chemistry rather than of disturbed emotions? Positive answers to that question are not unusual in the current biological climate of psychiatry and medicine. The approach to most psychiatric disorders has shifted dramatically from personal understanding to diagnostic and biochemical manipulation. If we could sort out the biological/psychosocial interface in the major disorders, perhaps we could view the whole problem in a better perspective.

Let us first consider the genetic predisposition for certain types of symptom formation, because that is the main reason a disorder is regarded as predominantly biological. We will soon see, however, that genetic trends toward certain symptoms are but one part of a more general genetic basis for many aspects of human nature; of special interest here are personality, behavior, and temperament.

Data to be reviewed later in this chapter show that the major psychiatric disorders have many symptoms in common, and are not as discrete as is suggested by the DSM categories. Nevertheless, a genetic predisposition has been demonstrated for the cultural symptom clusters known as schizophrenia, bipolar disorder, major depression, panic disorder, and alcoholism. A genetic trend toward antisocial personality [20] and somatization disorder [21] has also been suggested. Have specific genes evolved to enable *Homo sapiens* to think crazy thoughts, feel unrealistically good or bad, be morbidly despondent and self-deprecatory, or fearful, to drink too much, act irresponsibly, or complain of physical symptoms? Hardly. Such data simply show, as Dobzhansky says, that "persons who are similar or identical in genotype are likely to react more similarly to whatever environments they may meet than [will] persons with dissimilar genotypes." [22] The chain of family, personal, social, and cultural influences between a genetic susceptibility at the beginning of life and a psychiatric disorder later on is long and devious.

Just what is transmitted? No confirmed *premorbid* biologic marker has been established for any psychiatric disorder, though many have been proposed. Thus it is not known how a genetic diathesis is expressed or activated in the evolution of the illness. There being no answers, I can offer only conjectures. Let us consider two general points of view: (1) is there a biochemical fault or disease process of some kind? and (2) could the transmission be related mainly to the genetics of temperament?

Is There a Biochemical Fault or Disease Process?

There appear to be three possibilities:

A. *A major premorbid fault.* This would be a genetically determined dysfunctional biological system of sufficient magnitude to be a major factor in symptom formation in the relative absence of a significant psychosocial disturbance, thus predisposing the individual to react to a disturbance with unique and intense symptoms that would rarely occur in others. The dysfunctional system could result from a specific fault (neurotransmitter, enzyme, receptor, etc.), or from a disease process such as has been proposed for schizophrenia, or it could represent an extreme but otherwise normal physiologic variant, as described next.

B. *A physiological variant in the regulation of otherwise normal systems of emotional expression.* In this case the central and peripheral neuroendocrine systems in which emotions, particularly, are expressed normally (Ch. 11)—that is, the adrenergic and other arousal systems that are activated in emergency states and deactivated in withdrawal states—are normal in all respects except that the genetic threshold for the release of these reactions is set lower than usual, or the reactions are set to proceed with greater intensity and/or not to be self-limiting. The source of the disorder is primarily a psychosocial disturbance, but the biological expression of the ensuing emotions occurs more readily, more frequently, or more strongly because of the hyperreactive system. The reactivity, if plotted on a curve of normal biological variability, would be found at the more sensitive or reactive end of the curve. The neurological systems underlying other mental functions could be similarly affected.

C. *No biological abnormality of any kind.* The source of the disorder is psychosocial, and the emotional responses are normal in all respects, comparable to the autonomic discharge triggered in everyone by fear, anger, or anxiety, or to the withdrawal states of fatigue, grief, or feeling depressed. The genetics are normal.

Biologic Pathways and Psychiatric Disorders

Let us next consider such biologic pathways in relation to the major psychiatric disorders.

Schizophrenia and bipolar disorder. It is now generally accepted that dysfunctional systems of the A type (above) play a significant role in most patients with chronic schizophrenia, bipolar disorder, and perhaps also obsessive-compulsive disorder. [23, 24] Some aspect of bipolar biology may also play a role in certain patients with recurrent unipolar major depression. Nevertheless, the balance of "nature/nurture" forces in all these conditions remains unknown, and it presumably varies from illness to illness and from patient to patient.

In schizophrenia, for example, distinct evidence from family, twin, and adoption studies points to an important genetic contribution. [25] A susceptibility gene, however, has not been identified. [26] Incomplete penetrance and variable phenotypes characterize the transmission of the trait generally. [27] The 50-percent discordance rate among identical twins points to powerful nongenetic factors, which are equally important to understand. [28] How the genetics relates to the brain abnormalities demonstrated in many patients, [29, 30] particularly the affected twins of monozygotic pairs discordant for the disorder, [31, 32] is not yet known.

Schizophrenia is sometimes precipitated by turbulent situations, with no premorbid disturbance of personality or social functioning, and then remits. [33] A long-term remission of schizophrenia, or of the related syndromes of brief reactive psychosis or schizophreniform disorder, [34] suggests that psychological factors outweigh any latent genetic or organic components in such patients.

Thus schizophrenia, though well defined as a symptom complex, is poorly defined as a basic biologic or psychologic entity. It may well comprise multiple subsets with differing etiologies. How genetic, anatomic/biochemical, and psychological factors interrelate is not known. In the psychoses that remit, psychosocial sources predominate, and in many such patients there may be no significant premorbid fault. In most patients with chronic schizophrenia, however, there is presumably a primary fault of the A type that predominates over environmental forces.

Anxiety, panic, and depression. Feeling anxious, depressed, or, often, both, are the common feelings that pervade the emotional distress experienced by four of five U.S. adults in any one year. Such feelings are found in virtually all psychiatric disorders, regardless of how they are categorized. [35] Obviously, such universal feelings of distress—the nervous tension and acute emotional upsets, the anxiety and depression, of most patients—are normal emotional responses to life situations, as in C above.

Nevertheless, at the extremes of these responses, there is a distinct family clustering of major depression, and, though less noticeably, of clinical anxiety disorders, shared in various ways with depression. [36] The clustering in anxiety has been demonstrated mainly for the brief, intense attacks shown as panic disorder, not for the other, more common, persistent-anxiety syndromes. [37, 38]

Family clustering reflects a common environment, common learning genes, or both. Probably most family clusters of depression and/or anxiety are predominantly related to a family milieu of stressful interpersonal relationships. If so, the corresponding biology simply represents the usual reactions of normal physiological systems to emotional distress, conscious or unconscious, or to the excessive responses of inherently normal systems sensitized by previous, often repetitive, emotional trauma. In the latter situation, the biological responses would be found to be hypersensitive on provocative testing, but this would indicate an acquired trait, not a premorbidly abnormal regulatory mechanism.

If, however, family clustering includes a genetic factor in some families, as has been demonstrated in twin or adoption studies for both depression [39] and panic disorder [40], I propose that the mode of transmission is most likely a variant in the regulation of biological response to stress, as in B, not a primary fault sufficient to cause symptoms independently, as in A. The genetics of depression is restricted primarily to certain subtypes of major depression. Other forms of major depression, dysthymia, and depressive adjustment disorders appear to be affected negligibly if at all by direct genetic factors. [41, 42] And the genetics of anxiety applies primarily to panic attacks, not to generalized anxiety. [40]

There is ongoing controversy, but I argue that anxiety, panic, and depression are essentially psychogenic disorders in most patients, even in families with a genetic diathesis. The form, the intensity, or the frequency of the symptomatic response is modified or patterned by genetic factors, but the basic source of the distress lies in emotionally disturbing situations that occur early or late in life. The emotional responses may be immediate, may not evolve until provoked repetitively, or may be suppressed altogether only to reappear much later in life when triggered by situations that are often related to the subject's background but do not superficially appear to be so. When the emotional disturbance is sufficiently intense, it will be expressed physiologically, as will any emotion. The biology of the response may be normal (C) or accentuated (B), but what is transmitted in the latter is not a unique proclivity for personal problems or an inherent dysphoria but the capacity for an accentuated biological response to stressful situations. The key to understanding is the life situation that lies at the roots of the illness.

The psychosocial basis of anxiety and depression, as opposed to the "endogenous" point of view, will be argued further. First, however, let us consider another possible mode of genetic transmission that may be related to the above.

The role of temperament. Perhaps the search for specific genes, defective neurotransmitters, regulatory faults, etc., may be too narrow a research focus for the genetic transmission of anxiety, panic, depression, and alcoholism, which are so confluent with the distress and practices of daily life. Could the genetics lie in the wider context of the inheritance of temperament, personality, and behavioral traits generally?

The inheritance of these aspects of human nature has been well documented in studies of identical vs. fraternal same-sexed twins, [43] identical twins raised apart, [44] the temperament and development of infants and children, [45] and adult personality. [46] Similar findings are noted in many animal models of behavioral genetics. [47–49] Studies of the biology of temperament, closely related to the same biological systems in which anxiety and depression are expressed, are beginning to appear, [50, 51] though neither the genes nor the modes of expression are yet well known.

Thus temperament, personality, and behavior have a substantial genetic basis, though one that is modified considerably as the patterns interact with one another and with life experiences. [52] This being so, many psychiatric disorders, viewed as the responses of individuals with certain temperaments and predisposing behavioral patterns to certain kinds of life experiences, will also be found to have a genetic predilection. The more profound the response—panic disorder compared to general anxiety, major depression compared to adjustment disorder with depressed mood, problem drinking compared to social drinking—the more likely the genetic background will be demonstrable. How trait (personality) might lead to state (psychiatric disorder) has been suggested for anxiety, [48, 53, 54] alcoholism, [55, 56] and depression. [57, 58] Whether or not persistent mood disturbances, such as dysthymia or cyclothymia, or the personality disorders are acquired states, temperamental traits determined by more specific physiologic variants, or a mixture of all three, remains to be seen. Because of the extensive interplay of personality traits and life experience, investigation is difficult. Nevertheless, as summarized by Akiskal et al., "Future research may reveal more complex links whereby both personality and affective illness emerge as part of a multifactorial continuum, including familial-genetic loading, development vicissitudes, sociocultural background, sex effects, and life events." [58]

The evolution of depression or alcoholism in individuals may depend in part on different genetic or social patterns of temperament and behavior in their families. [59, 60] Population studies, however, show that men become alcoholic two to three times more often than women, [61] whereas women suffer depression two to three times more often than men. [62] This may indicate how cultural factors can override genetic diathesis as determinants of the eventual phenotype.

Men still have greater freedom to individuate, and to determine their own independent paths through life. They tend to suppress their emotions, and their drinking behaviors are more acceptable. This may explain in part why men are more prone to alcoholism. Women often find their greatest strength and meaning in relationships. On the other hand, they are often restricted in terms of personal growth and opportunity as they are placed in secondary or "put-down" roles from which it is difficult to escape in a patriarchal society. [63, 64] And they are more likely than men to have suffered the far-reaching, long-term effects of sexual abuse in childhood (Ch. 17). For these and many other reasons, it is not surprising that women are more prone to depression. [65, 66]

In conclusion, then, it seems unlikely, in the recent evolution of the human species, that the genetic basis of such ancient and stable brain systems as the limbic and subcortical areas of arousal and emotionality would undergo such specific mutations as would be necessary to constitute a primary biologic fault as the sole or main cause of anxiety, panic, depression, or alcoholism, independently of psychosocial distress. If such defects did evolve, how would they determine phenotypes of uniquely human values? The evolution of human consciousness and society, which pose such remarkable and unprecedented problems for human life, interacting with genetically based but normal variants of the neurobiological substrates of emotional expression, temperament, and personality, provides a more reasonable explanation for the heritability of these disorders, and would account for the absence of specific biological markers.

Panic and Anxiety: Emotional Distress or Brain Disease?

The arousal of vigilance, adrenergic discharge, muscle tension, hyperventilation, and other biological expressions of panic and anxiety that we see in patients are the same physiological responses to threat that have evolved in all higher animals. Yet many biologically oriented psychiatrists hold that panic and depression are endogenous disease entities in which the limbic, neuroendocrine, and other systems primarily activated in response to strong emotions or stress are so dysfunctional as to discharge spontaneously, and thus must be viewed (inappropriately and maladaptively) as "disease." It is implied, moreover, that such a dysfunctional system would then not only express itself in the adrenergic and other physiological expressions of arousal, or in the vegetative physiology of withdrawal, but also account for the associated feelings of fear, panic, failure, inadequacy, self-hate, and the like. Though we all learn that these feelings, as normal responses, are ways of defining our anxiety or despair, the biological-dysfunction emphasis does not account for them in their context of a person living out a unique life history and personality or a difficult personal situation. Instead, these responses are said to be pathological neuroendocrine function occurring for biological reasons independent of situation and personality. That view of primary endogenous pathology discounts the fact that learning, failed adaptations, inabilities to cope, and personal sensitivities either carried over from the past or recently triggered, whether conscious or unconscious, play a role in accounting for the anguish the patient feels and presents: it is implied that nothing human causes the anguish; suppression and psychodynamic features are irrelevant concepts; no biologically normal person would react that way. This view is taken not only by the biological psychiatrist; it can be a convenient one for the disease-oriented medical practitioner to take as well. But here we must ask if that makes sense.

If, for example, the primary action of the postulated endogenous fault were an adrenergic discharge or augmented muscular tension, would this precipitate a feeling of panic? There is considerable evidence that this would not be so. First of all, normal human subjects rarely experience an emotional response when injected with epinephrine or isoproterenol, though the adrenergic effects may feel somewhat "as if" an emotion were present. [67–70] Similarly, patients with pheochromocytoma [71], paroxysmal tachycardia, or other physical states that simulate the various aspects of adrenergic discharge, or healthy subjects who hyperventilate voluntarily, rarely experience panic, acute anxiety, or terror, in contrast to patients with panic disorder. Conversely, a sympathectomized cat manifests all its usual postural and other fear responses when confronted by a threatening situation, even though the adrenergic effects have been eliminated. [72]

Thus there are no inherent aspects of the adrenergic, hyperventilatory, muscular, or gastrointestinal components of a panic attack that would be expected to cause a subjective feeling of panic. Yet in patients with panic disorder the panic appears in conjunction with the physiologic arousal, whether induced spontaneously or by isoproterenol, sodium lactate, or other provocative tests that produce somatic but few emotional effects in normal subjects. [70] Why? On the basis of countless observations of patients with panic and anxiety, as well as many functional disturbances of all kinds, in whom the emotional source was eventually revealed and resolved, the most plausible explanation to me is that the source lies in the patient's latent anxiety acquired during previously disturbing, albeit suppressed, experiences.

In everyday life, for example, when someone suddenly bursts into tears or explodes in anger with what appears to be little or no provocation, we "know" that this person has been "holding it in," even though the individual may deny it: "I don't know why I did that. It's not me!" We do not regard the incident as "endogenous" and unrelated to life's realities. The commonsense observer realizes that the outburst is clearly caused by suppressed emotions that have escaped from control. Why, then, in medical practice, do we regard the appearance of anxiety or depression without obvious provocation as though it were a strictly biological event? Is there such a difference? Could panic disorder really be a unique condition in which the central issue is a "biological defect" [73] or "biochemical abnormality" [74] rather than a suppression of emotional disturbances that from time to time virtually everyone finds difficult to resolve?

It should be emphasized here that most patients seen in medical practice with functional syndromes cannot explain the symptoms when first questioned. The symptoms have appeared "out of the blue." There is nothing unusual about panic disorder in this respect. Patients are focused on the symptoms, not the source. When symptoms are physical, as in irritable-bowel syndrome, patients are aware of neither the personal source nor the corresponding emotions. If the symptoms are emotional, as in feeling anxious or depressed, the patient, though aware of feeling disturbed, is still not aware of the source. Even when patients do know about the source, they usually fail to connect the symptoms to the marital conflict, disagreeable job, or whatever the problem may be. Finally, even in the throes of a conflict, an apprehensive patient in the emergency room "can't breathe," trembles, and chokes, but makes no mention of rejection by his lover two hours previously. Unconscious suppression of emotions and their personal source is the rule for all functional syndromes in clinical medicine; a disturbed person who is fully aware of all aspects of an emotional disturbance—its source as well as its physical expression—is not likely to seek medical advice.

We need to keep in mind the immense variation in the suppressive forces that keep the source of an emotional disturbance from awareness. Mary S. (Ch. 3), for example, had a classic panic disorder, as defined in DSM-III-R. [75] The attacks appeared to be spontaneous, unexpected, and unrelated to any provocative events. How far the personal situation is explored in such a situation will vary with the orientation of the interviewer. Nevertheless, many physicians would suspect a sexual problem because of the evolution of symptoms in her recent marriage. The source here was indeed revealed in a more searching interview. In this case even a staunchly biological psychiatrist would grant that Mary's panic attacks were the symptoms of an emotional problem, and that there was no biological defect.

If, however, you encounter a patient whose personal integrity was undermined in childhood, much of which the patient neither recalls nor understands, then it will be difficult to sort out the source. The background could vary all the way from family dynamics that simply fail to nourish in some ways, [76] to parental separation, physical or sexual abuse, or other gross disturbances. [77] It can be extremely difficult to understand such a patient. Nothing unusual is noted about his/her current adult relationship during which the panic attacks first appear—the "sudden appearance of spontaneous panic," [73] "a special kind of anxiety never before experienced, even under stress." [74] Then too, the interviewer will draw a negative or unemotional response about the patient's childhood if the memories of abuse, for example, are sufficiently suppressed, as with Amy B. (Ch. 11). Thus it is not surprising that the panic (anxiety, or depression) itself is viewed as the basic pathology. Nor is it surprising that psychoanalysis or psychotherapy, though skillful and compassionate, may not readily unravel the source, to produce change. This takes time. Hypnosis with age regression in conjunction with a psychotherapeutic relationship may be effective. Few patients, however, are motivated for extended care. Without an understanding of the source and some kind of resolution of the corresponding emotional containment, it will be difficult for the patient to accept, or the therapist to provide, the special guidance necessary to replace the patient's many trepidations with self-confidence. Moreover, understanding, though it constitutes a significant beginning to the healing process, is not enough. The patient must learn by actual experience to feel good about self, to trust, to relate to others more effectively. The same applies to the background of, and recovery from, alcohol and drug dependency and many other chronic disturbances. That is why a residential program, Alcoholics Anonymous, group therapy, or other kinds of support systems in which the subject can work with and respond to others in a caring and secure environment, can in certain situations be more effective than (or a useful complement to) individual therapy. Amy's problems, for example, slowly resolved only with the intensive program of a weekly peer-support group with specially trained therapists over a period of two years.

The emotional source of panic disorder can be viewed in many ways. Symptoms may first appear in childhood, as expressed in separation anxiety, [77, 78] or in adults, when precipitated by many kinds of disturbing events. [77, 79, 80] The symptoms may appear to be spontaneous, but the basis for the adult reaction could have been formed in childhood, or it may be caused mainly by a current situation, as with Mary, though the problem is not at all clear at first. The background may be a chronic situation, a series of events, or even a single traumatic event to which the patient did not, could not, react emotionally at the time.

Then, too, insecure patients have often acquired many cognitive/perceptive styles of formulating life experience that are conducive to anxiety. A patient may have an overriding feeling of uncertainty, unpredictability, and helplessness, no distinct sense of being in charge of his or her life. A patient may have little capacity to perceive bodily feelings or emotions in self or others. A patient may have impossibly fixed and arbitrary goals for success and happiness. These and many other self-defeating attitudinal and behavior patterns entrench the problems.

The psychiatric literature of the past century is replete with case histories delineating the emotional source of panic and anxiety. Yet our understanding of the countless ways in which emotional integrity can be undermined has only begun to unfold. The very existence of the sexual and physical abuse of children, for example, and, therefore, its extent and impact, have only recently been recognized. Thus it is most likely, even in those patients in whom the source is not clear, that anxiety disorders begin in disturbing life situations. Though the immediate impact is often suppressed, especially in childhood, there emerges a steady state of residual fears and concerns, unique for each individual, but often associated with a loss of confidence and trust in self and others, impaired interpersonal relationships, a tendency to dependency, and a diminished capacity to be responsible for one's own life. From this steady state, often with no obvious distress, frank panic or anxiety can emerge with little provocation.

Though the sensitivity of the emotional systems in panic disorder may be due in part to a B-type genetic variant, in most patients it is probably more of an acquired state that predominates over trait. The reverberating circuits between the underlying emotions and their biological expression have been unduly sensitized by repetitive trauma. Otherwise, in the absence of trauma, and regardless of the genetic patterning of the biological circuits, neither the emotionality of the experience nor its somatic manifestations would have evolved. It is most improbable that a faulty neurobiological system of some kind could substantially reverse the entire normal biological sequence of an emotion: threatening situation → perception of threat → feeling of fear or other emotion → physical expression of the emotional response → appropriate action or constraint thereof. Nevertheless, from the endogenous point of view, the genetic patterning of the response is regarded as the overriding "defect" that constitutes the principal problem. This has led many physicians to regard the nature/nurture ratio here to be perhaps 5/1 rather than 1/5, which is, I believe, closer to the reality.

We touch here on an issue critical in the doctor/patient relationship. Do we regard, for example, the relation of adult panic disorder to childhood separation anxiety as "a shared pathophysiological dysfunction," [81] that is, an abnormal reaction of both child and adult? Or is the child's anxiety a universal instinctual response to parental separation [78, 82] that would understandably lead to adult concerns about relationships and accentuated reactions to stress or loss? Clearly, the way we seek to understand and help patients is governed by our thoughts about such questions. Ideally, we need to think in terms of an integrated model of panic and anxiety, incorporating the emotional source with its biological expression [37, 83, 84], regardless of the balance of forces.

If the underlying personal situation can be resolved, as with Mary, that is clearly the best approach, whether the intensity of the symptoms is due in part to a genetic diathesis or not.

In other patients, however, especially those with agoraphobia, such a resolution cannot be readily achieved. The source is remote, difficult to elicit. The panic experience is terrifying. The patient is repeatedly caught in a vicious circle of anticipatory anxiety and conditioned responses as the experience occurs again and again. [70, 85, 86] The patient makes every effort to avoid situations that may provoke symptoms, or from which escape or help is not possible should symptoms occur. [73] Nevertheless, the panic attacks can be blocked with tricyclic antidepressants, triazolo-benzodiazepines, or monoamine oxidase inhibitors, and the anticipatory anxiety and phobic components can be relieved by behavioral approaches. Thus, there is a practical advantage to the biological regimen, and it can be applied immediately.

Unfortunately, however, we often approach panic patients, with or without agoraphobia, as though the disorder were purely physical, and little or no effort is made to know the troubled person. The drugs serve as a barrier instead of an adjunct to the psychotherapeutic healing process.

My point here is supported by Katon, [87] who notes that about half of all patients who complain predominantly of nonischemic chest pain can be classified as having panic disorder; that is, they have chest pain and panic attacks plus at least three other typical somatic symptoms of anxiety. The author's understanding of the emotional source of panic is evident in his book. [84] Yet his paper on chest pain, like thousands of other reports in the current psychiatric literature, is restricted to an exclusively biological analysis. Panic disorder is described as a "brain disease" that can be treated pharmacologically. The reader could well infer that the disorder is not psychogenic. No suggestion is offered that perhaps the patient would be well if helped to understand the underlying personal situation, and to do something about it.

I have found, however (see Chs. 11 and 13), that most of my patients with nonischemic chest pain have appreciated the opportunity to share their personal distress. We could usually begin to understand the underlying emotional tensions, and improvement could be expected when we attended to core issues. This was true whether the chest pain was an isolated symptom or was associated with enough other nervous symptoms to be classified as a DSM panic or generalized anxiety disorder.

Noting that some patients with nonischemic chest pain have panic disorder, Katon confirms what Osler noted in 1892, [88] as have many others since then [89]: such pain is one symptom of an emotional disorder. But if panic is reclassified as a brain disease, we may be diverted into a deceptive tangent. Does this mean that patients with chest pain and three or more other nervous symptoms have a brain disease, whereas those with no other symptoms, or only one or two, have some other condition altogether? A better approach to *all* patients with this kind of chest pain (better designated as psychogenic chest pain), rather than counting the symptoms, is to focus on the underlying personal distressful situation and what can be done about that.

The Psychobiologic Unit

A patient (compare Orvieta T., Ch. 2) complains of a cluster of symptoms. She feels anxious and depressed and notes abdominal pains, headaches, backache, fatigue, and aches "all over." In a biomedical analysis, this illness can be separated into the two sets of emotional symptoms and the five physical symptoms: irritable-bowel syndrome, tension headaches, lumbosacral strain, a fatigue syndrome, and fibromyalgia. Each of the seven symptoms is an appropriate focus of clinical attention that has been described as a "specific" syndrome or disorder, with its own name and presumed physiology, and treated with "specific" antidotes. This provides a convenient means of diagnosis and treatment, especially if any one disorder dominates the clinical picture, but the symptoms often appear in clusters. Obviously, it is most effective in the long run to focus on the source of the disturbance—the frustrating life situation in Orvieta's case—whether one, or several, or all seven disorders are present at any one time. If the therapeutic focus always falls primarily on the medical pathology or psychopathology, as named in the classifications of disease, the clinician often fails to recognize the common denominator.

Similarly, in psychiatry, even in the major disorders that are genetically patterned so that one symptom is more likely to appear than another, the symptoms often evolve in clusters. Here too, the disturbance in each sector of mental activity (thought, perception, mood, behavior) is an appropriate focus of clinical attention that has been described as a "specific" disorder with its own name and physiology, and many such disturbances can be treated with "specific" antidotes. Again, this provides a convenient means of diagnosis and treatment, especially if any one disorder dominates the clinical picture. In that the disturbances are so often concurrent, however, it is apparent that each "disorder" is but the *symptom* of a common source of disturbance. In most patients, the source lies predominantly in their life situations, though the form taken by the disturbance is determined in part by an inherent biological pathway.

Consider the following observations:

Zigler and Phillips analyzed 35 symptoms in 793 patients divided into four groups (manic-depressive, psychoneurotic, character disorder, and schizophrenic). Their conclusion: "Although relationships exist between symptoms and diagnoses, the magnitude of these relationships is generally so small that membership in a particular diagnostic group conveys only minimal information about the symptomatology of the patient." [90]

The same was found by Freudenberg and Robertson: "The assessments of symptoms . . . confirmed very clearly the enormous extent to which symptoms overlap from one psychiatric diagnosis to another . . . [which] thus emphasizes the need for a dimensional and profile approach to the problems of psychiatric diagnosis." [91] They found, for example, that patients diagnosed as schizophrenic feel more depressed on scales of depression than do those diagnosed as depressive. These concepts are expanded by Schulterbrandt et al., who point out the close resemblance for most major categories of psychopathology—depressed mood, anxiety, somatic concern, emotional withdrawal, hostility, paranoia, conceptional disorganization, and motor retardation—whether the diagnosis is schizophrenia or depression. [92] Such clusters suggest that psychiatric disorders should be viewed, not as discrete entities, but as "hierarchies" of interrelated symptoms. [35, 93, 94]

In a recent survey of mental disorders in a community population, using the current definitions of the NIMH Diagnostic Interview Schedule, [95] minus the DSM exclusion criteria that arbitrarily determine their "specificity" (to be discussed shortly), a general tendency toward co-occurrence was noted. [5] The presence of any disorder increased the probability, often strikingly, of having almost any other disorder, even those that are not generally considered to be related. The odds that a subject with "schizophrenia," for example, would also have manic episodes, major depression, or panic disorder exceeded 28:1 for each of these three symptoms! Conversely, the odds that a subject with a major depressive episode would also have criteria for panic disorder or schizophrenia exceeded 18:1 for both symptoms.

Such data pose a formidable problem for the diagnostic model of psychiatry. The association of symptoms suggests that psychiatric disorders are better viewed as symptoms of a common etiology than as discrete entities that can be neatly distinguished, one from the other.

Each symptom is, of course, "specific," even though it is joined by other symptoms in a cluster. Paranoia is not the same as panic, any more than tension headaches are the same as hyperventilation syndrome, though these four symptoms may coexist in any combination. Classifying the dominant symptom is indeed important heuristically—for communication, for genetic, biologic, epidemiologic, psychodynamic, and prognostic studies, and for decisions about the most effective pharmacotherapy or kind of psychotherapy, for each symptom. It is helpful in many ways to distinguish, for example, panic disorder from generalized anxiety, or anxiety from depression, though these often occur concurrently. The difficulty here is that as DSM defines each symptom more precisely, a new paradigm results, and a thousand studies, mostly biological, soon appear, analyzing the symptom in all its ramifications. As this occurs, the symptom appears to be an ever more specific entity that has somehow lost its source in a human situation common to other symptoms.

Certain symptom clusters, most notably those diagnosed as schizophrenia or the major affective disorders, tend to reappear in similar form through the lifetime of a patient [96] or in first-degree relatives who develop a mental disorder, [97] though there are many exceptions. The genetic patterning of these and other disorders has been verified extensively. Thus there is a certain biological pattern to the way symptoms congregate, which dominates, etc. And particular physiological configurations have been suggested for each sector of mental activity, though the biology is readily confused when symptoms of psychosis, depression, and anxiety coexist.

Thus the specificity of symptom clusters *as diagnosed* has a certain validity, but the specificity is sometimes more apparent than real, particularly when it results mainly from arbitrary rules of classification.

A patient, for example, has psychotic ideation, manic episodes, a major depression, panic attacks, and somatization disorder, [5] as well as substance abuse. [98] Obviously, this patient does not have six separate disorders, coincidentally concurrent, any more than Orvieta had seven unrelated disorders. How, then, is this patient labeled? The presence of psychosis preempts the diagnosis. So the patient is said to have "schizophrenia." In other words, the consistency of diagnosis in such patients, though multiple symptoms are present, is in part an artifact of the rules and customs of diagnosis. If psychotic ideation were not one of the symptoms, the cluster would be identified by one of the other names.

Similarly, most depressed patients are anxious, often more so than patients who have been diagnosed as having an anxiety disorder, [99] but anxiety, categorized separately, is not even listed in the DSM affective categories as a related disorder. Thus depression usually preempts the diagnosis when the two kinds of dysphoria coexist.

When one disorder follows another, the second could in part be precipitated by the first. A delusional state could in turn lead to panic attacks, or alcoholism, for example. In most cases, however, a more rational explanation is that multiple disorders, especially when they are not known to follow one another in any set sequence, are conjoint symptoms of the same underlying psychosocial/biologic disturbance.

Because there is no way to define schizophrenia or any other psychiatric disorder biologically, as most organic diseases can be defined, the diagnosis is always a sorting out of symptoms, even though each symptom may have certain significant genetic, biologic, and therapeutic aspects. The limitations of a taxonomy of symptoms are indeed made explicit in the prefaces to DSM-III and III-R. The authors emphasize that the manuals are "descriptive"; the disorders are viewed as "manifestations" [100] or as "behavioral signs or *symptoms*" [101] (italics mine). The manuals do not presume to classify "etiology."

Nevertheless, to be useful the manual must seek specificity insofar as this can be imposed on the symptoms. This is done in two ways. First, human functioning as a psychobiologic unit is dissected into separate categories of cognitive/perceptual, affective, anxious (its own separate category), behavioral, and physical symptoms. Each major symptom category is then subdivided into subcategories. Finally, to maintain the separation, multiple symptoms are segregated by arbitrary exclusion criteria provided throughout the text, according to which symptoms appeared first, persisted the longest, or take precedence for other reasons. Every physician, considering a patient with a psychiatric diagnosis, should realize just how convoluted the diagnostic process can be.

Under "Schizophrenia," for example, we are instructed: "The differential diagnosis [from Mood Disorder and Schizoaffective Disorder] can be difficult, because mood disturbance, particularly with depressive symptoms, is common during all three phases of Schizophrenia. If episodes of marked mood disturbance are present and are confined to the *residual* phase, an additional diagnosis of either Depressive Disorder NOS or Bipolar Disorder NOS should be considered." But, "If the total duration of all episodes of a mood syndrome are *brief* relative to the duration of Schizophrenia (active and residual phases), then the mood disturbance is considered an associated feature of Schizophrenia, and no additional diagnosis need be made. If the total duration . . . is *not brief*, then a diagnosis of Schizophrenia is not made, and Schizoaffective Disorder and Mood Disorder with Psychotic Features must be considered." [102]

I hesitate to be critical of such exercises because I cannot conceive how any manual could better provide specificity, considering the inherent problem here. The logic of the argument, however, is reminiscent of that of the physicians at the bedside of Christopher Robin [103]:

> they asked if the sneezles
> came after the wheezles,
> or if the first sneezle
> came first.

The manual goes on to describe schizoaffective disorder "as one of the most confusing and controversial concepts in psychiatric nosology." [104] What is confusing, of course, is not the symptoms but a taxonomy that attempts to confine the disorder to a single category. It should be neither confusing nor surprising that the two kinds of disturbance coexist, which indeed they usually do. If DSM were truly descriptive, according to its stated purpose, there would be no problem about describing a hallucinatory or delusional state with depressed mood, and the profile would go on to include all aspects of the disturbance. That would be an accurate description of the illness, but it would be a list of symptoms, not a "diagnosis."

Thus, many diagnoses, coming to rest like roulette balls in DSM slots, create an illusion of specificity. The very fact that DSM pursues specificity so consistently, despite the disclaimers in its preface, is what leads most practitioners to believe that psychiatric diagnoses are more descriptive of basic entities than of symptoms. If you survey *diagnoses* made according to DSM exclusion criteria, you will indeed find specificity. If you survey *symptoms*, [90–92] or diagnoses based on cardinal symptoms without the exclusion criteria, [5] you will find a plethora of symptoms but far less specificity.

I find it helpful to regard every person as a *unique, psychobiologic unit* of temperament, personality, cognitive/perceptual system, emotions and intuitions, mood, and behavior. The mental functions are intricately interconnected with each other, with the physiology of brain and body, and with the distinctive family and social constellations to which each individual belongs. Every person thinks, acts, feels, etc., in a continuum. The organism functions as a whole. If any aspect is impaired, or if the equilibrium is disturbed in some way, the integrity of the unit suffers, and any aggregation of its interdependent components can be disturbed accordingly.

We would understand individual patients better in many ways if we would surmount the DSM partitions and develop a profile of evaluation. Perhaps then we could focus more on the personal source of the problem and less on the diagnosis as the foundation for our whole approach.

Instead of the "diagnosis," I find it far more effective to consider the psychobiologic unit as a whole. The clinical problem then boils down to the source of the disturbance, its symptomatic profile, and what can be done to improve the source, the symptoms, or both. The person with the illness is the central focus of attention. Included in the symptomatic profile, of course, are those symptoms that merit special genetic, biologic, or pharmacotherapeutic considerations. But that is not the main issue in most patients. If, however, I focus on the diagnosis as the key to understanding, my attention readily shifts from the ill person to the "disease," and it is likely to stay there.

My early training in psychodynamics first drew my attention to the person as well as the disorder. But my medical training still had me fixed to diagnosis until I encountered such singularly effective therapists as Carl Rogers [105] and Virginia Satir [106] and was struck by the absence of psychiatric terminology in their work. Most of their clients did not have the major disorders of psychiatry, but neither do most disturbed patients seen in medical practice. I also noted how I resisted the attempts of my own personal counselors and friends to label me as depressed or compulsive, though I was often both. I felt much like the crab in the parable of William James: "Probably a crab would be filled with a sense of personal outrage if it could hear us class it without ado or apology as a crustacean, and thus dispose of it. 'I am no such thing,' it would say; 'I am MYSELF, MYSELF alone.'" [107]

So I started recording brief profiles in my appraisals to indicate the cause in relation to the symptoms—all the symptoms—just as I did for organic and psychosomatic conditions.

For example, the eventual profile worked out for Joseph (Ch. 1) was:

Nervous reaction related to death of wife and ensuing loneliness [general diagnosis and immediate cause]:
   · No significant values for life other than the relationship [cognitive background].
   · Nonspecific dizziness [physical symptom].
   · Reactive depression [affective symptom].
   · Withdrawal from social activities [behavioral symptom].

Note how uninformative is a diagnosis restricted to "depression" or "dizziness of unknown etiology."

For the usual purposes of office psychotherapy, most psychiatrists do indeed think more in profiles than of specific diagnosis unless they encounter an insurance form, a more distinctly disturbed patient, the need for pharmacotherapy, the diagnostic mandates of hospital admission and discharge, or they write a medical paper.

The task of describing the patient's disturbed psychobiologic unit to fit the rules of psychiatric taxonomy is often laborious. Yet because we are trained as doctors, the resulting diagnosis is reassuring, because it gives us confidence that we know what we are doing. This it does, to a degree, as long as we recognize its limitations and perceive the diagnosis as but one part of a creative clinical formulation individualized to the unique background, personal needs, and expressions of the disturbance in each patient.

Everyone shares the same basic needs, as outlined in Chapter 5, but some people have found better ways to meet those needs than have others. As strange and dysfunctional as the psychiatric disorders may seem, they are usually ways of reacting to or getting around difficult life situations. The emotional distress may be expressed directly (anxiety, depression) or indirectly (psychosomatic symptoms). The patient may have found a way to block out the distress (alcohol, drugs). Some fears and concerns take errant forms (delusions, paranoia). Difficult situations can be avoided altogether (dissociative disorders). Personal gains can be achieved by disregarding the rules of society (antisocial personality). Self-esteem can be salvaged in various ways (mania, narcissistic or histrionic personality, believing that one is God). One can avoid or gain control over difficult work, military, or personal situations (conversion reactions, psychogenic pain disorder). Even schizophrenia or bipolar disorder can often be understood more clearly in some patients when viewed in the context of the family and subsequent life situations that provoked the expression of the latent genetic diathesis.

It may well tax our prevailing modes of biological conceptualization to view psychiatric disorders in this way, but if we do, we are more likely to approach our patients with greater depth of understanding. The medical model of psychiatry, as necessary and useful as it may be, need not dehumanize the most uniquely human of all clinical conditions.

Psychiatric Disorders: Is Feeling Depressed a Disease?

Our present knowledge of the genetic/biologic aspects of major depression provides an opportunity for a truly biopsychosocial approach. Because the biologic focus so often predominates, however, the result is quite the contrary: feeling depressed comes to be regarded as a kind of "disease" that has little to do with problems of the human condition.

This chapter presents a critique of the disease concept. Depression is fundamentally a psychological expression of uniquely human concerns. Feeling seriously depressed can precipitate a series of biological disturbances that intensify the dysphoric experience. The biology of major depression, however, should not lead us away from understanding the personal situations, personality factors, views of self, and outlook on life that cause people to feel depressed.

The purpose of the critique here is not to minimize the immense value of understanding the biology of depression and its treatment, but rather to restore a balance to our thinking about this inherently human problem.

᭙ The concept of depression as disease has in many ways displaced our view of depression as a fundamentally human problem. I focus here on depression because it is a common experience, [1] and because the biological focus has in so many ways dehumanized our thinking about psychiatric disorders in general. The disease concept stems from the neurobiological concomitants and genetic predisposition of major depression, the actions of antidepressant drugs, and the appearance of depression in the absence of obvious precipitating situations. The cause/effect sequences of the emotional and biological components of depression remain controversial, and the ensuing observations are intended to suggest that the basic cause is psychosocial. The biology of depression is the result, not the cause, of feeling depressed. Genetic factors in major depression act not by initiating the biological response but by accentuating its intensity.

The Spectrum of Feeling Sad, Discouraged, Despondent, Depressed

The prevalence of moderately to maximally severe "depressive symptoms" ranges from 13 to 20 percent of the total population of the U.S. and England at any one time; the prevalence of the subset of feeling depressed that psychiatrists would diagnose as major unipolar depression is 2.3–3.2 percent of the adult male population and 4.5–9.3 percent of the adult female population of industrialized nations. [1] If we consider the range of uniquely human concerns from feeling inadequate, insecure, sad, or discouraged to feeling hopeless and worthless, in conjunction with the prevalence of the whole spectrum of "depressive symptoms" and the data cited in the first paragraph of Chapter 8, it is clear that such a common condition is not a primary biological disorder like hemophilia, which bears no causative relation to life situations. Depression is an inherent problem of human consciousness and our reflective nature.

At one end of the spectrum are bereavement and the discouraging marital, occupational, and other situational problems of everyday life "not attributed to a mental disorder." [2] Here also are the common states of psychogenic fatigue (Ch. 13) that abound in general practice, and many kinds of withdrawal, fears, or failure to embrace life fully, though there may be no complaints of fatigue or despondency. An example would be an adolescent moping around his or her room "with nothing to do." Such a person does not feel hopeless and helpless, yet suffers from what might be viewed as an incipient "evolutional melancholia."

Next up the scale of severity are the adjustment disorders with depressed or anxious mood, or mixed emotional features, the least disruptive dysphorias to be defined in DSM as "mental disorders." [3]

At the next level is dysthymia (or depressive neurosis), [4] chronic depressions of mood, closely allied with depression-prone personality characteristics, that begin in early life and persist for years. The mild to moderate impairment of social and occupational functioning in these patients is related more to the chronicity of the depressive syndrome than to its severity. Such states have also been viewed as depressive personality, [5] characterologic depression, [6] or intermittent depressive disorders. [7]

Because anxiety is so often associated with depression, episodic dysphorias less severe than major depression are also designated by Research Diagnostic Criteria as minor depressive disorder with significant anxiety, or as generalized anxiety disorder with significant depression. [7]

Finally, at the far end of the spectrum, is major depression, [8] a distinctly abnormal and incapacitating mood complicated by biological dysfunctions that indeed accentuate the devastation of the whole syndrome.

Depression can appear for the first time at any level of severity, and any stage can shift to another of greater or lesser intensity, or abate altogether, suddenly or slowly. Each gradation can be defined, though the definitions shade off one into another, as would be expected. Depressive episodes appear at all stages of the life cycle, from the anaclitic depressions of infants separated from their mothers, [9] through the depressions of childhood and adolescence, [10] to those of the aged. [11]

Depression, viewed in this way, is a continuum, a spectrum phenomenon. [12] If so, depression is not primarily a biological state. It is a feeling, a state of mind, an emotional appraisal of self in relation to one's life situation. Unlike anger, fear, or anxiety, emotions that evoke an immediate biologic response phylogenetically evolved to protect the organism, the "giving up" of depression is a feeling that evokes very little biological response unless the feeling is intense, protracted, or pervasive, or associated with anxiety and other emotions. In individuals who feel discouraged, just plain "tired, no energy," or mildly to moderately depressed, there may be few if any of the distinct biological responses that characterize major depression. The biology is mainly a withdrawal of the physiologic basis of arousal. Alternatively, the subject's concerns are expressed in the form of psychosomatic functional disorders, or in the usual expressions of sadness, anger, or anxiety. As noted, it is mainly at the far end of the spectrum that the profound biological responses of major depression are provoked. Although major depression can evolve in the absence of a demonstrable genetic vulnerability, it is here that the genetic factors appear in some patients.

If genetic vulnerability to major depression is regarded as a biologic potential or capacity to develop this kind or intensity of emotional reaction in response to disturbing psychological, social, and cultural situations, as was suggested in the preceding chapter, then the genetic component, if present, can be viewed as but one of many factors in a continuum of depressive reactions. [13] If, however, the genetic component is viewed as a specific biologic defect that can be the sole or main cause of feeling depressed, then depression is a dichotomy, with "biological" depressions at one pole and "psychological" depressions at the other. This distinction may apply in part to some unipolar depressions found later to be related to bipolar biology. But if one views the spectrum of depression as a whole, noting the commonality of its core feelings regardless of degree, a causative biological essence seems unlikely for most patients, even those with major depression or melancholia. If it were so, what would be the common factor connecting the neurotransmitter, neurohormonal, hypothalamic, circadian rhythm, and other physiological dysfunctions of major depression? And how would a biological defect in any one system inversely cause the whole constellation of reflections about self that constitute the essence of depression?

A sedative, such as reserpine, [14] can precipitate depression in some patients, more commonly in those with previous psychological difficulties, [15] indicating that sedation and depletion of central stores of catecholamines and indoleamines can retrogradely cause a vulnerable subject to feel depressed. But until we have a premorbid vulnerability marker for depression, the reserpine effects can hardly be construed as a model for what occurs naturally.

Thus the biology of depression, when it appears, is regarded here as the result, not the cause, of feeling depressed. In major depression the intensity of the biological response, combined with the desultory view of self that initiates the process, can envelop the patient in an autonomous syndrome, the response accentuating the feeling of depression, and the feeling accentuating the response. This debilitating complication, fortunately amenable to antidepressant medication, does not alter, however, the importance of the patient's personal concerns as the prime mover of the whole syndrome. Melancholia can be defined, as can retarded or agitated, situational or "endogenous" depression, and the other grades of primary depressive symptoms outlined previously. Each subtype can be characterized by certain genetic, biologic, therapeutic, and prognostic variables that are clinically useful. They are, nevertheless, viewed here as variants in the depressive continuum. [16]

Self-esteem, achievement, a sense of being valued by others, and confidence in one's own capacity to be responsible for self, to grow, and to be fulfilled, are distinctly human values. So are their opposites, the quintessence of depression—feeling worthless, hopeless, helpless, mired. Such universal personal concerns cannot be explained away as the simple penetrance of a genetic trait or as the strangely human symptoms of a primary biological dysfunction, nothing more.

The Biology of Major Depression

The dysfunctions of neurotransmitter, neurohormonal, hypothalamic, circadian rhythm, and other physiological systems in major depression have been well documented. I will not attempt a summary here. The implication of much of this work, although not usually stated explicitly, is that the biodysfunction is something more than the final expression of a latent biological reactivity to psychosocial distress. It is regarded as perhaps the primary event, at least a necessary if not sufficient cause of the depression, rather than the natural effect of feeling depressed. There are no clear data to substantiate such an implication, nor is there yet a known premorbid marker to indicate the biological vulnerability by which a genetic predisposition could be expressed. Let us consider this question.

In early studies of the hypercortisolemia demonstrated by the dexamethasone suppression test, nonsuppression, for example, was thought to be a marker that distinguished the "melancholic" or "endogenous" type of major depression from less severe depression and other psychiatric disorders. [17] Subsequent studies showed it to be far less specific, and nonsuppression was also found in mania and generalized anxiety disorder. [18–20] Nonsuppression is also common in anorexia nervosa, [21] bulimia, [22] weight loss in healthy obese subjects, [12] alcoholism, [24] primary degenerative dementia, [25] and miscellaneous nonacute hospital patients. [26]

Most important for our consideration here is that hypercortisolism is an adaptive response to many kinds of physical and emotional stress, both in animals and in human beings. [27, 28] Depression is one kind of emotional distress.

I cite these data to make a point. Depression, mania, and anxiety are *affective*, that is, *emotional* crises. Because emotional distress normally activates the hypothalamic-pituitary-adrenocortical (HPA) axis, it could be anticipated that hypercortisolemia would be evoked most often by those disturbances of the psychobiologic unit with the most emotional turmoil. The core of depression—that one has not been up to life's possibilities in one way or another, that the opportunities have been wasted or have come to naught, that little can now be done about it—is overwhelming. That is how the patient feels, whether it makes sense to anyone else or not. The biologic response is consistent with the desperation of the emotional state. Sachar had suggested that the hypercortisolemia was specific to depression because it was found whether the patients were anxious and agitated or not. [29] This belies the profound emotional impact of the depressive affect per se as a sufficient stimulus for the HPA response. Thus hypercortisolemia is the result, not the cause, of feeling depressed, as it is in many other kinds of physical or emotional stress. Similarly, I believe, other markers will be found to be part of the normal adaptive physiology of stress and arousal, on the one hand, or of fatigue, exhaustion, and withdrawal, on the other, or intermediate states thereof.

Another example is the shortened rapid eye movement (REM) latency

(SRL), that is, the time from falling asleep to the first period of REM sleep. This was also regarded as a specific marker, indicative of the unique sleep abnormalities of major depression. [30] SRL was soon noted, however, in other psychiatric disorders: schizophrenia, [31, 32] mania, [33] obsessive-compulsive disorder, [34] and borderline personality. [35] It is found in narcolepsy. [36] It appears during the jet lag of westward air travel. [37] It can be induced in normal volunteers in several ways without causing depression; some normal subjects appear naturally to have SRL, whereas depressed patients may have normal sleep features. [38] SRL appears readily in normal subjects during two and one-half days of bed rest in an environment without diversion or cues as to time of day. [39] Obviously, such sleep patterns can be induced by many conditions, both normal and abnormal, that disturb arousal systems in one way or another. As with hypercortisolemia, the sleep disturbances are epiphenomena of depression—the result, not the cause, of feeling depressed.

The principal biological effects of major depression involve the central neurotransmitter systems that normally transmit the messages of the organism's need for arousal or for vegetative functions, rest, and restoration. Most likely, both the genetic vulnerability to panic disorder or depression and the main actions of antidepressant drugs lie in the regulation of these systems.

Depression, however, is a complex affect, usually including elements of arousal as well as of giving up or withdrawal. It is not a concrete entity readily separable from other disturbances of the psychobiologic unit. A simplistic genetic/biologic hypothesis is unlikely. Because the relative activation or deactivation of adrenergic, cholinergic, and other biogenic amines varies over time and from patient to patient, it is probably not possible to formulate a precise neurotransmitter theory of depression.

In general, the core biology of depression is perhaps best viewed in terms of some kind of an imbalance of cholinergic/adrenergic systems, [40, 41] if described physiologically, or of the endophylactic-trophotropic (parasympathetic) and ergotropic (sympathetic) central systems, if described anatomically, as by Hess. [42] The emphasis has varied from catecholamine depletion [43] or cholinergic dominance, [44] to catechol activation [45] or other types of "dysregulation." [46]

We see that the details and interrelationships of the neurotransmitter systems in arousal, sleep, and withdrawal are not at all clear in depression. Nevertheless, as emphasized previously, these systems are ancient and stable, and, like the neuroendocrine axes, circadian rhythms, and other central functions that are closely coordinated, the responses are most likely those of normal physiological systems. Gold et al. provide a provocative parallel between the general adaptational responses to stress and the syndrome of depression. [45]

In some patients the response may be accentuated because of a genetic variant in reactivity. In any person, however, with or without such a variant, if the emotional disturbance is sufficiently profound, the biologic dysfunctions can be provoked. A vicious circle is then established. The personal anguish evokes a further accentuation of the biologic response, and the latter, mediated through limbic, hypothalamic, pontine (locus ceruleus), and other brain-stem systems, results in a further disturbance of sleep and appetite, loss of intellectual functions, physical energy, sexuality, and capacity to experience interest or pleasure or to respond to surroundings, all of which evokes a deeper negative affect, and so on.

William James attempted years ago to define emotion as its physical expression, little more. [47] That is where we are now with the concept that there would be little or no feeling of depression without the neurotransmitter or other dysfunctions. Cannon, however, demonstrated years ago that the core of emotion is the appraisal of the threat, not the physical expression of the emotion or the ensuing fight or flight. [48] In terms of depression this means that the sense of failure, loss, or whatever the personal source, and the appalling reflections about one's desultory state, are the primary problem. But just as tears accentuate a feeling of sadness, or hyperventilation and palpitation feelings of panic, the biologic responses to depression accentuate the feelings that initiated the process in the first place.

Human emotions, of course, are complex. Patients are often not fully aware of their source, especially in depression. Tricyclic compounds or monoamine oxidase (MAO) inhibitors normalize the neurotransmitter dysfunctions and thereby break the vicious circle of the more severe and, therefore, biological forms of depression. Understandably, the physician, who is no more aware of the psychological chain of circumstances that culminated in the depression than is the patient, comes to view the biology and physical symptoms of the depression as the essence of the problem, rather than the basic emotions which lie at its source. Antidepressant symptom relief does not prove that the sequence of events began with a biological defect.

The Psychological Basis of Depression

Each stage of life is associated with an advance from one major developmental phase to another. Each change inherently constitutes a psychological loss of past relationships, experiences, and opportunities, and a challenge for what lies ahead. [12, 49] Depression can result from dismay about any important aspect of one's life: misgiving about what one has or has not done about what has happened so far, and doubts about the future. Current investigations focus on a breakdown of self-esteem in relation to difficulties in, or losses of, significant interpersonal relationships, or to personal failures in terms of the standards by which one lives. For those who remain dubious about the psychological basis of depression, I recommend reading Arieti and Bemporad, [50] Klerman, Weissman, Rounsaville, and Chevron, [51] Beck, Rush, Shaw, and Emery, [52] or Burns. [53, 54] Their case histories are eminently convincing. The concepts are clear, readable, and helpful to patients as well as doctors in understanding and working through the underlying problems. There are, of course, many other ways to understand situations in which individuals are mired and become depressed. Each person is unique. There is no one prevailing problem common to all depressions, but, as summarized by Arieti: "I have never treated for a considerable length of time a case of depression about which I could say that there was no psychological factor involved . . . that his depression came from nowhere and its origin had to be sought exclusively in a metabolic disorder." [55]

The cause of depression may well be obscure if one focuses only on "environmental events," [56] "psychosocial stressors that have occurred in the year preceding," [57] or "contributory situations." [7] Asked about what situations may have provoked the depression, the patient often says, "Nothing." Asked a specific question, "How is your marriage?" the patient says, "OK." It is only when you meet husband and wife together, or explore the patient's story in greater depth, that the psychodynamics begin to unfold.

We make a great mistake here, and in psychiatry and psychosomatic medicine generally, if we think exclusively in terms of acute situations or crisis intervention. The cause of depression or any kind of emotional illness is often a steady or slowly progressive state unchanged for years: doubts about one's capabilities, a limited sense of self-esteem, guilt about one's past conduct, an unhappy marriage in which one can foresee no possibility of change or escape, a mundane job, untapped potentials for personal development, unattainable standards for success or happiness, a dependent personality and failure to be assertive about one's own needs and wants, an inability to assume full responsibility for oneself or to make important strategic choices, fears of making changes, and a host of other attitudinal, personal, and social situations having nothing to do with recent antecedent events. The difficulties that characterize these states evolve throughout life. A latent sense of insecurity acquired in childhood, for example, though long since suppressed during a successful career and the multiple achievements of adulthood, persists, nevertheless. It may take very little to trigger a symptomatic breakdown. A simple loss or failure can resurrect deep feelings that have lain dormant for years. Or one begins to question the meaning, purpose, or values of one's own life.

In the psychoanalytic formulations of Abraham and Freud, depression can represent "hostility toward others turned inward." In many patients I believe that depression is better viewed as despair, or even anger toward the self alone, for not making appropriate changes that could have been made long ago. One finally comes to realize how one's own behavior has adversely affected the lives of other people, or how one could have embraced life's many opportunities more positively.

I do not mean here to question the complexity of the problem, the difficulty of change, or the value of biologic therapy. I do believe, however, that both doctor and patient need to appreciate that there *is* a psychological basis to depression. If this can be understood, and changes made, in spite of the difficulties, the patient is the richer for the experience.

Psychotherapy and Depression

Controlled studies consistently substantiate the efficacy of psychotherapy for depression. [58] In general, psychotherapy appears to be somewhat more effective than pharmacotherapy, [58] or roughly comparable, [59] in overall studies of patients depressed enough to be in psychiatric care. Combined therapy is found to add very little, [58] or to be somewhat more effective, [60, 61] than either pharmaceutic or psychotherapy alone. Antidepressants may be more effective in relieving symptoms, especially the vegetative decline of acute major depression, and preventing relapse, whereas psychotherapy has a more evident long-range effect on problems of living: work, interests, social functioning, interpersonal relationships. [60]

Antidepressants are usually considered essential in the treatment of major depression. It is important to keep in mind, however, that about one-third of all patients with manifest clinical depression, two-thirds of these with dysthymia, and most patients with episodes of relatively mild depression do not respond to antidepressant drugs (see the later section on drug specificity). Thus, psychotherapy may be the only effective approach, especially for the majority of patients with the depressive symptoms (functional syndromes and nervous tension) seen in medical practice.

With or without referral for psychotherapy, general physicians can be of great help to depressed patients through their inherent capacity to be fully present, to listen empathically, to support and encourage, to accept the patient and the problem with understanding as well as perspective. The physician can also note the possible relationship of the depression to life transitions, the menopause, the aging process, or states of disease. Depression is the patient's way of looking at his/her situation; feeling depressed is understandable, and recovery is anticipated. When patients feel understood and accepted as they are, they can begin to accept and view themselves with compassion, and to start from there to build confidence again.

The physician can explain the ubiquity of depression and how, if appropriate to the patient, it often affects those with the most idealism and the highest demands upon themselves. There may be many ways to emphasize the patient's strengths and restore self-esteem. The discerning physician may also be able to interact more specifically, such as noting obvious ways the patient could be more assertive, be responsible for self, focus on certain necessary choices, etc. A conjoint interview with patient and spouse or significant family members can be particularly informative. The patient may be loaded with an immense baggage of self-reproach about past failures, faults, or behaviors that have adversely affected other people. Such judgments may or may not have a valid basis. The past cannot be undone, of course, but if what has hitherto been secret can be shared, openly and honestly, with someone who can be compassionate about the humanity, frailty, and present struggle of this person to "set things straight," this can often provide relief for the current depression and open the way to a more positive future. Depressed patients are in urgent need of a caring but objective person with whom to share their problems.

"Endogenous" Depression?

For many years of psychiatric practice, if a depression appeared to develop independently of recent disturbing events, it was assumed not only that it came "from within" and was, therefore, "endogenous," but also that the "within" was biologic, not psychologic. In that the term was applied mainly to major depression, it was also used to indicate severity. In this way "endogenous" depression was viewed as a primarily biologic disorder, in contrast to "reactive," "situational," or "neurotic" depressions, which were less severe, primarily psychologic, disorders. In the continuum described above, (1) depression (primary, unipolar), regardless of intensity, is viewed as a predominantly emotional state with a psychosocial basis, though not necessarily related to recent events, and (2) the biology of major depression is considered to be predominantly secondary to feeling depressed, though genetic factors affect the form and intensity of the biologic response.

"Endogenous," therefore, with any of its former meanings, is not a tenable concept. The depression comes "from within," if you will, but the "within" is fundamentally psychosocial, not a biologic fault. The origin of the concept is, of course, understandable: many observers find it hard to believe how such a devastating disorder with obvious biologic components could otherwise appear in a previously healthy individual without any obvious precipitating situation. In this regard, however, it is important to realize that the same problem applies to most of the other emotional disturbances and psychosomatic disorders described throughout this book. They, too, often appear without obvious cause (Chs. 8 and 11).

In the evolving history of psychological thinking it has become clear that many major depressions with pervasive autonomous anhedonia and vegetative symptoms are "situational." [62, 63] A term was needed to describe such depressions, regardless of etiology. Klein proposed the term *endogenomorphic*. [64] This implies, however, that the depression, though provoked psychologically, would not occur without a premorbid biologic vulnerability. A better term would be simply *psychosomatic*, to indicate that the emotional distress is expressed physically, as is any emotion.

For the reasons described above, *endogenous* was dropped altogether from DSM III in 1980. [65] In practice, the term should be abandoned, as recommended. Nevertheless, it remains in common use to indicate the biodysfunctions, the somatic expressions, of depression. Such usage is strange indeed. Anxiety has not been traditionally described as "endogenous" even when the adrenergic discharge and hyperventilation are extreme and the psychosocial basis obscure. We do not refer to tension or migraine headaches, or the physical dysfunctions of any other functional syndrome, as "endogenous." We do not describe mirth or sadness as "endogenous" because of laughter or tears, though such expressions are both genetic and somatic. Why, then, do we distinguish depression from the other emotions with such a singular designation?

If depression (or panic) represented the simple penetrance of a depressive genotype in the absence of emotional concerns, the concept would make sense. Thinking in "endogenous" terminology, however, is misleading, inevitably limiting the physician's attention to but one aspect of what should be a more comprehensive approach.

The Continuum of Anxiety and Depression

In DSM [66] and ICD-9-CM, The International Classification of Diseases, [67] depression is classified as a disorder of mood, whereas anxiety is categorized as an entirely different kind of mental disorder. The separation of depression and anxiety as unrelated entities is inappropriate and misleading. So is their former characterization as "psychotic" and "neurotic," respectively, still found in ICD-9-CM. Anxiety is a disturbance of mood or affect, as much so as depression, and it can be just as disabling.

Though feeling depressed is different from feeling anxious [68] and can be so defined, as it is in DSM, the two aspects of dysphoria lie along a continuum of affective disturbance in which they are often interfused and difficult to separate. [69–71] Historically, many psychiatrists, regardless of their general orientation, beginning perhaps with Kraepelin, [72] have considered anxiety and depression as closely related. [73] Following DSM guidelines, judgments can be made about whether disturbed patients are predominantly depressed or anxious, and the judgments confirmed by statistical analysis. The scales used to measure the two moods and their associated symptoms, however, usually show considerable overlap. [73–75] Depression can clearly predominate, as in the retarded type of major depression, or anxiety can predominate, as in acute panic attacks, but in most chronically disturbed states they are appropriately considered together.

But I find no difficulty in distinguishing anxiety and depression. They are indeed different emotions. My argument here is with those who view them as "two different syndromes," [73] whereas I prefer to regard them simply as closely allied emotional responses to life situations.

When any of us face life's problems, especially the experience or possibility of loss, failure, or disruption of some kind, or of not realizing basic needs or cherished hopes, or of barriers to personal growth, freedom, or expression, we may keep cool, learn what we need to do, solve one problem at a time, and feel OK about ourselves and our process, though quite aware of the difficulties and concerned about the outcome. On the other hand, an appraisal of our situation, at both cognitive and emotional levels, partly conscious and partly unconscious, combined with a latent feeling of impaired self-esteem and self-confidence, can readily cause us to feel more distinctly troubled, often without knowing just why. This evokes far more uncertainty, insecurity, dread, foreboding, and other concerns, than we can comfortably handle, especially if allied to feelings of fear, anger, guilt, or shame. The resulting distress, a sense of threat with dubious outcome, is experienced as *anxiety*. The feeling of anxiety is usually associated with some possibility of getting through, around, or out of the situation, either by just hoping that things will somehow turn out OK or by pursuing a more active struggle, resistance, or avoidance. The same distress, when one feels that the problems are not likely to change, and one does not know what more to do about them, can be associated with inertia, giving up, resignation, the effect seeming hopeless, no longer worth the effort. This is experienced as *depression*. Darwin put it simply: "If we expect to suffer, we are anxious; if we have no hope of relief, we despair." [76] Anxiety and depression, therefore, describe different poles of the distress emanating from difficult life situations, and shaped by one's personal experience, personality, temperament, problem-solving styles, and countless other factors. The fears and struggle of anxiety shade into depression as they become dispirited. Whereas anxious subjects may focus on external events as unpredictable and beyond their control, depressed subjects often dwell on personal responsibility for what has happened.

It is very difficult to analyze these two emotions. The tentative description here is but one point of view, but it may help to focus on their common source, whereas a reductive analysis to two separate syndromes leads to a focus on the symptoms instead of the cause.

It is not surprising, then, that these shades of feeling often coexist. Of the 27 percent of American adults in a random household survey who reported high levels of psychic distress during the preceding year, 46 percent reported both anxiety and depression, 36 percent reported anxiety only, and 16 percent depression only. [77] Most patients with major depression are found to be distinctly anxious or agitated (the motor equivalent of anxiety); only about 14 percent are of the retarded type with no apparent anxiety. [78, 79] Patients diagnosed as depressed may have more anxiety, as measured on appropriate scales, than do those diagnosed as anxious. [74] Many studies have demonstrated the frequent association of panic disorder, persistent anxiety, and major depression, either simultaneously or one after the other. [80–82] When the personal distress underlying the many psychosomatic functional syndromes of medical practice is analyzed in terms of mood, both anxious and depressive aspects are noted. [83]

From this perspective, if psychoactive drugs are to be prescribed, does it matter whether the patient is predominantly depressed or anxious? Are there specific "antidepressants" and "anxiolytics"? Many studies have demonstrated a remarkable dispersion of the effects one thought to be characteristic of the two drug classes. In most states of mixed anxiety/depression other than major depression, insofar as the drugs are demonstrably effective, the benzodiazepines are found to reduce the depressive symptoms as well as the anxiety, [84] and the tricyclics are found to reduce the anxiety symptoms (often more effectively than the benzodiazepines) as well as the depression. [79, 84–86] The popular use of the benzodiazepines in medical practice has more to do with their safety and fewer side effects than with any specificity of action. They may not be as "anxiolytic" as are the tricyclics, which, in addition to their use in major depression, are the drugs of choice for panic disorder [87] and, according to recent studies, for generalized anxiety disorder. [85]

Thus the "anxiolytics" and "antidepressants" are by no means as specific as implied by these idealized designations. Except for major depression, panic disorder, and obsessive-compulsive disorder, for which "antidepressants" are specifically indicated, the decision to use any drug or, if so, which drug, in most disturbed outpatients depends less on the preponderance of one affect over the other than on global effectiveness, safety, toxicity, the likelihood of dependency, and other considerations in relation to the patient's personal situation and needs for relief.

In summary, if we regard anxiety and depression as distinct syndromes and the drugs as specific antidotes, we are likely to focus on a dissection of the psychobiologic unit as the primary goal of the doctor-patient relationship. Wrong! I suggest that in medical practice generally, it makes little difference whether most "nervous" patients are viewed as predominantly anxious or depressed, whether psychosomatic functional symptoms indicate a "masked" anxiety or a "masked" depression, or whether the symptoms are due simply to stress without any dysphoria of either type. Though pharmacotherapy may be helpful, it is often not clearly effective. What *is* important is to recognize that the patient is under stress or emotionally disturbed in some way, and then, whenever possible, to focus on the central issue, the patient's personal situation, and what can be done about that.

The Specificity of Antidepressants

We have seen that the tricyclic agents are not so specific; their psychoactive effectiveness is found at both poles of the anxiety/depression continuum. They can reduce the pain of certain chronic pain disorders, particularly headaches, diabetic neuropathy, atypical facial pain, postherpetic neuralgia, and fibromyalgia. [88, 89] Clomipramine and related tricyclics are effective in obsessive-compulsive disorder. [90] Other uses are beginning to appear. [91] The effects in disorders other than depression occur in the absence of any evidence of depressed affect, and the timing of effects, dosage, and other aspects differ in many ways from antidepressant effects. How the common denominators at central sites of action result in such apparently disparate psychoactive effects remains unknown. It is clear, however, that the effects are better described as antidysphoric than as antidepressant. In that the effects of feeling depressed on neurotransmitter systems, the neuroendocrine axes, and circadian rhythms are similar to those of many other kinds of physical and emotional stress, the diverse and diffuse effects of tricyclic agents are not at all surprising.

How effective are the tricyclics in depression? They presumably act by altering certain biological effects of the more profound disturbances. Thus a 70–80 percent response rate can be expected for major depression, [91] and at most about 30 percent for dysthymia, [92] although most observers find the tricyclic effects in patients with "depressive personality" [63] or "characterological depression" [93] to be negligible. How the nonresponse to tricyclics in some reports of "neurotic depression" [94] or of "the less severely depressed and functionally impaired patients" [59] relate to the favorable response noted in the reports of "nonendogenous" mixed anxiety/depression summarized in the previous section is not clear. No studies of "adjustment disorder with depressed mood" have been reported, presumably because there is no effect.

Morris and Beck provide an overview. They cite 106 well-controlled double-blind studies comparing tricyclics and MAO inhibitors to placebo in the treatment of "manifest clinical depression"; 65 percent showed the drug to be more effective than placebo; 35 percent did not. [95] If one-third of these studies are negative, then obviously the effects noted in the others, which showed simply a *statistical* advantage over placebo, were absent or minimal in many patients. The improvement, of course, is sometimes striking, but others have commented that the "effects were generally small." [94] Georgotas put it realistically: even if the depression meets appropriate DSM criteria for responsive subtypes, pharmacotherapy often has little to offer "other than satisfying the magical expectations of both therapist and the patient." [96]

We can now view the problem in perspective. The tricyclic drugs are mainly effective in affective disorders when there are significant components of panic, anxiety, or the biological concomitants of major depression. In many, if not most, of the 13 to 20 percent of the population who feel depressed, the dysphoria is not intense enough, or it has not triggered a biological response of sufficient magnitude, to be affected by the drugs. Because so many patients who feel depressed do not respond, or respond but slightly, it is apparent that the drugs are not, strictly speaking, antidepressant. Their effects are mediated primarily through the biological effects of feeling depressed; they have very little direct effect on the feeling itself. They are not mood elevators, except by the slow indirect pathways of ameliorating the secondary biologic dysfunctions that complicate the more profound disturbances.

Nevertheless, when the biologic dysfunctions of depression do occur, the drugs are often useful in reversing the process. As the autonomy of the depression, with its physical and mental inertia, abates, the physical symptoms improve, and the patients become more active and responsive. In so doing, they feel less hopeless and helpless and can begin to cope more effectively with the cognitive and emotional sets that initiated the depression in the first place. The patient may then become responsive to psychotherapy, which was not possible in the autonomous stage. Therefore, many psychiatrists, though strong advocates of psychotherapy, believe that the problem of major depression should be presented to patients in terms of the medical model, to ensure their participation in a healing plan combining pharmacotherapy and psychotherapy. [97, 98] In patients with major depression who do respond to the drugs, the tricyclics can also prevent relapse. [99]

For these many important reasons, the tricyclics and MAO inhibitors deserve their respected place in our therapeutic armamentarium. Their designation as "antidepressant," however, has led to a widespread use in patients where the drugs are not effective, converted a uniquely human problem into a kind of "disease" that is alleged to be far more specific than it really is, and overly medicalized our thinking about psychiatric disorders generally. The drugs should be designated, not as antidepressants, but as "neurotransmitter regulators," or whatever their actual biologic action is determined to be, just as digitalis is designated as "inotropic" or "chronotropic," but not as an "anti-congestive-failurant."

The critique here is not to minimize the value of "antidepressants" as useful adjuncts to a comprehensive approach to major depression, but to decry their use as the sole approach to patients in whom they are of little value. They are used much too often as substitutes for a comprehensive doctor/patient relationship. When drugs are used as substitutes, no attempt is made to understand the patient's underlying situation, even in a general way. Nor is the patient informed that some kind of personal situation is the likely cause of symptoms. Sometimes the patient is not even advised that the purpose of the prescription is to relieve "depression." In that circumstance, the patient cannot begin to understand or work through the personal issues that have caused the depression and will cause it again if no changes are made.

In summary, feeling sad, discouraged, despondent, depressed are common, inherent problems of human life and consciousness. When sufficiently severe and protracted, such dysphoria can be expressed in a more autonomous mood known as major depression. The depression often reflects a loss or failure in terms of one's value system of needs, relationships, right behavior, or goals for success and happiness. Though the source of depression is primarily psychosocial, a major depression may result in secondary biological disturbances that add to the apathy and inertia of the mood itself and can be reversed to some extent by tricyclic compounds and MAO inhibitors. The drugs are useful adjuncts to the therapy of such patients. The same drugs are ineffective, however, in most patients who feel depressed, or who present with the common functional syndromes of medical practice, because the underlying dysphoria has not provoked reversible central nervous system dysfunctions. All depressed patients are in urgent need of personal understanding, acceptance and support, and, usually, some revision of their views of self, their needs, relationships, attitudes, goals, and/or behaviors, that led to the breakdown.

CHAPTER 10

Barriers to Person-Centered Care

The demands of disease, the difficulties of emotional problems, the appeal of the medical model for both doctor and patient, and the exigencies of time and payment plans constitute formidable barriers to person-centered care. In this chapter I play devil's advocate to summarize why many doctors find such care to be so difficult. We must appreciate the impact of these barriers before we can begin to make changes. Specific suggestions about working with the time problem are also offered here.

The Physician's Point of View

The Demands of Disease

Regardless of what we may seek to accomplish, or what our patients expect of us in terms of person-centered care, the detection and treatment of organic disease is our sole and absolute responsibility. We could overlook the psychosocial basis, or even the correct diagnosis, of functional bowel syndromes, for example, over and over again, and no one would notice, but we cannot miss a single carcinoma. This responsibility weighs heavily. If we fail, we expect no quarter from our patients, our colleagues, or our own consciences. Beyond all that lies the specter of malpractice.

The problem is compounded by the proliferation of medical knowledge. Optimal disease management has become an insuperable challenge. It is difficult enough just to acquire the necessary basic principles and techniques, to say nothing about learning how to understand human problems. The study of disease dominates our training and the medical literature for good reason, and we can barely keep up with what is new. So we are never satisfied that we have enough scientific understanding to do a first-rate job.

These concerns constitute major barriers to person-centered care, and they explain the reluctance of many physicians to diagnose functional disorders. The illness remains a "clinical problem" until all disease has been ruled out. Even then the search may continue, and the final diagnosis will often be ". . . of unknown etiology." Some doctors, concerned about their "duty" to detect disease if at all possible, virtually never diagnose an illness with physical symptoms as a psychogenic disorder.

The Vagaries of Emotions

Contrasted with the disease problem are the difficulties of emotional disorders. Understanding people is not always easy. Even if we do understand, or think we do, what can *we* do about *their* personal problems? Is it not *our* responsibility to do something to make our patients feel better? And what can the patients do? Can they really change? Change is not easy either. Nor is intimacy. Both physician and patient may be uncomfortable with feelings, disclosure, frailty, and personal responsibility. We are not trained to deal with feelings; we are trained to diagnose and treat. So we are quite comfortable with the medical model, which effectively depersonalizes the encounter. And it is easy for us to act. We have an immense armamentarium of things to do, and we are trained to assume responsibility. The patient is not.

The Covert Advantages of the Medical Model

Both doctor and patient are concerned about what is wrong and what can be done about it. Doctors, like all healers, are expected to know these things. The focus, therefore, is on what the doctor knows and does rather than on what patients know and can do for themselves. The medical model fills the bill precisely, for there is a name and a treatment for every kind of illness. That is what the patient expects; that is what the patient gets; and that is what the doctor wants to provide. If doctors do not *do* something, the question may be raised that they perhaps have not earned their fee. Understanding and counseling are not enough. A diagnosis and a treatment constitute what many regard as the main purpose of medicine.

The medical model is, of course, essential for scientific medicine. But there are covert advantages to the model, as there are to any other system of healing. The healer can always fall back on the disease model, in which he or she practices, identifies a disordered part, and does something about it. Healers are never at a loss, whether they understand a person in relation to an illness or not.

In medicine, for example, if the patient has epigastric distress, and peptic ulcer has been ruled out, the diagnosis is often dyspepsia, but the treatment is the same. If underlying nervous tension is apparent, then the psycho-physiological component of the reaction is recognized, and a tranquilizer may be added. If the clinical picture is dominated by the nervous tension, and the epigastric distress is but one of several symptoms, then the psyche is classified instead of the stomach. The diagnosis is anxiety state or depression, and the treatment shifts predominantly to psychoactive drugs. The point is that the medical names and treatments apply to different levels of the disorder, but the underlying personal situation that is the cause of the illness is bypassed in each transaction.

The names and treatments keep the doctor in control. If epigastric distress is labeled "hiatus hernia"; cold hands, "acrocyanosis"; or muscular pains, "fibrositis"; what can the patient say? The doctor has total jurisdiction over these insidious entities. The diagnosis and the treatment comprise a "battery"—to borrow the baseball term—sure to "win the game." And the prescription is the signal that the visit is over. The medical model gives the doctor control over the duration of the encounter as well as the whole illness.

Doctors who say instead, "These are nervous symptoms; let's see if we can understand why," may be in for trouble. They run the risk of losing control. Their patients are now involved in the interaction. They may appreciate the physician's overture and the opportunity to share their problems, or they may be surprised or, worse, resist, desist, argue, get mad, depart, etc. Whatever happens, it takes more time, at least at this visit. An interview cannot be terminated at a poignant moment of sharing, so such moments are avoided. As noted by Magraw: "If the doctor were going to work this through with the patient, *time, energy, and personal involvement* would be required. These are all things in short supply." [1]

Thus it is abundantly clear that there are appropriate and responsible professional reasons why physicians do what they do, and do best, and that is, first and foremost, to diagnose and treat disease.

The Patient as Unwitting Partner in a "Conspiracy"

Meanwhile, most patients are also focused on the malady. They hope that it turns out to be something simple that the doctor can take care of readily. They are not immediately prepared to assume responsibility either for being ill or for getting well. Even if they were, they would usually prefer that a medical solution would obviate the necessity of personal change. No matter how bad the habit, how unnecessary the stress, how inappropriate the behavior, patients are invested in life as it is. They wouldn't do what they do if it did not seem to serve some useful purpose or pleasure. What they do is their identity. They are not sure they want to change, could, or who they would be if they did.

So the medical model has a compelling attraction for both parties. The doctor wants to take responsibility for taking care of the illness, and the patient doesn't. The two forces play on each other, pushing the doctor to do more and more and the patient to do less and less. Patients who *do* want to accept more responsibility, and *do not* want to be treated unless it is essential, rarely say so. So the physician can only assume that the patient expects to be treated. The *therapeutic imperative* as an aura overrides the interplay of both parties in the medical encounter.

This approach to treatment mirrors the prevailing cultural attitude that science and technology can solve most problems. Scientific medicine, when expected to solve all medical problems, represents the quintessence of this belief. Every pain seems to merit a procaine injection; every cold, an antibiotic; every qualm, a tranquilizer. Whether we give "shots," when ineffective or unnecessary, because we feel the patient expects us to do so, or the patient expects the shots because we or another doctor gave them before, is moot. A vicious circle is established for which we must take responsibility. But it is tempting to fall into line with the popular culture and do what we believe our patients expect us to do.

When significant personal problems are involved in causing the illness, there may evolve a covert conspiracy of silence about the real issues, which are never made explicit. Because the medical model appears to suffice for all the care necessary, both parties are satisfied with the transaction. Even in psychological disorders, the crisis may pass, and symptomatic treatment is enough to see the patient through. Magraw says: "What each is really up to at this point is the employment of the familiar psychological defenses of avoiding pain, unpleasantness, and effort for the moment, regardless of the fact that such action will inevitably cause more distress in the future." [1] Even when the suffering continues, year after year, neither doctor nor patient questions the process. The disorder is simply regarded as a chronic condition that is difficult to treat.

The patient, however, who has never been presented with a clear choice about alternatives, is an unwitting accomplice to the conspiracy. It is the doctor who is trained to understand the illness, not the patient. It is clearly the doctor's responsibility to break down the barriers described above which stand in the way of such understanding. The demands of disease and the inherent problems of the medical model need not be impenetrable barriers to person-centered care.

The Organization of Medical Practice

In many ways we are now bound by the impact of the cost of medical care, a marketplace health-care system, third-party payment and regulation, and often too many patients. The result is tight office-visit schedules, whether imposed upon us in group practice or by a prepaid health-care system, or self-imposed in independent practice. Furthermore, technical procedures command much higher fees than office time spent with patients. All these factors constitute greater incentives for seeing more patients, which results in more special procedures, than for spending more time with one patient. Obviously, the expeditious solution to these problems of practice is simply to get the medical data, do the procedures, diagnose, and treat.

Nevertheless, what many patients need most is more time, time for understanding the clinical problem, whatever it is, time to ask questions and have their questions answered, and time to participate wisely in treatment choices. They need time for education, support, counsel, for many things far more important than the diagnostic/pharmaceutic decisions that can be completed so quickly. It takes time to understand a complex medical problem—diabetes with uremia and hypertension, for example—and to instruct the patient in the necessary care. It takes time to review the many factor other than disease that combine to cause a chronic backache, and to advise the patient about exercise, posture, lifting, etc. It takes time to review the risk factors for coronary artery disease and to help the patient with nutritional counseling, cessation of smoking, and other pertinent issues. It takes time to understand the personal background of psychosomatic and psychiatric disorders. A 15-minute office visit may be insufficient for these and many other situations. The time problem can be solved in several ways:

1. *The physician can provide the care personally, take the time, and charge for it.* The visit is scheduled for 30, 45, or 60 minutes, repeated if necessary, and the patient is charged accordingly. Insurance policies that provide for office visits may allow for this. We are concerned here with an overview of the patient's personal situation in relation to the illness, rather than with psychotherapy. If the need for extra time is explained to uninsured patients, many will respond positively to the physician's offer, regardless of the additional cost.

2. *The physician can focus on the central issues in the time available.* A patient is being followed, let us say, for dyspepsia, migraine, hypertension, menopause, anxiety, or depression, any condition in which underlying personal issues may be significant. The diagnosis has already been established. The nurse has recorded the blood pressure and other data. There is no in-

dication for a repeat physical examination. The therapeutic and side effects of medication can be evaluated in two or three minutes. In the remaining 12 of the 15 minutes scheduled for the visit, the physician can focus on the central personal issues, rather than on medical maneuvers such as listening to the heart and lungs unnecessarily. Castelnuovo-Tedesco refers to this as the twenty-minute hour in his excellent book on brief psychotherapy for medical doctors. [2] It is the quality, not the quantity, of the time that matters.

A physician at the bedside of a dying patient, for example, can cover the medical problems in a quick perusal of the nurse's notes and a brief examination. The remaining few minutes of the visit, committed to a genuine friendly exchange, one person with another, may mean far more to the patient than the whole edifice of medical science.

I know several skillful emergency-room specialists who are quite able to clue into the personal background of psychosomatic illness in new patients within a few minutes, yet cover the medical database as well. The busy doctor can also keep to a schedule by shunting time from patients with easily managed disease (upper respiratory tract infections, many skin conditions) to those who need time the most. Another way to make time count is to have patients complete routine history forms so that the doctor can shift time from the collection of mundane data to a more effective focus on the subtleties of the illness (Ch. 14).

The shortage of time is indeed a barrier, but not the barrier it is often said to be. The physician motivated for person-centered care can be efficient and develop a capacity to be alert to, recognize, and focus on the central personal elements of an illness expeditiously. Granted the time problem, however, there are still other ways to provide the care, as we shall see next.

3. The physician can work effectively with allied health professionals and patient-support groups. When the physician has barely enough time for the diagnostic and therapeutic basis of modern medicine—a 60- to 80-hour work week is not uncommon—person-centered care is impossible without help.

The doctor's own personnel—nurses, nurse practitioners, physician assistants—can be trained to provide the detailed instruction and support necessary for child and maternal care, coronary disease and coronary risk-factor management, diabetes, congestive failure, allergy control, chronic obstructive pulmonary disease, backache, headache, disabling arthritis, and many other conditions. Or the doctor can establish effective relationships with nurse specialists, nutritionists, physical therapists, health-promotion and disease-prevention clinics, health-education specialists, respiratory therapists, and other professionals who are trained to help patients with specific problems.

We need to be familiar with the services available in the community. Too often our practices are much too insular. We lack the time and the experience to provide the personal support needed by a cancer patient, for example, but there may well be a support group in the hospital or community. Hospice is another valuable source of support. Furthermore, a group that includes other patients often provides a kind of support the patient can receive in no other way. The classic model is Alcoholics Anonymous. Trained counselors or support groups are often available for mastectomy, enterostomy, paraplegia, and many other specific disease states; for weight reduction, nutritional advice, smoking cessation, and health promotion generally; for child care and parenting skills, pregnancy and delivery, death and dying, and grief; and for the specific problems of battered women, sexual assault, adults molested as children, the families of alcohol-dependent individuals, and families in which abuse of children has occurred. Person-centered care results simply from our awareness of such services, and appropriate referral.

4. *The physician can refer patients for psychosocial evaluation.* The most difficult referral problem for most physicians is for evaluation of the patient's psychosocial situation in relation to the illness. Getting such help is more feasible in teaching clinics where a clinical social worker or consulting psychologist/psychiatrist can see the patient right in the doctor's office area. One busy general practitioner in our area arranged to have a clinical social worker consult regularly in his own private office. [3] In most group clinics or health-maintenance organizations where psychological services are available, the patient can be seen in the same building. Such arrangements are acceptable to most patients. Many resident physicians, however, are reluctant to call upon anyone, even the clinical social worker attached to the clinic. In private practice, referral is especially difficult for most doctors.

The reluctance has to do with all the barriers discussed in this chapter. Physicians may feel, at a deeper level, that if the referral is truly appropriate, then they ought to be doing more of this themselves. The very act of referral may be unconsciously construed as an adverse reflection on their customary (medical-model) approach to illness. It is always more reassuring to feel that what one does *not* do is not necessary! For the same reason, the doctor with this point of view will not have begun to elicit the underlying personal situation during the medical history. Whereas a more extended psychosocial interview, by either the doctor or a consultant, can flow readily out of such a history (Ch. 14), referral is difficult when the patient is poorly prepared to recognize the need. The patient will perceive the referral not as a means to help the doctor provide better care but as a rejection.

What is needed here is a doctor who is confident of his or her ability and prepared to provide comprehensive care. An effective relationship is established with the patient through empathic history-taking and careful physical examination. The doctor plans to continue the medical care but feels strongly that a psychosocial evaluation is necessary to understand and help the patient through the illness. Because of the doctor's schedule and training, however, it is explained that s/he is not in a position to do the interview personally but customarily works with X, who does it very well.

Ideally, the doctor has a working relationship with the person to whom the patient is referred. In the doctor's own office, an informative psychosocial survey can often be accomplished by a nurse practitioner or physician assistant. For outside referral, liaisons can be established with a marriage, family, and child therapist, clinical social worker, psychologist, psychiatrist, or medical colleague experienced in psychosomatic disorders.

The purpose of the interview is simply to identify the underlying problem areas in relation to the illness. The better the understanding, the more effective can be the plan for getting well. Decisions can then be made about what the patient may be able to do about the problem and what the patient's personal physician can best do medically. The referral is a consultation, not a transfer of care.

It should be understood by the patient, as well as by the colleague to whom the referral is made, that this preliminary overview is limited to one or two visits (one hour each) unless the patient is already prepared for more extensive counseling. A referral to psychotherapy may be threatening to some patients. The physician's confidence in the colleague and in his/her decision to make the referral is helpful. The patient's commitment need be only at a level appropriate for medical patients to accept at an early juncture in their care. Further counseling, by either the primary physician or a consulting colleague, may well evolve from the initial interview(s), but that is a later decision.

In the Stanford Clinics, when I had made a presumptive diagnosis of psychosomatic illness in Spanish-speaking patients, I would ask the staff translators, who had translated the medical history for me, to interview the patient independently in their own way to identify the underlying personal problems. They are not trained for such interviews, but they are indeed familiar with the language and the culture, and they do not introduce a white-coat barrier to such sharing. Clinics that serve large minority populations often employ trained health aides for this purpose. In medical practice, unlike psychiatry, the underlying problems in any culture are usually more "social" than "psychological," although the two aspects are always mixed. While the problem can often be identified by an empathic listener, this surely has its potential problems. One doesn't know the messages that are actually transmitted.

This chapter has sought to provide a summary of the barriers to person-centered care as they are described to me by many physicians and patients. The barriers are real enough, but at the same time they can too readily be used as excuses for avoiding person-centered issues. All of the barriers can be surmounted by a physician motivated to do so.

The time limit, for example, is often cited as the main barrier. Note that Orvieta T.'s doctor (Ch. 2) saw his patients on a 15-minute office-visit schedule, as most doctors do. We saw how he stuck to a standard medical-model approach because "there was no time for more." Nevertheless, he then proceeded to see the patient eight times a year for three years, a total of six hours (and $600 at $25 per visit), but after all this, she was no better. That her life situation was the cause of her illness should have been suspected in the first few visits, simply by the multiplicity of symptoms. An understanding could have been achieved in the next two visits, thereby obviating most of the subsequent visits, lab tests, and X-ray examinations and simplifying the treatment plan considerably. Even referral for a psychosocial survey would have involved at most two hours, or $200, a fraction of what was eventually paid for all of the visits and workups.

It cannot be said, therefore, that there was not enough time. There was plenty of time. The physician did not use the available time to explore the central issues, but chose instead to prescribe for symptoms, one at a time. That is the fundamental barrier that stands in the way of a meaningful doctor/patient relationship.

PART II

*Emotions and
Emotional Symptoms*

Cognitive/Emotional Dissociation:
A Common Cause of Illness

Mammalian emotional systems evolved to augment and integrate behavioral responses to immediate needs and threats. Thus the "emotion," which describes the kind of response, is both purposeful and physical. Its function, biologically, cannot be separated from the action it reinforces. The human species, however, can block the biological purpose of emotions with cognitive controls that can suppress not only the many ways in which emotions are expressed but also the appropriate behaviors necessary to respond more directly to the needs or threats that activated the response in the first place. Such inhibition, however, cannot abolish the subjective feelings of distress. Denied tears or fists, or resolution of the disappointments, unfilled needs, conflicts, or effects of the neglect, abuse, or other trauma from which they arise, the emotional feelings remain suppressed. Though dissociated from conscious awareness, they continue to disturb personality and behavior in many ways, and constitute a major cause of psychosomatic and psychiatric illness. In this way, the underlying emotions come to be viewed, by both doctors and patients, as undesirable, disruptive, mental forces. Nevertheless, if the emotions can be reexperienced and appreciated in relation to their source, the conflicts resolved, the damaged personality revitalized in some way, the underlying needs recognized and filled at least in part, healing can occur. The emotions can then again be perceived as purposeful and inherently physical in terms of appropriate actions and behavior.

Understanding the process of cognitive/emotional dissociation and its possible resolution is essential to an effective outcome when such forces are involved.

∾ Any physician would recognize that Mary S. (Ch. 3) had an emotional disorder. If, however, the source of the disorder is not detected, the symptoms (described as panic, anxiety, or hyperventilation) seem to represent a failure of emotional control of some kind, a neurotic pathology or biological fault. In this way emotions, at least in patients, appear to be undesirable, primitive, disruptive mental forces that cause psychosomatic and psychiatric illness. Suppression is the usual therapeutic goal.

Yet the evolutionary function of emotions is to augment and integrate total behavior in response to immediate needs. Thus emotions are inherently purposeful, and, because they unite prevailing needs or threats with appropriate actions, they are inherently physical.

How, then, do emotional responses appear to be so *mental* and *disruptive* in the lives of human beings, whereas they are invariably *physical and appropriate* in the lives of other species? In the answers to these questions lie the unique nature of human emotions, how they cause symptoms, and why they are the key to understanding and helping patients through emotionally induced illness.

Human emotions can indeed be disruptive. Fear, shame, sadness, anger, and other negative emotions cannot be readily discharged in situations where the threats, regretted behaviors, losses, or conflicts cannot be changed. Anger results in violence. If caused by long-standing situations beyond the subject's control, such as parental abuse or neglect, poverty, prejudice and discrimination, injustices and impaired opportunities of many kinds, the alienation and hostility may persist for a lifetime. The anger is projected to other individuals or to society in general in cruel, violent, and criminal behavior. Obviously suppressed human emotions, unlike the direct emotional responses of other species, which are discharged in immediate actions, can be very destructive.

In medical practice, however, we rarely see the people who act out aggressive behavior. Nor do we see many people, except in psychiatry, who are emotionally disturbed but quite aware of the nature of the disturbance or its source. What we see most commonly are emotionally induced physical symptoms, anxiety, or depression, caused by feelings that have become so dissociated from awareness that the patient is no longer in touch with their source and cannot act toward resolution. How does this happen? To answer the question, we need first to consider some behaviors of animals that illustrate the evolutionary purpose of emotional responses.

Emotional Behavior in Animals

Imagine a cat sunning on a lawn, not hungry, threatened, uncomfortable, or in heat. It remains alert but perceives no external or internal cues requiring any special action. If a friendly dog appears, the cat responds with a mere turn of its head. If the dog threatens, we see the cat with hunched back, hair on end, hissing. If the dog attacks, the cat flees, or, if cornered, fights back with howls and claws. Cats playing games with a spool, or purring on one's lap, display still other kinds of emotional behavior.

The postural, vocal, and motor behaviors represent a total commitment of the cat appropriate to each situation. Its instinctive, intuitive, experiential appraisal in terms of its own welfare is converted into correspondingly varied moods and actions. Presumably, the cat does not "reflect" on its feelings of fear, playfulness, or contentment apart from the gestalt of its unified experience. Nevertheless, these remarkable differences in the quality of the integrated behaviors constitute the *emotional* aspect of the response.

In animals, *emotional* means nothing more than the type and degree of investment in ongoing activity. An emotion is not something that can be separated from the corresponding action. While the cat lay on the lawn, its muscles relaxed, its sympathetic nervous system idling, its "emotionality" was one of quiescent comfort. As the dog appeared, threatened, and attacked, immediate adjustments of arousal, of autonomic and muscular activity, occurred, but the cat's total behavior was integrated at each moment. In this way, the cat is always *emotional*, and the emotions are always *physical*. Is it the cat or its body that expresses the response? Obviously, they are inseparable. Can humankind separate body from emotion? Here lie the key differences that result in the problems of psychosomatic medicine.

The components of an emotional response include an appraisal of the prevailing situation, [1, 2] a subjective feeling, and an objective response. The appraisal includes both a perception of the sensory data (hunger, sight of the dog) and a sense of what the situation means. The meaning is both cognitive (need to find food, danger) and affective (discomfort, fear, rage). The feeling or affective component is the bridge that unites the appraisal with the ensuing action. In animals the appraisal, the feeling, and the action are immediate, automatic, and fused.

The resulting behavior includes both an expressive attitude and appropriate action. The attitude is communicated by postural, vocal, and other means. This alone may constitute a sufficient response to handle the situation. The cat hunches and hisses, or the opossum plays dead, and the enemy retreats. The attitude assumed is also the beginning arousal for whatever further action may be necessary.

A common evolutionary basis for the expression of emotions in human and animal species was demonstrated by Darwin in 1872. [3] Human emotions are complex, but observations on commonalities in facial expression across species, particularly nonhuman primates, across human cultures in infants and children, and in those born blind, indicate a major genetic contribution. [4]

This, then, is our biological heritage. The central nervous system loci that organize the intuitive appraisal and emotional discharge in animals serve the same function for human beings. These loci include most of the phylogenetically old cortex described long ago by MacLean [5–8] as the paleomammalian cortex, limbic system, or visceral brain (hippocampus, amygdala, cingulate gyrus, and their connections). Originally allied with smell, the limbic system integrates and interprets experience in terms of quality and intensity, a "language" not of words but of feelings. [6] Of special importance in the final common pathway of emotional expression are the subcortical areas of the diencephalon (thalamus, hypothalamus), the pons (locus ceruleus), the medulla (reticular activating system), and their connections. For our purpose here it is not necessary to review how this elaborate integrated system functions. [9–16] To understand psychosomatic medicine we need know only that these brain centers *below the threshold of conscious thinking and control,* integrate organismic responses through appropriate discharges to the musculoskeletal and autonomic nervous systems and to the hypothalamic-pituitary-endocrine axes. Without these primordial functions, neither the individual nor the species would have survived.

Emotional Behavior in the Human Species

Eventually, evolution resulted in an unusual animal with a neocortex superimposed on the older cortical and subcortical areas. This allowed the new species to represent reality with signs and symbols, define logical categories, and to reason with its own propositions. Its experience is abstracted in systems of names, rules, and goals that govern its behaviors. We live by cognitive constructs about how we ought to be, ought to think, and ought to feel! [17–21] These precepts are indeed important, because our welfare depends upon our ability to adapt to a complex society. Nevertheless, they are human abstractions, not biological imperatives. So we no longer just live our lives as did our animal progenitors. We plan. We hope. We often live in the future, our choices tied to the past. In many ways we are not even receptive to the salient aspects of present experience. [22]

In spite of the remarkable evolutionary gains of the neocortex, its cognitive format embroils us in a variety of problems that are difficult to avoid. We develop strong investments in the values by which we learn to live. [23] These values constitute a positive force in our lives, [24] but can be devastating when we fail to live by or attain the same standards. [20, 21] In this way, human emotions have cultural and cognitive as well as biological determinants, with many idiosyncratic personal variables. Our emotions are by no means restricted to the primitive sexual, aggressive, and other urges emphasized by Freud. Moreover, the beliefs, habits, and constructs that govern our lives, acquired early in life, often conflict with one another and with the basic human needs outlined in Chapter 5. Thus, emotional investment is divided: some is discharged in ongoing activities appropriate to one set of goals; some is retained when actions appropriate to other needs are denied by supervening but contrary rules of behavior. Cognitive/emotional polarities are inevitable.

The division of an emotional response into its appraisal and behavioral components, therefore, represents a strictly anthropomorphic analysis. No such division occurs in animal behavior in which mind/body unity is maintained at all times. The mind of *Homo sapiens*, however, fixed on one system of goals, not only restricts competing behaviors but also attempts to eliminate the feelings that would otherwise empower them. We try to *disembody* the emotion (though our facial expression may give us away)!

We have varying success in bringing off this ingenious human trick. The cognitive controls can be so dictatorial that the suppressed feelings may be barely noticed, or denied. Even an alternative appraisal of the situation may be blocked. The entire emotional experience can be bypassed and thereby eliminated from conscious awareness. Nevertheless, if the unfilled needs or unresolved conflicts and their attendant emotional feelings have sufficient importance, they will be noticed by something like the "hidden observer" demonstrated by Hilgard in his studies of hypnosis, and retained at dissociated levels of mental activity. [25] There the feelings retain their primordial connections for emotional discharge.

Because the functions of the limbic system and subcortical areas preclude communication in verbal terms, [5] the feelings that remain are difficult to define without being tautological. *Anger*, for example, can be described only in terms of situations that make one angry, just as *red* can be described only in reference to objects of that color. Feeling does include, however, an intuitive summation, a kind of vector that includes how situations are likely to affect a person, one's previous experience in similar situations, what might be done about it, what may result if one does or does not act accordingly, and how all this might satisfy or hinder one's comfort, security, needs, values, goals, hopes, fantasies, at different levels. The feeling includes unconscious as well as conscious elements. It may or may not be congruent with a cognitive appraisal of the same situation. Feeling also includes an awareness of the incipient changes in autonomic activity, muscular tension, and breathing before overt changes occur.

If the feelings erupt later in an unguarded outburst, the individual, identified all along with the mental forces that sidetracked the emotional response in the first place, may react with dismay at the surprising, alien, and disorganizing force from within. The feelings cannot be perceived as the core of an appraisal and action appropriate to one set of needs but denied by another. When a feeling reappears in any guise, divorced from the action for which it was originally intended, it does indeed appear as a "mental" force with no clear purpose. The emotion that nature evolved as a quality of integrated behavior has been abstracted as a thing in itself.

Cognitive/Emotional Dissociation as the Cause of Clinical Symptoms

Usually, the feelings cannot be disembodied forever. Denied verbal or emotional expression, with no resolution of the underlying problem, the feelings are shunted into other channels. Nature forces a mind/body connection denied by the cognitive interventions.

Evelyn C. was a 40-year-old, married homemaker who was referred for evaluation of a diffuse anterior chest pain that had dominated her life for three years. She struggled to do her housework but had no energy for any other activity. The referral diagnosis was angina pectoris, based on borderline ST-T abnormalities on the resting electrocardiogram and 1-mm. depressions on the exercise EKG. (This patient was seen before the advent of coronary arteriography.)

The pain, however, was not typical of angina. It was quite severe, present most of the time, and neither related to exercise nor relieved by nitroglycerin. Because she appeared tense, with other symptoms of panic and anxiety, it was our impression that she most likely had psychogenic chest pain, perhaps mediated through muscular tension in the chest wall.

During the customary workup, the student physician with whom I was consulting explored possible sources for stress in three follow-up visits. She spoke dispassionately of herself, her husband, their children, her sexuality, early life, interests, worldview, and future hopes. Although a few problems, such as we all have, were revealed, no clear understanding was reached concerning the source of the incapacitating emotional tension that had to be present to explain the intensity of the pain, if indeed it was an emotional pain. If seen today, she would have an arteriogram; with that found negative, many doctors would simply diagnose "non-ischemic chest pain," and reassure her that "it" was "nothing serious."

Meanwhile, her desperation became more difficult to contain as the pain steadily increased. The climactic moment came on the fifth visit, when her husband brought her to the clinic in a state of frenzy. Her previous equa-

nimity had suddenly vanished, and her anguish poured forth in a fit of un-controllable, convulsive sobbing during which she blurted out the contained emotions of 15 years of marriage: unfilled needs, resentments, frustrations, a torrent of feelings never before expressed or experienced.

The key point here is that for all these years Evelyn's cognitive mind, trained as it was in her own family background, had directed her to perceive only what it *thought* she should perceive: how she *ought to be*—a good person, wife, and mother, whose main purpose was to serve a nice husband, family, and home. As her emotional outburst subsided, her husband was brought in to share her feelings. He was at first surprised and overwhelmed. Unlike Seymour (Ch. 5), he was, however, a loving husband who was prepared to accept his wife's feelings, appreciate the sharing, and to respond. They did, in fact, have a good relationship and family situation, but she had never learned to express to him what she was really feeling, what she wanted, needed.

All of her symptoms disappeared that very day, and, in this remarkable case of contained emotions—it is by no means usually possible to reveal and change the source of such a problem so readily—the symptoms did not recur in 20 years of follow-up. She quickly regained her energy, obtained a full-time job, and realized more and more the full potential of her relationship with her husband and children.

Irene F. was a 56-year-old psychologist whom I knew socially. She was referred to me as a patient for a similar kind of chest pain, but here there were no other symptoms to suggest a nervous condition. Though she was quite sophisticated about emotions and symptoms in her clients, and appeared to respond readily to my queries about every phase of her life, I was unable to form any idea about the emotional cause of her pain. I would never have uncovered it if I had not happened to see her again at a dinner party during which I noted how her husband interrupted and dominated her again and again, though this did not appear to upset her in any way. The next day I confronted her with my own anger at her husband's behavior and her apparent willingness to put up with it. Suddenly, like Evelyn, her control vanished as she screamed, clutching her chest with both hands, "I can't stand it, I can't stand it, it gets me—right in here!"

The essential mind/body unity of emotions has been known since antiquity. Aristotle: ". . . all the affections of soul involve a body—passion, gentleness, fear, pity, courage, joy, loving, and hating. . . ." [26] How emotions can be suppressed from conscious awareness, yet profoundly affect behavior, mood, thinking, and body, was the major contribution of Breuer and Freud as far back as 1895. [27] Many observers since then have delineated the psychological process and connected it with the ordinary psychosomatic and psychiatric symptoms of medical practice, with unique insight. The primal connection of mind and body is reflected endlessly in what we read, see, and experience in ourselves. Yet this ancient wisdom, scientifically documented in a voluminous literature for almost a century, often has little impact on medical practice. Doctors have difficulty understanding the emotional basis of illness. Patients with commonplace psychosomatic symptoms are convinced they are diseased. Emotions continue to be regarded as suspect; emotional symptoms, as shameful. Why does this view of a split between mind, emotions, and body prevail with such conviction?

The Major (Cognitive) and Minor (Intuitive/Emotional) Hemispheres

The answer lies partly in the division of neocortical, limbic system, and subcortical functions outlined above. The division of the neocortex, as it evolved, into the nonverbal, imaginative, intuitive functions of the minor hemisphere, also beyond the control of the verbal, rational, cognitive mind of the major hemisphere, completes the story. Ideally, the division is a great advantage. The "I" has access to two kinds of mental functioning by which one can think logically or intuitively in whatever mode or combination of modes is best suited to the presenting situation. The major hemisphere (left hemisphere in right-handed people, right hemisphere in most left-handed people), however, is truly dominant. That is the problem. Because it controls language, symbols, and handedness, and because it processes information in a sequential, logical, largely verbal, reasoning analysis (the way we actually think consciously most of the time), it literally dominates awareness and behavior so completely that it becomes identified as the real *me,* or *self.* But as Levy et al. point out so well, "The propensity of the language hemisphere to note analytical details in a way that facilitates their description in language seems to interfere with the perception of an over-all Gestalt, leaving the [major] hemisphere 'unable to see the wood for the trees.'" [28]

As demonstrated by Sperry and his colleagues, [28–33] this is the function of the minor hemisphere. It can see the "wood" because it processes information in maplike wholes or three-dimensional representations of spatial configurations, which the major hemisphere cannot readily do. The minor hemisphere also thinks intuitively; that is, its solutions to problems are based on multiple converging determinates rather than a single causal chain of logical sequences. [34] With limited access to language, it primarily uses nonverbal representations and "reasons" by nonlinear modes of association. An emotional feeling is one type of intuitive response, a summation of multiple factors as they relate to the individual's welfare, as described previously. Thus the minor hemisphere can read out the emotional impact of situations that the cognitive mind may be unable to read because of the latter's governing constructs about how things "ought to be." In one of Sperry's experimental subjects (whose cerebral commissures had been divided to limit epileptic seizures uncontrolled by medication), the minor hemisphere, recognizing an emotionally charged situation that could not be perceived by the major hemisphere, releases an emotional discharge (blushing, exclamations, facial expressions). It knows, feels, and acts, but has no words to explain.(29)

The integration of the functions of the two hemispheres, limbic system, and subcortical areas of intact brains is not fully understood. The two hemispheres are connected, after all, by the corpus callosum, though their respective functions often appear to be separated by a practice of use (major) and disuse (minor), if not by an anatomic/physiologic disconnection. [34] The functional separation appears to be confirmed in experimental observations on subjects who have difficulty experiencing and communicating their own emotions. [35] We have much more to learn about the anatomic/physiologic basis for the cognitive, intuitive, and emotional discord of normal subjects with intact brains. It is clear, nevertheless, that quite different kinds of mental activity are going on in everyone continuously. The two that concern us here are designated as cognitive mind and intuitive/emotional mind. They are often dissociated. Depending on the situation, either one of them can dominate, with little or no awareness of the other. In daily life, cognitive mind usually has control of consciousness.

Actually, most mental activity is automatic. If I decide to go to the grocery store, for example, I am not aware of processing innumerable proprioceptive, vestibular, and visual impulses, or of sending efferent messages to muscles. I am not even aware of driving the car as I think about other things. Levels of conscious awareness vary constantly. Cognitive mind does little more than supply strategic direction to life, but it seems to itself to be doing everything. It would be paralyzed if it had to keep track of the infinite coordinating details that the silent areas of the mind handle unobtrusively.

We have seen how cognitive mind often guides actions in emotionally charged situations according to its own precepts, ignoring or detouring around those aspects it does not choose to deal with. Urgent, basic, long-term needs and conflicts are often neglected, and languish unattended for years. Freud described the process as *repression*, which implies that conscious mind or the *ego*, here called *cognitive mind*, considered but rejected an alternative action. This indeed occurs, but perhaps more commonly the process is better regarded as *dissociation*, as described by Hilgard. [25] Cognitive mind is so absorbed with its own ideas that it does not even notice the alternatives. It is barely aware of the mass of feelings and memories stored either by its own deeper recesses or by its restrained mental partners who communicate in such strange ways. Because these areas do indeed process the input as it is received, they are best described as *co-conscious*, active but silent, unnoticed by the busy cognitive mind which usurps the whole of consciousness with its own concerns. The silent areas are *unconscious* or *subconscious* only as viewed by the cognitive mind which has control. The dissociative disorders of psychiatry, such as multiple personality, constitute just one type of expression of the relative independence, or dissociation, of cognitive and intuitive/emotional appraisals that characterize so much of the emotionally charged mental activities of everyday life. [36]

How Cognitive/Emotional Dissociation Affects Our Lives

The intensity of the dissociated disturbances is augmented in many ways. The habitual suppression of negative emotions reinforces the process continuously. An additional disturbance is the subliminal resentment of one's own fear of open expression, and of the family or marital systems that appear to demand that the emotions be held in check. Meanwhile, the personal problems multiply as nothing is done to change the ongoing situation. The resulting cognitive/emotional polarities affect our daily lives in countless ways. The constant monitoring of behaviors necessary to maintain suppression constrains what otherwise could be a joyous, spontaneous personality. Sadly, a common corollary of inhibiting "bad" feelings is the inhibition of "good" feelings as well. Evelyn's anger almost succeeded in destroying the very love its containment was supposed to protect. Her loving side could not be reexperienced until the negative side had been released.

Evelyn and Irene learned early in life not to express negative emotions, perhaps not to *have* negative emotions! This comes from a very common child-rearing indoctrination in our culture that demands conformity and a kind of peace in the family, from the point of view of the parents, but fails to nourish self-esteem in the children with an appreciation of their own unique qualities, and a sense of reality about themselves and their feelings. This is not to suggest that children should be allowed to act out negative feelings, that every feeling is appropriate to the situation on which it is projected, or that emotional control is not essential to daily living. But children need to be able to share their feelings comfortably, whatever they are, and have the feelings acknowledged as real and understandable, whether they can be acted upon or not. Feeling OK about oneself is essential to the process of becoming fully human. Otherwise, a lifelong cognitive construct of withholding emotions spawns an endless series of polarities with corresponding personal and clinical problems, throughout life. A generalized emotional impoverishment results. [37] Because of the restricted personality, the individual may even find it difficult to experience and express that which is most sublime, loving, and compassionate. [38]

In medical practice, we see suppressed emotions most commonly expressed as physical symptoms. The functional disorders are also caused by stress and a host of other problems in the absence of any cognitive/emotional polarities, but contained emotions are a very common constituent. The form taken may be that of psychophysiologic reactions, as with Evelyn and Irene, or of acting-out behaviors—the conversion reactions and psychogenic pain syndromes to be described in the next chapter.

The Dilemma for Patients and Their Doctors

In functional illness, cognitive mind (that is, the patient identified as cognitive mind) notices the symptoms but has no way to read the message. Bypassing emotional issues so often, cognitive mind considers itself and the person it controls as relatively unemotional. Furthermore, it regards the body—which it orders around all the time to carry out its will—as its very own and cannot believe that it could be affected by anything so ephemeral as emotions. Cognitive mind cannot imagine what has happened when the body feels sick. So a doctor is consulted.

Now we can perceive more clearly the dilemmas posed by functional disorders for both doctors and patients in medical practice.

The physician must be wary that the consultation is not restricted to one cognitive mind communicating with another. The medical history obtained by talking reveals only the biased point of view of the patient's verbal mind which has difficulty describing the mood, even the symptoms, and describes the life situation in terms of its own limited constructs, as did Evelyn's cognitive mind in the first three interviews. It is often unaware of the emotion, its source, and the relation of all this to the symptoms. Even if it is aware of a conflict, it fails to perceive the conflict's relation to the illness. "I know there is something wrong," it says to the doctor. "Find the disease."

Meanwhile, the doctor's cognitive mind, busy with differential diagnosis, especially of organic diseases, may now have inactivated its own silent, intuitive, emotionally responsive potential. If so, the doctor may fail to notice either the clinical inconsistencies between the patient's symptoms and the disease postulated, or the patient's nonverbal expressions, which indicate that something else is amiss. "Yes, there must be a disease," the doctor agrees. "I'll find it." The result: an unwitting conspiracy of two cognitive minds to avoid the basic problem.

If the suppressed feelings do not emerge as physical symptoms, they may break out directly as uncontrolled but unfocused emotional expressions, or take the form of anxiety, depression, and/or other psychiatric syndromes. Again, cognitive mind may be unaware of the original feelings, their source, or their relation to the symptoms.

The real problem is to translate the somatic, mental, and affective messages to get back to their source. If this can be done, the relevance of the corresponding emotions will be clarified. This can be difficult. (Suggestions for a beginning to this process are outlined in Chs. 14–17.)

The therapeutic encounter can evolve in many ways. Talking with the patient about possible problems may be sufficient. The feelings may be just under the surface, as with Mary (Ch. 3), and a deeper emotional breakthrough, such as occurred with Evelyn and Irene, is not necessary to reveal the core problem. At the other extreme, even an extended period of psychotherapy may accomplish very little until an alternative approach hits upon the key issue. Sometimes in an interview the patient's emotional mind will release a transient emotional expression as the source is touched upon, only to be denied by cognitive mind as it regains control. This provides the interviewer who notices the breakthrough a unique opportunity to help the patient begin to understand the polarity that causes the symptoms. Evelyn's breakthrough involved a sudden and total reversal from her identity with the cognitive side of her mind to an experience of the emotional. Fortunately, her feelings applied appropriately to her current situation, and resolution was feasible.

When the situation revealed cannot be changed readily, as was the case with Ann (Ch. 5), at least the problem has been identified, and the patient can begin to consider possible options. If the problem is not identified, the alternative is an extended illness "of unknown etiology." Most patients improve symptomatically when the source is understood, even though there may be no immediate resolution of the underlying problems.

Although they did not with Evelyn and Irene, suppressed emotions acquired early in life may affect many aspects of life and subsequent relationships to which they do not properly apply. Consider the plight of Amy B., a four-year-old girl who is sexually abused repeatedly by her father, and threatened if she tells. At one level she knows that something is wrong. It hurts, and she feels bewildered, upset, ashamed. On the other hand, she is dependent, needs her parents and their love, and, like most children, will find some way to accommodate cognitively to her childhood situation. To do this, the bad feelings, and even memories of the abuse, go underground. She grows up believing she is somehow a bad person, and gets involved in a series of self-destructive behaviors, including unsatisfying, promiscuous sexual episodes. Sex, but not caring, is one of the few things she knows about human relationships. She suffers from periodic physical and emotional symptoms related to anxiety and depression, and she is unable to respond sexually to her husband. These many problems prompt her referral to a sexual-abuse treatment center. There she eventually recalls how she used to imagine herself hiding in the closet while her father abused her body in the bed. In this way the cognitive/emotional split is finally revealed and slowly resolved over an extended period of counseling and involvement with a support group of peers who had also been abused as children.

It could be argued here that the cognitive adjustments to the inescapable conflict of childhood were essential at that time but disastrous thereafter. To approach her life and marriage more effectively, she must first reexperience, discharge, and work through the hurts, realize that she was an innocent victim, and learn to view herself positively, to take care of herself responsibly, and to be more self-assured in relationships. Resolution often hinges on an integration of both the cognitive and the emotional sides of the conflict.

In seeking to understand the polarities discovered in your patients (or, for that matter, in yourself, your friends, or family), consider that either the cognitive or the intuitive/emotional "readout" may be "good" or "bad," "right" or "wrong." Each must be judged in reference to the situation from which the split arose, and to which it is applied. Anger may be "right," to the extent it is based on a legitimate grievance that warrants change. Anger may be very "wrong," when projected inappropriately on a spouse, children, or society, even though its origin in childhood abuse is understandable.

A rational analysis and an emotional response are, after all, different ways of viewing the same situation. Each is valid in terms of its "own reasons." One stays with a job or a marriage, for example, for good reasons, although for other reasons one feels unbearably stuck and restricted in the same situation. While cognitive mind dictates what it thinks *ought to be*, emotional/intuitive mind reads out the same situation more realistically by knowing in its own way how *it really feels* at another level. Intuitive wisdom is sometimes wiser. On the other hand, strong feelings—real enough for the individual who holds them, but destructive, nevertheless—can be fixed on wishes, fantasies, and irrational beliefs, [39] or projected onto another situation.

Both the governing construct and the resulting emotion may be "right," as in Evelyn's case, where "being a good wife" and "feeling frustrated," respectively, expressed different but realistic aspects of the same situation. When the emotion, which had gone underground, was experienced and dealt with, both the illness and the underlying situation resolved.

In contrast, both the governing construct and the resulting emotion may be "wrong." The constructs "I am worthwhile only if I succeed" or "if others think well of me" lead to depression when one fails or is rejected. The depression is "right" only in terms of the arbitrary constructs on which it is based. Both the construct and the resulting emotion are "wrong" in terms of the subject's well-being. In this situation, it is the construct, accepted as basic truth for so long that it is no longer questioned, that has gone underground. The patient is aware only of feeling depressed, but the depression calls attention to a conceptual problem that must be revised to abolish the affective disturbance. This is the basis of cognitive therapy. [19–21] Jerome Frank points out how much of the patient's assumptive world (as he describes the constructs by which one lives) is unconscious. [18]

Emotional pain can, of course, be relieved in many ways by changing the way one views a situation. That is one purpose of humor. The situation is viewed as absurd rather than tragic, and one laughs instead of cries. Or, as described by Victor Frankl, a prisoner in a concentration camp survives better by switching focus from the cruelty and injustice of the situation to one's personal strength and forbearance. [40] Many problems in life, especially chronic disease, force upon us a need for change. Then, what begins as a need for adjustment may evolve into what can also be viewed as an opportunity for a new line of personal development. Most everyone can cite examples of this process.

The Ideal: An Integrated Personality

A major purpose of this extended discussion is to emphasize that divisions of cognitive and intuitive/emotional functions are inherent in human consciousness. Ideally, the two minds work together as one. Some people are fortunate enough to encounter no major problems, or they learn to resolve problems as they arise. The individual remains sensitive to varying needs at different levels and satisfies them sufficiently to remain in reasonable harmony, no need denied too much or too long. Intuitive mind notices no particular needs or conflicts to monitor. If it does express itself, cognitive mind listens, receives the message, and responds appropriately. But few people are able to do all this effectively. Cognitive/emotional dissociations are inevitable. When symptoms result, the help of a physician or counselor is essential.

Psychopathology is often too pejorative a term to use in describing the universal process of emotional containment that underlies most functional and nervous disorders. Freud, unfortunately, despite his great insights into the unconscious and sexuality as forces in human life and a cause of symptoms, tied emotions to drives of libido and aggression, a limited and mechanistic view to say the least. He went on to divide the personality into a somewhat simplistic trinity, introduced an abstruse jargon, and theorized excessively about correlating behavioral qualities with childhood sexuality. Freud was often right, within the limits of his insights, but we still view emotions as primitive, and symptom formation as a pathology called *neurosis*. Freud's influence was profound, and affects our views today. But human emotions are often either corollaries or reciprocals of our most cherished values, needs, or goals, depending on how those are realized or thwarted. Emotions express who we are as much as our cognitive constructs do, often more so. They must be considered together. Viewing emotions as "primitive" may lead us to reinforce the patient's inhibitory forces. While trying to be helpful with symptomatic drugs we may unwittingly entrench emotional containment.

Consonant with the cognitive/emotional polarities discussed here is the figure/ground concept of gestalt psychology and gestalt therapy. [41] Our perceptions are experienced not as pieces but as whole configurations, one thing at a time. This is illustrated by the well-known picture in which you see either a white chalice with a black background or two black faces in profile with a white background, but you cannot perceive both simultaneously. The object of perception is the *figure*; the rest, which you cannot perceive for what it is though it is there, is the *ground*. In Evelyn's case, the cognitive construct about how her personal situation ought to be was the figure; her anger about the same situation was the ground. In depression, the emotion (feeling depressed) is the figure; a dissociated cognitive construct about how one's situation ought to be is often the ground.

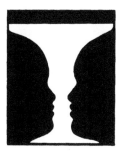

In either case, both the cognitive and emotional—reciprocal perceptions of the same situation—must be reexperienced, reconsidered, and reintegrated in order to reach a more effective resolution for the individual, in conjunction with the corresponding needs of the other important persons in the patient's life. Something about the patient, or the situation itself, needs to be changed. A formidable challenge! It could be said, nevertheless, that the ultimate goal for patients with emotional disorders is to find a way toward such a resolution.

It is not the job of physicians or counselors to tell patients what to do, but it *is* our responsibility, whenever possible, to clarify the nature of the illness.

The ultimate, integrated *I*, or self, is not easy to define, but the ideal *I* constitutes a supervening, coordinating core of consciousness that brings about an effective collaboration of the cognitive, emotional, somatic, and spiritual aspects of experience. [42] It is, after all, the many combinations and permutations of all these elements that make life so exciting at times, so challenging at others. No one aspect or subsystem should command the whole. [43]

Emotionally Induced Physical Symptoms

The barrier that too often blocks a comprehensive approach to patients with functional disorders is the difficulty we experience in establishing an early, correct, and positive diagnosis of emotionally induced physical symptoms. We are not well trained to recognize this kind of illness (especially psychogenic pain disorders). In this chapter, key attributes of the two major types, physiological disturbances and somatoform disorders, are reviewed. Understanding their characteristics is essential for accurate diagnosis and an effective therapeutic plan.

ৎৎ We have seen that strong emotions, if not discharged through appropriate actions to ameliorate the source of the problem, cannot simply be contained and thereby obliterated. The distress will find expression in other ways. Clinically, it may appear as anxiety, depression, or other psychiatric disorders. Or it appears as physical symptoms—the subject of this chapter. The physical symptoms take form in two ways: the psychophysiologic reactions, such as tension headaches or hyperventilation syndrome; and the somatoform disorders (formerly known as conversion reactions), [1] such as the pain syndromes suffered by Ruth (Ch. 1) and George (Ch. 2).

Most functional disorders seen in medical practice are one or the other of these two types of reaction. Both are common. To establish the diagnosis, we need to understand the nature of, and especially the differences between, these two kinds of disorders, just as we learn to distinguish one kind of anemia from another. But we are not so trained. That is why the symptoms are often regarded as "nonspecific," "atypical," or "uncharacteristic." *Atypical* means only that the symptoms do not match those of the organic diseases postulated in the differential diagnosis. The symptoms are *typical,* nevertheless, but typical of a functional disorder, not of disease. After all, symptoms, whatever they are, characterize the unique illness of each patient. That is what we need to discover.

It is quite feasible to make accurate primary positive diagnoses of functional disorders *from the symptoms alone* if all of the symptoms are elicited just as they are. All that is needed is to be open to the realities of this half of medicine, and to learn by following all patients carefully enough and long enough to find out what is really wrong or not wrong. Only by actual clinical experience can we learn to correlate symptoms with the basic clinical problem, whatever it is. In the diagnosis of functional disorders, the symptoms are all-important, because the workup will be negative, and it may be difficult to elicit the confirming evidence of the underlying personal problem. Ruling out organic disease is important, but it is a roundabout and usually ineffective route to a positive diagnosis. The most informative data are the symptoms per se, how described, and the physician's understanding of the underlying mechanisms. This is strictly a problem for the primary physician. Patients with physical symptoms rarely consult psychiatrists, and they do not readily accept referral.

The general characteristics of emotionally induced symptoms are described in this chapter, and the differential diagnosis of specific symptoms, as against organic disease, in the following chapter.

Definitions

There are two distinct differences between what will be called here *psychophysiologic reactions* (PPR) and *somatoform disorders* (SD). The symptom of a PPR is caused by the activation of a physiologic pathway; the symptom of an SD is not. For example, tension headache is thought to be caused by the tension of muscles in the head and neck; irritable-bowel syndrome, by disturbances of gastrointestinal motility. But in a somatoform disorder, such as hysterical paralysis, the anatomy and physiology of the nervous system are perfectly normal; the symptom results from a kind of unconscious "acting out," a projection of distress expressed as symptoms that simulate a physical disorder (hence, "somatoform").

Somatoform disorders serve a purpose. Through the illness, the patient avoids facing a conflict or a need that cannot be realized, or indirectly solves the problem, fills the need, or communicates distress, more effectively than by direct confrontation. All of this serves to salvage self-esteem while reducing the emotional tension associated with the real underlying problem.

The soldier with a sudden paralysis is removed from the battlefield. The injured person with a superimposed psychogenic pain disorder gets out of work and receives a better settlement in the ensuing litigation. The individual in marital conflict receives attention and sympathy instead of indifference and criticism. The symptom is usually a communication to which others *must* respond.

The typical PPR serves no such function. The busy executive with dyspepsia, the college student with diarrhea during final exams, and Mary (Ch. 3) with panic disorder derive no advantage from their symptoms. The PPR is a physiological outflow from subcortical and limbic systems that organize emotional expression beyond the range of cognitive control. Whereas an SD often serves as a communication to someone else, the PPR is primarily a communication to oneself, if one is willing to listen to the messages from one's own body. Accumulated stresses culminate in a PPR that forces the subject to stop and notice whether she/he wants to or not. I may want to go on working 14 hours a day and sleeping 6 hours a night to finish a project, but headache says, "No! Enough is enough." In this way nature appears to have more "sense" than the patient!

Psychophysiologic Reactions

This term was abandoned in DSM-III, for several reasons. [2] First, the term was rarely used, either by psychiatrists or by medical doctors, who called the disorders by their medical names. Second, the disorders, though they are often psychogenic as the term implies, can also be caused by other factors. Migraine headaches, for example, though sometimes an expression of emotional distress, can also be precipitated by dietary tyramines, alcohol, or intense work and lack of sleep, without the presence of a psychic disturbance. Irritable-bowel syndromes and painless diarrhea or constipation can be related to diet, smoking, bowel habits, laxative abuse, or other factors, though emotional distress is often the most significant.

In the diagnostic system of DSM-III, the physical condition is recorded by its medical name, such as irritable-bowel syndrome, in one section (Axis III), and the diagnostic phrase, *psychological factors affecting physical condition*, is recorded in another (Axis I), if such factors are deemed significant. This system is rarely used either.

It is unfortunate that the term *psychophysiologic reaction* has been abandoned. The result is a medical practice in which the functional disorders are often viewed as discrete diseases, rather than as *reactions*, without sufficient attention to the underlying personal and environmental factors, whatever they are.

In this chapter I will use the term *psychophysiologic reactions* to emphasize their *physiologic* nature (as distinguished from that of the somatoform disorders) as well as their *reactive* nature. The therapeutic goal is to identify the stress or whatever factors cause the reaction. The conventional prefix, *psycho-*, will be understood here to include all personal factors, emotional and otherwise, which could be modified to prevent the reaction.

Somatoform Disorders

This term was introduced in DSM-III (1980) to replace the terms *conversion reaction* and *hysteria*, as they were formerly designated. Such disorders do indeed represent a process of *conversion*; that is, the underlying distress is *converted* into an illness. The literature can be confusing, however, because emotions are converted to symptoms in a psychophysiological reaction as well as in a conversion reaction, albeit in different ways, and the terms are often used loosely. The more specific term, *somatoform*, cannot be confused, and I will use it here. It is properly restricted to (1) conversion at a mental rather than a physiological level, and (2) conversion as including the concept of purpose. Here I will use the term *conversion* mainly to refer to the mental process by which somatoform disorders are formulated.

There are several types of somatoform disorders, three of which will be discussed in this chapter. One of these is *somatoform pain disorder.* [3] This specific term replaces the former *psychogenic pain disorder*, a term that was ambiguous because a painful physiological reaction such as tension headache can also be psychogenic. In somatoform pain disorder, by far the most common SD, the experience or perception of pain, or the projection of pain to the body, however it is viewed, can occur in the absence of activated pain receptors, as described so thoroughly by Engel. [4] There need be no muscle tension, hollow viscous spasm or distension, vasodilation or constriction, congestion or inflammation, no disease or injury of any kind. Somatoform pain can also occur as the re-experience of pain at the site of a former pathology, or as an accentuation of the pain of a current or recent pathology.

In some pain clinics, where the focus is less on the psychodynamics than on the reorientation of the chronic pain patient from the sick role to healthy behavior, the terms *somatoform* or *psychogenic pain* are not used. Instead, the same process is characterized as *pain behavior.* [5]

The second of the somatoform disorders is *conversion disorder.* [6] Unfortunately, this term is retained in DSM-III-R but restricted to specific somatoform symptoms other than pain. These include the symptoms that simulate neurologic disease, such as paralysis, aphonia, seizures, akinesia or dyskinesia, blindness, anesthesias and paresthesias. Here I will refer to such symptoms more specifically as pseudoseizures, conversion blindness, etc.

Finally, there is *somatization disorder* (formerly Briquet's syndrome), [7] which is defined as a chronic condition with multiple symptoms of many different kinds in many body systems.

The Prevalence of Psychophysiologic Reactions and Somatoform Disorders

The frequency of functional disorders in medical practice was the subject of Chapter 4. Usually, however, the literature provides little data on type of disorder. This I did with 400 consecutive patients I personally examined in the Stanford General Medicine Clinics. These patients represent a broad spectrum of problems, from acute walk-in emergencies to complex diagnostic problems referred for consultation. Patients with difficult problems, especially undiagnosed psychosomatic illness, gravitate to teaching centers, and because of my interests I was called to see more of these patients than were my colleagues. Thus my findings are weighted toward the psychological. Nevertheless, certain observations are instructive, because all physicians see a similar spectrum within the respective categories. That had been my experience, too, in prior private practice.

The illnesses that prompted the examination have been divided into (1) primarily psychosocial disturbances, and (2) illnesses caused by organic diseases, including those that may be in part psychosomatic, such as hypertension (Ch. 7). The psychosocial group was then subdivided into primarily psychological symptoms (anxiety, depression, psychosis, alcoholism, simple insomnia) and primarily physical symptoms. The latter were in turn divided as well as one can into primarily PPR or SD, using the two definitions cited above. Pain is noted when it was the dominant symptom. The findings:

	Number of Patients			
Nature of illness	Total	Male	Female	With pain as dominant symptom
Due to organic disease	199	93	106	58
Due to psychosocial distress	201	71	130	116
Psychophysiologic reaction	99	36	63	49
Somatoform disorder	75	21	54	67
Psychological symptoms	27	14	13	0

Pain is usually regarded as primarily due to organic disease. The data here show quite the contrary. The percent of pain as the dominant symptom in each subgroup was found to be:

Illness due to organic disease: 58/199 (29 percent)
Psychophysiologic disorders: 49/99 (50 percent)
Somatoform disorders: 67/75 (89 percent)

Or, viewed in terms of the entire study, 174/400 patients had pain as the dominant symptom. Of these, the pain was psychophysiological in 28 percent, somatoform in 39 percent, and caused by organic disease in only 33 percent.

Another striking observation is not that functional disorders are common but that somatoform disorders are so much more common than generally realized. They seem to be rare only because we are unwilling to consider the diagnosis. Note that somatoform pain disorder is by far the most frequent kind of conversion (89 percent of the 75 patients). In another study from the psychiatric consultation service of a general hospital, the frequency was reported as 56 percent of the SDs seen. [8] The difference may be explained by the reluctance of physicians to refer, or of patients to accept referral, for psychiatric consultation in chronic pain syndromes.

Somatoform pain can be localized or generalized, and it can be ascribed to any area of the body. In the medical clinic series, somatoform pain was ascribed to the abdomen and/or pelvis; to multiple sites, the whole body, or widespread contiguous areas; and to other sites of the head, extremities, back, neck, and genitalia. In our series, emotionally induced chest pain was considered to be psychophysiological because of its frequent association with the adrenergic discharge and hyperventilation of anxiety, thus excluded from the somatoform group. Because patients with industrial injuries and chronic back pain are customarily referred to orthopedic or neurosurgery clinics, we saw only three patients in whom what we considered to be somatoform pain was restricted to the back. The relative absence of industrial injuries in a medical clinic may also explain the preponderance of women in the somatoform group, because the process of conversion, when it occurs in men, often settles on the accident process.

The frequency of somatoform pain has escaped notice over the years for several reasons. Physicians have always been reluctant to make the diagnosis. The earliest reports of conversion symptoms were of pseudoneurologic syndromes only. The definition of hysteria in many recent reports has been restricted to somatization disorder in which pain is but one of many symptoms. Even in the psychiatric literature, the frequency of somatoform pain is not always recognized.

In the Stanford survey, a "classic" pseudoneurologic syndrome was found in only one patient (pseudoseizures). Paralyses, blindness, etc., may be seen in neurology or other specialties but rarely in medical practice. Hemianesthesia is a common finding in somatoform disorders if you test for it, but, surprisingly, it is rarely a complaint of the patient. Full-blown somatization disorder as defined in DSM was found in only nine patients, two of whom were men.

Note also that PPR and SD are common in both men and women, though more frequent in the latter. The difference, as often reported, may be more apparent than real. A stoical-appearing male, like George, will virtually never be diagnosed as "hysterical." So the men masquerade as injured or diseased. On the other hand, doctors often regard women as "emotional," and therefore make a diagnosis of conversion, or send women patients to psychiatrists whose reports are biased by the select referrals.

Distinguishing Characteristics of Psychophysiologic Reactions and Somatoform Disorders

The Physiologic or Projection Pathway to the Symptom

Typical PPRs are tension and migraine headaches; psychogenic chest pain (see Ch. 13); certain esophageal motility disorders, psychogenic vomiting, dyspepsia, irritable-bowel syndromes, and functional diarrhea or constipation; muscle tension generally, a significant factor in painful syndromes throughout the body, particularly chronic backache and fibromyalgia; psychogenic vasovagal syncope; the syndromes of adrenergic discharge, hyperventilation, dizziness, chest pain, and/or muscle tension and tremor associated with anxiety or panic; and the dysfunctions of neurotransmitter, neurohormonal, hypothalamic, circadian rhythm, and other physiologic systems in major depression. The mechanism of psychogenic fatigue and weakness is not clear; presumably, the loss of energy represents a diminished adrenergic support stimulus, as in depression, but the personal conflicts that engender the reaction may introduce a superimposed somatoform factor. Many disturbances of appetite, eating, sleep, and sexuality, though they can be direct expressions of mental states, can also be viewed as the psychophysiologic effects of depression or other nervous disorders.

The physiologic pathways of a PPR are often those that normally transmit the organism's need for emotional arousal and expression, or for withdrawal, vegetative functions, rest, and restoration, as the case may be. Here, however, the arousal systems are activated without their purposeful "fight or flight." These include the neuroendocrine systems, the vagal peptic reactions found so universally in all kinds of stress, [9] hyperventilation, which occurs normally in excitement, and the variants of general "energy," muscular tension, weakness, or fatigue, similar to those of everyday life.

The pathways may represent a counterforce: the throat muscles tighten to block crying, or the chest muscles tighten to contain anger. The reactions are also determined by idiosyncratically vulnerable sites, such as in migraine or irritable-bowel syndrome, or the PPR may be superimposed on a disease process like asthma or hypertension. The particular symptoms of each person can be shaped by many biological and genetic factors.

My classification of PPR as physiologic disturbance revises to some extent previous definitions in which emotionally induced physical symptoms were divided into conversion reactions of the voluntary muscles and sense perception, on the one hand, and physiological reactions of the involuntary or autonomic neuroendocrine systems, on the other. [10] The difficulty with that dichotomy is that the physiology of emotions normally includes skeletal muscles and the autonomic nervous system simultaneously. The chest muscles participate in laughter, crying, and hyperventilation, and muscles everywhere are alerted for action in alarm and relaxed in vegetative states. Thus PPR, here defined more broadly as a disturbance of altered physiology in any system, includes hyperventilation, tension headaches and muscle tension pains anywhere, and the muscular inhibition that can occur in psychogenic weakness and fatigue, all of which involve skeletal muscles.

The SD is a purely mental phenomenon, with parallels to hypnosis. Both the emotional basis and the process of symptom formation in an SD are dissociated from conscious awareness, but mind/body unity reappears as a symbolic or "metaphorical" projection, connection, or disconnection, with the body. Cognitive mind may not direct messages to (paralysis, aphonia) or receive messages from (coma, anesthesia, blindness) the body, or what mind experiences as pain has no concurrent active somatic source (somatoform pain disorder).

The definition of SD as the physical expression of personal distress *without activation of a physiologic pathway* is both specific and useful. To understand a patient with somatoform pain in which there is no inciting stimulus to pain receptors, the concept is essential. Otherwise, the search for a disease mechanism may be endless and ineffective, if not also damaging to the patient.

The site of a somatoform symptom can be determined psychologically or superimposed on biological events. The disorder may be clearly symbolic, as Freud suggested: facial pain as though one were slapped in the face, a sudden paralysis of both lower extremities in combat, or the need to withdraw from an untenable situation that provokes "hysterical" coma.

The illness may mimic the real or imagined symptoms of another person who is important to the subject. In health professionals, it may mimic the illnesses of patients they have seen.

More often, however, the SD settles on a fortuitous medical event. George B. sprained his ankle, but because this event happened at a difficult time in his life, it evolved into a complex somatoform pain disorder. If he had injured his back, the symptom would have been back pain. The original injury acquires symbolic significance, though it did not begin that way. The process of conversion can settle at the site of any disease, injury, surgery, or other physical pain, whether current, recent, or long-since healed. Somatoform pain is often transposed physically to the most vulnerable site in the patient's previous pain experience.

Any pain has an emotional component, but the previous pain may have had more specific emotional connotations. This may explain pelvic pain as a site of conversion pain in women: menstrual cramps and childbirth *are* painful, the only normal physiological events that are; at the same time, the area is highly charged emotionally (Ch. 1). Thus the evolution of psychic pain here has both biological and psychological roots.

Sometimes anxiety flows so readily through physiological channels that the resulting PPR serves the functions of the conversion process directly:

Martha O. was 65 years old, unhappy, unmarried, and dependent. She had mucous colitis with 10–15 loose mucoid bowel movements daily for many years, confining her to the family home where she lived with married brothers and sisters. Her health was good, weight stable. Sigmoidoscopy, barium enema, and innumerable other studies were negative. The diarrhea responded poorly to all treatments. One day while visiting her gastroenterologist in a teaching hospital, she mentioned some recent chest pain. EKG showed only T-wave inversions. She refused hospitalization. Because this questionable and uncomplicated myocardial infarction had appeared before the advent of the coronary care unit, and because she lived one block away from the hospital, her doctor asked me, the resident, if I would watch her at home. I visited her daily, noting (1) her total lack of dismay about the possible heart attack and its clear use as a means of communicating her needs to the rest of the family, and (2) that she had but one formed bowel movement every morning. After three weeks of the conventional bed rest of that time, I congratulated her on the uneventful recovery and suggested that she begin sitting up in a chair. That very day she had 12 loose stools again, and the process went on indefinitely!

If the illness caused by any injury or disease, even a psychophysiologic reaction or psychiatric disorder, provides some advantage, otherwise difficult to come by—more attention, or money, or freedom from facing self or external situations—the conversion process may be superimposed. When the disability is excessive and unusual, especially when litigation is involved, we should suspect the possibility.

Conversions are but one aspect of the problem of illness: there is, after all, no standard way to be sick. Illness is subjective. The illness initiated by any disease or injury is often determined more by the patient's life situation than by the pathology per se. Consider the reverse of conversion, the patient who denies or minimizes the illness:

Richard D., 45, was self-employed, working his own farm by himself, 12 hours a day. He limped into the clinic, his face showing no pain, but his gait clearly guarded. The present illness: "This pain in my back began eight months ago. When I get into this position [demonstrating], it shoots down the back of my right thigh to the outside of the leg, and it's kind of numb there. It's hard to work the tractor. I'm okay if I stretch out like this."

Physical exam showed an absent achilles tendon reflex, hypesthesia, atrophy, and extreme pain on straight leg raising or flexion of the back from standing. I advised that he had an obvious herniated disk and recommended immediate hospitalization for study and probably laminectomy. His response: "Well, I guess I should, but I'd rather wait until the summer work is over. I'm not so bad I can't get through the busy season."

Contrast this patient with George. Richard's ratio of disability to disease ("disability quotient") was 1:10; that of George, 10:1. In terms of the figure/ground concept of Ch. 11 (p. 177), Richard's figure was the farm; the pain was the ground. With George, the pain was the figure; his life situation, the ground.

In this way, the concept of conversion helps us to understand intractable illness superimposed on otherwise manageable medical conditions. Similarly, we can appreciate a denial of disease or depression, as for example when it gets in the patient's way. Idiosyncratic reactions to illness are virtually universal. One can hardly have a common cold without ignoring, overreacting, imputing meanings to, or in some way modifying one's reaction to this simple event.

Somatoform Pain Disorder: Making the Diagnosis

The diagnosis of a conversion disorder simulating neurologic disease is not difficult, because the absence of a physiologic defect can be demonstrated. The pupillary responses and evoked potentials on EEG are normal in conversion blindness; no encephalographic abnormalities appear during pseudoseizures; etc. Somatoform pain disorder, however, poses a more difficult problem, because the absence of an activated pathway can only be inferred. There is no way to be sure that there is no physiological disturbance or even a disease process. Many physicians doubt that such a nebulous entity exists at all. Nevertheless, the evidence for it is pooled from many observations, each of which helps to establish the diagnosis:

1. The emotional basis. The symptoms disappear if the underlying problem can be solved, as was the case with Ruth. Chronic pain syndromes following injury often disappear when a final settlement of the litigation is concluded. On the other hand, if the patient is suggestively "cured" by surgery or drugs, without changing the life situation, the symptoms will disappear only to recur or shift to another site (Janet, Ch. 1).

2. Other SDs. Concurrent or previous signs or symptoms of classical conversions (hemihypesthesia, pseudoseizures, multiple pain syndromes without a clear organic basis) demonstrate that the patient can act in this way, and support the diagnosis of pain as a possible conversion.

3. The pain is unusually sustained. The pain is often both severe and unremitting, unlike that caused by disease or a PPR that might cause pain in the same area. In the Stanford series, somatoform pain had been present longer than a year in three-fourths of the patients. There is no objective evidence of organic disease, however, or the postulated disease, even if present, would not cause such protracted pain. This combination of findings is the most reliable indicator of somatoform pain disorder.

Carcinoma of the pancreas, metastatic disease to the spine, a brain tumor, and other major diseases can, of course, cause continuous pain in the absence of any signs of disease on physical, routine lab, and X-ray examinations. But disease sufficient to cause *continuous* severe pain can usually be ruled out by ultrasound scanning, computerized tomography, magnetic resonance imaging, laparoscopy, exploratory surgery, or other modern techniques.

In like manner, an SD can usually be distinguished from physiological disturbances, such as migraine or tension headaches, that are intermittent. The setting of the illness also helps to separate the two kinds of reactions. If the headache, for example, is continuous, day and night, month after month, the patient disabled, her mother taking care of the baby, the husband kept at a distance (actual case history), then this is a somatoform pain disorder, not a tension or migraine headache.

In the 58/199 patients in the Stanford study with pain as the main symptom of organic disease, about half had transient or intermittent pain (gout, angina, muscular-strain backache, herniated disk, biliary colic, etc.); the other half had persistent pain (ischemic foot ulcer, compression fracture, Paget's disease of the spine, rheumatoid arthritis, cancer, etc.). *In all but one of these patients, however, the cause was obvious after a reasonable workup.* The exception was a 72-year-old woman with a headache who was found to have temporal arteritis on arteriography after a biopsy was negative. This is not to say that cancer or other disease never crops up to explain a chronic pain of several months' standing in a patient with a negative examination and extensive workup. But this occurrence in medical practice is rare indeed. The physician usually suspects organic disease because of the age of the patient, the character of the pain, its appearance in the absence of any evidence of nervous tension, past or present, and other features. The entire setting of the illness usually serves to distinguish organic from psychogenic pain. When organic disease is the dominant cause, it can usually be demonstrated without difficulty.

Chronic pain should not be such a diagnostic problem. It is an enigma partly because we are unwilling to look at its psychological components or recognize the ubiquity of functional pain disorders. To reiterate: two-thirds of the patients with pain in our medical clinics had no apparent organic disease.

4. The symptoms are incompatible with pathophysiology. Often the site is a contiguous region (axilla to knee on right side only, for example) with several innervations rather than the specific areas associated with disease. In the painful areas, cutaneous responses to pain stimuli, which would be normal in most disease states, may be accentuated or absent altogether. These and associated characteristics were delineated in a remarkable series of 430 patients with somatoform pain disorder treated by Walters of Toronto in a brief period of 10 years—43 such patients per year! [11]

5. Too many pain syndromes simultaneously. A patient is not likely to have, by pure coincidence, *pain* in the head (? migraine), left shoulder (? bursitis), epigastrium (? ulcer disease), lower abdomen (? diverticular disease), and back (? arthritis). Such a combination could represent a psychophysiological as well as a conversion process, but their concurrence suggests an emotional basis. Separate diseases are unlikely.

6. Too many pain syndromes serially. A patient is not likely to have, by pure coincidence, a painful chronic disease in the right lower quadrant until the appendix and right ovary are removed, then in the midline until the uterus is removed, then in the left lower quadrant until the remaining ovary is removed, and finally in the right upper quadrant (? gall bladder disease). Better to check the surgical and path reports to be sure the pathology was sufficient to explain the symptoms.

7. Negative physical exam in relation to the symptom. A patient has full fluid range of back motion, or totally relaxed nontender pelvis while complaining bitterly of disabling backache or pelvic pain. To be reliable, this finding must be combined with other aspects of the illness, because patients with disease can have negative examinations, and a patient with psychogenic pelvic pain may double up on the table. A negative exam, however, in conjunction with other data, helps to establish the correct diagnosis.

8. Nerve block. This procedure relieves organic pain, but not somatoform pain distal to the block. Such a study must be carefully controlled by saline injections. In pain clinics, if the pain persists after the block, it is often classified as "central."

The Somatoform Disorder: Function and Process

The somatoform disorder must be understood as communication, and as a drama that can absorb both doctor and patient as unwitting actors. Though its symptoms are real enough, its conversion process rarely works well.

The SD as Communication

The conversion process can be understood as a form of acting, albeit at a precognitive, dissociated level of consciousness. The symptoms are a communication, as described so comprehensively by Szasz [12] and others. [13–14] The subject may be quite verbal, but words would be ineffective. Body language is eloquent, and forces the issue. It is unlikely, for example, that George thought through his predicament consciously, but even if he had, he could not say to his boss, "I hate it here and don't want to work so hard, but I need to be paid for a year until I find something else to do." Nor could he say to himself and his wife, "I can't face my impotence." Nevertheless, all these needs were filled as his sprained ankle slid over into a somatoform pain disorder.

A woman may not be fully aware how much she is disturbed by her husband, marriage, or sex, but even if she were, she would find it difficult to say, "Dear, you upset me, I need more attention, and I'm not going to have any more sex." But if she gets a "disease" (pelvic pain), her feelings are expressed, though very indirectly, she does get more attention, and sex is avoided. Her husband is sympathetic instead of angry. In your office the patient does not appear tense and denies any feelings of nervous tension. There is "no problem," she says. She describes her husband as concerned: "He knows how I suffer."

The clinician has a direct lead into the conversion process by viewing it as a communication. As soon as an SD is suspected, the fruitful questions to wonder about are: What are the patient's needs? What is the inner meaning of the message? Who receives it, and how? What situation forces the problem to take this form? Can the needs be filled in a better way? The message is often best decoded by interviewing the receiver as well as the sender, and observing them together.

Sometimes there is no specific recipient; the message serves a function for the patient alone.

Andrew T. was a 60-year-old, single accountant. He was in therapy for depression, with a psychiatrist who referred him for an intractable neck pain that disabled him for all activities except his daily job. He wore a neck collar continuously, and applied a self-rigged traction device every evening in his small apartment, where he lived alone.

The examination was completely negative. He had a full range of motion, no root signs or symptoms, and normal X-rays. A somatoform pain disorder seemed likely. But what function did it serve?

The social history disclosed that he grew up in a remote rural area, an only child, with no companions whatsoever. At school he was painfully shy and socially inept. I soon discovered that he had never made any real friends with anyone of either sex. I decided I had better back off from this brief interview that had revealed such a bleak personal situation. As I did so, I thought I noticed his eyes moisten. I asked what he was feeling, and he said, "Nothing, I don't feel anything," and then, parenthetically, "My tear ducts dried up—I never cry."

My interpretation: It was far better to live with the pain of a disabling disease than to face the enormity of a life of such intolerable loneliness. The symptom served as an excuse to himself and anyone else who might ask about his activities.

I discussed the problem with his psychiatrist, who planned to ease him, if at all possible, into a boardinghouse or some kind of group activity. I do not know the final outcome.

The symptoms, often with years of suffering, can also serve to atone for real or imagined guilt. [4] Though others must respond, the meaning of the illness is more a means of self-imposed expiation than a specific demand on others.

The Patient and the Doctor as Unwitting Actors in a Drama

In the conversion process, the patient does not consciously "decide" to have an illness, any more than you "decide" to be one kind of person with your patients and another with your superiors, your subordinates, your spouse, or your lover. The behavioral changes "happen" automatically. In the process of conversion there is no planning or willful malingering. If the process is described as "somatization," or "retreat into or resort to illness," it must be clearly understood that such phrases do not imply cognitive control. Otherwise, the terms can be inappropriately judgmental.

The acting process will seem less mysterious if we realize how universal it is. Even animals do it. The horse falters as it is directed away from its home stables, but gallops on the return trip. The grouse feigns a broken wing to distract an intruder while the chicks escape.

There is an actor in everyone. It begins as soon as an infant discovers that crying brings mother for tender loving care as well as for relief of hunger or other distress. At that early stage, distress due to activated pain receptors is embellished with distress due to emotional needs, with crying the communication for both. The emphasis readily shifts from the pain stimulus to the emotional. Crying, as the expression of pain or other distress, is a universal summons for help. Almost everyone recalls, from childhood, crying a little harder or having a little more stomachache, if need be. Later in life, when the crying component of the *pain or emotional needs* → *crying* → *response of others sequence* is blocked, it is not difficult to imagine how pain once again becomes the focus of the distressed person. As one extremely anguished patient put it to me, "I have pain." "Where is it?" "I can't say." "But if you have pain it must be someplace." "It's everyplace." "Do you mean to say that you're feeling very disturbed and that is the best way to describe it?" "No. I feel pain. *It is pain.* Pain is the only way to describe what I feel." The refocus on pain is especially understandable if the distressed person has suffered a previous organic pain experience for which some unexpected but much needed personal support was received.

The fascinating aspect of the conversion process is that parts are acted, a drama unfolds, a game is played, but none of the players is fully aware of the process, including the doctor, who can easily win the Oscar for best supporting role. It is easy to get drawn into the action surrounding the brave patient's "disease." The medical games that ensue are well described by Sternbach. [15] Every doctor who works with chronic pain syndromes should read this text.

To avoid this predicament, the physician must be constantly alert to the possibility of an SD. When conversion is suspected, the doctor must act accordingly, throughout the history, the physical exam, the workup, and subsequent discussions, as will be outlined further in Part III.

The Patient's Split Personality

Throughout the interaction it is important to keep in mind that the patient with an SD is dissociated. You believe that you are examining a sick patient with symptoms. The patient does not seem to know much about what might be going on at an emotional level. But this patient is actually an alternate personality, dissociated from the physically well but emotionally distressed real person, who does know. The "sick patient" is doing the talking, but the real person is watching the interaction silently and unobtrusively in the background. Both are present at the interview. The real person knows about the sick personality, but the latter is not aware of the former. The dissociation of consciousness that characterizes the conversion process is incomplete.

The fact that there are here both one who "knows" and one who "doesn't know" what is really going on was the major contribution of Szasz. [12] This is identical to the process, described by Hilgard in hypnosis, where the subject has a "hidden observer" who notices what is *really* being done at one level while the subject appears to feel or be something else at the hypnotized level.

[16] Thus we need not be intimidated by the unconscious. It is not always as unconscious as Freud suggested.

The doctor should represent the healthy but troubled person [17] who knows what is going on, as well as the patient who feels sick. The doctor is concerned, of course, that the patient who appears to be sick might really have a disease. But if you talk only to the sick patient, which is what doctors generally do, you may be talking to the wrong person for years (previous care of Ruth and George). Talking indirectly to the hidden, healthy, but troubled person may very well crack the conversion barrier, or elicit the source of a PPR in a patient with suppressed emotions, depending on the extent of the dissociation.

As you begin the interview, you are obviously talking with the "sick patient." Knowing, however, that the emotionally distressed person is listening, you guide your remarks accordingly. After all, you need to know the life setting of any important illness, whether organic or functional, how it affects the person and his/her relationships, etc. As you seek to understand this, the distressed person will notice your comprehensive approach. This person is quietly judging you—whether you are really listening, can be trusted to respond empathically to emotional disclosure and to approach the conversion process with compassion. And you will be tested by indirect clues that the distressed person slips into the interview (Ch. 14).

Meanwhile, you do not know the extent of the dissociation. The conversion, for example, may have already served its purpose, and the real person would like a face-saving way of discarding the sick personality. Or the conversion has failed to accomplish its purpose, and the real person would like to be free of the suffering, which, though identified with the sick-patient personality, affects them both. Or the emotionally distressed person feels an intense need to share the real problem in spite of its tentative solution by the illness. Perhaps there is a better way to resolve the problem?

In these situations, the distressed person may be groping for an opportunity to enter the interview. This can happen quietly in an interview with the first physician who listens receptively (Ruth), gradually over several interviews (George), suddenly and dramatically (Evelyn, Ch. 11), or in any number of other ways. One of my patients blurted out the truth as she was leaving the office after 20 years of care; she had been well aware of the underlying problem the whole time, but had been ashamed to talk about it. For many distressed persons, however, to lose an illness that has satisfactorily solved a major life problem can be truly threatening. The physician thus proceeds with restraint. Some illnesses will not yield to extended, caring, and competent psychiatric care. A modified medical and behavioral program is the most that can be done.

Since becoming aware of the value of including both participants in the split personality of the interview, I have encountered four patients with somatoform (hysterical) coma. This can be suspected immediately in any unconscious patient looking otherwise well with a normal airway in the supine position. I quickly confirm the diagnosis by the normal vital signs and a brief physical exam, but I let it be known by my general demeanor that I am not reacting as a doctor to a medical emergency. I sit quietly, holding the patient's hand, doing nothing for a few minutes. Finally, ignoring the coma, I say quite definitively, "You have been unconscious long enough, wake up! The time has come to wake up!" Each of the four soon sat up. Such "coma" may, of course, represent a withdrawal from a disturbing situation that has since passed. In any event, the switching off of the symptom confirmed the diagnosis at the outset. The second advantage: with the person awake, but now aware that the coma had had something to do with the prevailing situation, I was able to elicit the basic problem then and there. The theory is essential to the practice.

Another patient with an anxiety state suddenly stiffened and shook, eyes rolled back, with what I took to be a pseudoseizure while I was taking the medical history. Having read Hilgard, I assumed that the fit was equivalent to a hypnotic trance. I have no experience with hypnosis, but I quickly decided to respond accordingly. First, I did nothing for two minutes. Then I said to her that I would shortly give a signal, at which moment the convulsion would stop, she would open her eyes, look at me, and tell me what was really wrong. This she did: "It's my job. I hate my job!" she exclaimed.

There is an important corollary here: don't teach the patient how to simulate disease! The somatoform disorder is primitive at first, but it is quickly assimilated into the medical model by the questions asked and the doctor's diagnostic and therapeutic responses. This is most poignantly true when the doctor responds to psychogenic pain with the first codeine prescription or pelvic operation.

Pain is obviously the most effective somatoform disorder. It is purely subjective. No one can deny the patient's experience. It is disturbing to see another person suffer. Pain is the quintessence of suffering. Other people must respond. The physician's basic drive is to relieve suffering, and s/he can't be sure about the conversion process. Even when conversion is suspected, physicians may be unwilling to "stick their necks out" and deal with it psychologically or behaviorally. This they defer to pain clinics or psychiatrists if it really becomes necessary. Thus physicians, doing their very best to help, may unwittingly complete the conversion process by their responses. It is far better, and much easier in the long run, to turn off the process as close to the beginning of the encounter as possible. Early diagnosis is essential, preferably as the "present illness" is elicited, so that the remainder of the medical history can be modified accordingly (Ch. 14).

Are Somatoform Symptoms Real?

If Ruth's pain disappeared when her marriage improved, George's pain disappeared when the litigation was settled, and the comatose patient wakes up on command, was the symptom *real*? Yes, as experienced by the patient's conscious cognitive mind, the symptom is very real indeed. Ruth and George appeared to suffer, just as did the patient who could describe her anguish only as pain. A comatose patient does not respond to painful stimuli, lumbar puncture, bladder catheters, or IV fluids. These procedures, nonetheless, were performed repeatedly for one week in a city hospital on one of the four somatoform coma patients mentioned above, during a previous episode of the patient's somatoform (hysterical) coma.

In patients with psychogenic pain, intense dissociated emotions are converted into the experience of pain. Pain is an *affective* experience, as well as a sensation caused by activated pain receptors, and the patient's experience is what is real. Organic pain is experienced at or near the site of disease or injury. It is never disembodied. Likewise, the subjective experience of somatoform pain disorder is usually referred to the body just where the patient says it is, though the distribution may be peculiar. The patient's or the doctor's *interpretation* of the pain as a sensation caused by peripheral disease may be unreal, but the *experience itself* is real. When we consider a pain to be "real," meaning only that it is caused by organic disease, we fail to distinguish between the interpretation and the experience. The patient's suffering may be intense, often more than would be experienced from disease, because there is no limit to this kind of pain. As Fordyce suggests, it is just as real as the saliva in Pavlov's dogs when the bell rings. [18] Pain is always real unless the patient is knowingly lying, but conscious malingering is rarely a component of the somatoform disorder.

The Conversion Process Rarely Works Well

On the few occasions when an SD really does succeed in converting a personal problem into an acceptable illness, one that "works" in a way that deals with the patient's stressful situation, the patient may gain weight, radiate health, look perfectly OK, and be relaxed on physical exam, while at the same time describing the pain in lurid detail. Such patients are the exception, not the rule. Of the 75 patients in the Stanford survey, "la belle indifférence" was noted in only five (two of them men). Though the symptoms may be charged with the driving emotion, SDs are rarely associated with histrionic personalities, contrary to a prevailing misconception. Most patients are miserable. Their personalities can vary, however, from dull to imaginative, from seductive to anything but. Usually, the message is received with mixed feelings by an ambivalent spouse, or a message—like Andrew's neck pain, disguising loneliness—is sent out to a world that doesn't respond at all, except for the doctors who can be asked to help. The "conversion" may accomplish nothing more than to be a face-saving device that shifts the responsibility for dealing with a difficult situation from self to the "disease." The patient's psychic pain has only been partially displaced by physical pain, with all the anguish of the basic emotion but without really resolving it. The patient suffers physically *and* emotionally.

The Conversion Process Is Often Monosymptomatic

In most SDs, one symptom, usually pain, dominates. Other background symptoms may be found if you ask. In the 75 patients, we found:

One dominant symptom, or one at a time	43
One dominant symptom, with a few minor symptoms	13
Multiple symptoms, all prominent	19

These data are contrary to the findings of previous reports of patients referred to psychiatrists, in which the diagnosis of "hysteria" was restricted to the multisymptomatic syndrome now known as somatization disorder. [19–21] This syndrome, characterized by many persistent symptoms in many systems in the absence of organic disease, is said to occur only in women, appears prior to age 30, and is associated with other psychiatric, social, sexual, menstrual, and personality disorders. Of the 19 patients with multiple symptoms in the Stanford survey, only nine (two of them men) fit the DSM definition. Even in this syndrome, pain is the dominant symptom, as indicated by the common history of many operations, usually performed to relieve pain (17 was the record in our series). The surgeon is either unfamiliar with the diagnosis, does not notice the other symptoms, or fails to question the wisdom of the previous operations. In spite of the multiple symptoms, the correct diagnosis is not always made.

The data cited here show clearly that the diagnosis of SD should not be restricted to the less common, more flagrant, multisymptomatic disorders. Many conversions are essentially monosymptomatic pain disorders in stable-appearing individuals. This combination can lead an unwary physician away from the current diagnosis far more readily than do the multisymptomatic disorders in obviously nervous patients.

How Emotionally Induced Symptoms Are Described by Patients

I can recall only a few patients who began a visit by saying something like this: "I've been under a lot of stress lately, and probably that's the cause of my headaches [or any other symptom]. But I thought I had better have it checked out to be sure there is nothing else wrong." To the contrary, most patients who consult doctors do so because they have failed to connect the stress with the symptom, and they provide no immediate clue about the source.

An emotionally induced symptom, however, whether physiologic or somatoform, may provide its own clue. Because it represents an emotional conflict, it often has a characteristic intensity. The patient is distressed by both the illness *and* the underlying situation. The patient may appear to be unusually concerned, demanding, frustrated. Something more than factual information is imparted to the account.

As we have seen, the patient with a somatoform disorder is both a participant in the formation of the symptom and an observer thereof, albeit at different levels of consciousness, and the dissociation is incomplete. Therefore, a certain confusion is inherent. The patient cannot be objective, and describes the symptoms with great difficulty. [22] Both the intensity and the patient's quandary may be quite unlike the usually objective descriptions of the symptoms of organic disease.

The same may be true of psychophysiologic symptoms, but that is less likely. The patient's account of a periodic physiologic reaction to stress—headache or dyspepsia, for example, especially if its meaning is known to the patient—can be quite objective. Even when physiologic symptoms are more strongly charged emotionally, the patient is an observer of the symptom, not an actor; that is, s/he is in no way a participant, unconsciously or otherwise, in the "choice" of symptom, and gains little or nothing from being sick. Thus physiologic symptoms are usually described more accurately than are somatoform symptoms.

For the same reasons, it is generally easier to talk with PPR patients about their underlying problems. They may not be prepared to change in any way, and cannot believe that obvious stresses have much to do with the illness, but they are less defensive. They are more likely to understand and accept the doctor's comprehensive approach than patients with SD, who are fearful at one level of losing the disease.

The patient's difficulty in symptom description is particularly characteristic of somatoform pain disorder. The patient cannot describe the characteristics of pain that every doctor learns to ask about in physical diagnosis. Constancy is the hallmark of somatoform pain, but even this is difficult to elicit unless you ask certain questions, "How often do you have the pain?" "A lot." "I mean do you have it most of the time, some of the time, or once in a while?" "That's hard to say." "Is it there when you first wake up?" "Usually." "If you wake up during the night is it there?" "I guess it is." "Can you recall times when it was gone altogether?" "No, I guess I can't." Careful questioning, for example, may reveal that pain which appeared to be premenstrual is really continuous all through the month.

Somatoform pain may be described simply as pain, sometimes as "throbbing," "burning," "fullness," "aching," "shooting." It can be described in extravagant metaphor, simile, or other unusual terms. Compare this with Richard's crisp description of sciatic pain.

In seven of the 75 illnesses classed as somatoform, the symptoms were bizarre enough to be viewed as somatic delusions. Such a complaint would be "coated, hairy tongue," "my head and neck so swollen I can't stand it," or "insects crawling in my skin." Somatic delusions often occur without other evidence of psychosis. [23]

A checklist to detect that an illness is probably psychophysiologic or somatoform, and not caused by organic disease, might be as follows:

1. *Are the symptoms described with the usual objectivity of an undisturbed patient with the disease suspected?* The patient with angina pectoris, for example, usually provides a concise and consistent description of the pain—when it first appeared, how often, what brings it on, how it is quickly relieved by standing still. Every episode of pain is about the same. The patient often belittles the symptoms (a "little gas"), and does not appear to be unduly disabled.

Recall that Evelyn's chest pain was quite severe, often present, but she could not say when. There was no clear correlation with exercise, etc., and its onset was obscure. The pain waxed and waned, varied from localized to diffuse, and spread to different areas. It was disabling, more or less, though she did what she could with homemaking activities. The pain clearly dominated her attention far more than would the usual angina.

There are exceptions, of course. In general, however, the way the symptom is described is a distinct clue to the correct diagnosis.

2. *How much relief is expected?* Patients with angina, rheumatoid arthritis, peptic ulcer, a herniated lumbar disk syndrome, and many other chronic painful organic diseases rarely request narcotics. In contrast, many patients with psychosomatic pain disorders are habituated to codeine or related drugs. The demand for relief may be diagnostic. Before prescribing narcotics, which may now be, or can soon become, a problem of drug dependency and thereby another barrier to getting well, consider the question: *Is the need for narcotics about that of the average undisturbed patient with the organic disease suspected?* If more than this, could the patient have, instead of a "low pain threshold" or "functional overlay" to disease, an emotionally induced symptom with little or no disease at all?

3. *Is the course of the illness that of an average undisturbed patient with the organic disease suspected?* Patients with ankle sprains are usually well in a few

weeks. George was not. The doctor legitimately asks: What was unusual about this sprain? But the more important question is: What is it about this person that results in disability?

All doctors are familiar with this problem. Because of our focus on treatment, however, an inappropriate disability can be overlooked, as I have done many times, until it has become entrenched much too long. Visit after visit, the patient describes the symptoms, not the disability. We believe we are treating a disease or an injury, not a troubled person. Unless we ask about the patient's work and other activities, or are presented with a disability form, we fail to recognize this important clue to emotional factors in the illness.

4. Can all of the patient's symptoms be explained by the organic disease proposed as the cause of the illness? Recall that Ruth, though focused on her pelvic pain, also looked and felt nervous, and complained of headaches. At one time, she could not move her legs, a typical conversion disorder. Her physicians, also focused on the pelvic pain, failed to connect the other symptoms with the illness. Many patients are referred for medical consultation in which the established or suspected organic diagnosis, even if valid, could not in any way explain *all* the symptoms. When this happens, it often turns out that the diagnosis is inappropriate for the one symptom that has attracted the most attention.

Any kind of functional syndrome can involve but one or a very few physical symptoms, and an SD particularly will occasionally displace the underlying dysphoria so completely that no nervous tension is apparent. Usually, however, there are other expressions of emotional and physical distress. In one series of 134 consecutive patients with somatoform disorders, the physical symptom was associated with an anxious or depressive affect (30 percent), incipient schizophrenic disorganization (14 percent), or fairly obvious ego-identity problems in many of the adolescent patients. [8] There are, of course, any number of interrelationships between an underlying personal problem and its affective, cognitive, and physical manifestations.

In the more chronically disturbed patients, the physical symptoms tend to be multiple, severe, persistent, disabling, and resistant to treatment. They are often associated, past or present, with smoking, or with excessive use of coffee, alcohol, or psychoactive drugs. Disturbances of sleep, appetite, weight, sex, and energy levels are common. In the medical history are found an unusual array of illnesses, doctors, diagnoses, clinics, prescriptions, and operations.

The medical history often indicates the doctor's dilemma. In spite of overwhelming evidence to the contrary, each episode of illness in the past history is recorded as an independent medical event, and so is the present illness.

To make a definitive clinical judgment, *all* the symptoms, both physical and emotional, past and present, must be carefully elicited, explained, and integrated.

Any one of these four checkpoints can alert us to the likelihood that emotional factors are significant. There are exceptions, of course, but, taken together with all the other data, these considerations can often lead directly to a unified view of the illness.

The Spectrum of Patients with Emotionally Induced Physical Symptoms

Doctors often refer patients to me with the comment: "He is the salt of the earth (or she is such a wonderful person)—there must be something really wrong!" Nevertheless, it is often the "good guys" who get the symptoms, for the very reason that they do indeed "do the right thing" and keep their emotions in check. So there is a wide spectrum of patients, from those who are quite stable but suffer a depression late in life, or have symptoms only under extreme duress, to those who grew up with impaired self-esteem and suffer chronic nervous tension with multiple symptoms most of the time.

Mario L., 51, complained of continuous epigastric pain for three months, the only symptom. Nothing about him suggested either nervous tension or serious disease. The medical history was completely negative, with the sole exception of a single illness 25 years previously in which he was paralyzed from the waist down for three months. He did not know what diagnosis had been made, but he slowly recovered on his own after discharge from the hospital. I suspected the current pain problem to be a somatoform pain disorder, as I do whenever pain is continuous, though cancer of the pancreas could cause a similar pain. The "paralysis" was a possible clue. So was his unwillingness to discuss in any way his life situation, which is unusual, in my experience, because most patients, disturbed or not, appreciate your interest. So there was no way to know what the situation might be.

The present exam and limited workup, including a GI series, was negative. I sent for the old records. At the time of the paralysis, the reflexes were normal, as was the lumbar puncture and all other studies. The discharge diagnosis was transverse myelitis, though there were no supporting data. After discharge, there appeared in the chart a mound of correspondence about disability due to an alleged injury that had never been mentioned during the hospitalization. Still, no one had tumbled to the obvious diagnosis of a conversion disorder.

Combining these data with the present illness, I concluded that a somatoform pain disorder seemed even more likely, but a psychological approach, which I prefer, was out of the question. So I advised him that I was sure he had nothing more than a kind of "spasm," perhaps due to some kind of stress, though I knew not what and suggested it would improve with an antispasmodic. The pain disappeared that night and was still absent on followup three months later.

Note that this stalwart-appearing male patient on the well end of a wellness/sickness spectrum was ill but twice in his life, each time with a straightforward SD. In each illness the symptom alone was enough to suggest the correct diagnosis, but only if one had considered the possibility.

Somatoform symptoms, like psychophysiologic reactions, vary considerably in frequency and severity. They may recur in the same or another form but only during periods of stress, or the same illness may disable the patient constantly for years. Sometimes the patient is regarded by the family as chronically ill but commendably brave and stoical as she/he carries on with most activities without complaining, in spite of the suffering. In times of stress, however, the symptoms break through, and the patient needs special attention. Such a patient "wins the game" both ways.

Is it important to distinguish the two kinds of emotionally induced physical symptoms? Yes and no. It can be very helpful. It may be next to impossible to diagnose or heal an SD without recognizing the actors or the function the SD serves for the patient. On the other hand, it is not always possible to distinguish the two kinds of reactions, especially when the conversion process is superimposed on a psychophysiologic reaction. In any case, to be well the patient must deal with the underlying emotional problem. The mechanism of symptom formation may not be important, as long as the disorder is recognized as psychogenic and the source of distress is identified.

Janet's pelvic pain, for example, was mainly somatoform, for many reasons, but at times it could have been due in part to the bowel spasm of irritable-bowel syndrome, the dysmenorrhea of adenomyosis, or, on one occasion, the rupture of a corpus luteum. As in many chronic pain disorders, the precise mechanism of pain cannot be established with certainty, but this need not be the sole focus of medical attention. When significant disease has been ruled out, it is most effective to explore the illness not as a discrete entity but as a problem caused by several factors, some physical, some psychosocial, all of which have to be worked through in the plan for healing. The same can be said for chronic backache, persistent abdominal pain, recurrent headache, the syndrome of chronic fatigue and weakness, and many others.

Functional disorders are generally distinctive, and rarely simulate disease. A positive primary diagnosis can be made early in the encounter if everything about the patient—all the symptoms and how they are described—is noted and collated. The database is often present in abundance. Diagnostic errors are rare if all possibilities are considered, the necessary workup completed, the findings reviewed with discretion, and the patient followed carefully. A not-uncommon error in practice is to explain illness as disease, when it is not, from a biased database in which the evidence for a psychogenic illness has been unwittingly but systematically excluded.

Functional Syndromes: Differential Diagnosis

Several common chronic or recurrent symptom complexes may be misconstrued as organic disease entities when they are actually functional syndromes. Their differential diagnosis is considered in the ten sections of this chapter.

❧ Knowing that jaundice is either hemolytic, hepatic, or obstructive, our first goal is to identify the correct category. Similarly, knowing that the three most common types of recurrent anterior chest pain are anginal, esophageal, or psychogenic, the first step again is to identify the correct category. If we are familiar with the relative frequency and distinguishing characteristics of each type of pain, we can move directly toward a positive diagnosis, beginning with the "chief complaint."

Clearly, we need to be aware of the many ways that functional syndromes can resemble, yet be distinguished from, disease. Unfortunately, however, in conventional texts of differential diagnosis, the functional syndrome is sometimes omitted altogether, though it may be the most frequent cause of the symptom, as with long-term persistent pelvic pain (Chs. 1, 6). Or it may be appended at the end of the differential, as though an afterthought, with no mention of its frequency or distinguishing features, such as psychogenic chest pain.

A discussion of every symptom complex that can pose such diagnostic dilemmas is beyond the scope of this book. I have focused instead on ten common chronic or recurrent problems that can be particularly enigmatic. Here the physician needs to be particularly alert to the likelihood of a personal source for the illness, and to anticipate (not obviate) a negative or misleading workup. Otherwise, the workup may well lead into nonresolution, or an erroneous diagnosis.

Every symptom begins sometime, of course, but the differential diagnosis of symptoms of recent onset, such as headache, or acute or subacute pelvic or chest pain, in which the first and predominant concern is organic disease, is quite different from that of chronic, persistent or recurrent, syndromes. Only the latter are discussed here.

Diagnosis is often straightforward, but distinguishing functional disorders from systemic disease can indeed constitute a diagnostic problem. If so, in addition to the history and physical exam, the basic workup (though it is difficult to provide a general guideline for screening) may appropriately include a complete blood count with differential smear, urinalysis, blood-chemistry screening panel, sedimentation rate, thyroid function tests, and chest X-ray (or tuberculin test in young patients). Most other studies are ordered more specifically to detect or exclude the disease in question. Whether the illness is functional or disease-induced, resolution is critical, and the workup, positive or negative, is often important. The process can go astray, however—and here I reiterate—if the physician fails to consider the possibility of a functional disorder from the very beginning.

Psychogenic Chest Pain

The three most common causes of recurrent anterior chest pain are, again, coronary artery disease, esophageal dysfunction, and emotional distress. The "atypical" chest pain of anxiety, to be described in this section, is the most characteristic form of psychogenic chest pain, but emotional distress can also constitute the basis of certain esophageal-motility disorders and microvascular angina.

Some physicians recognize psychogenic chest pain readily.[1] Others do not, and simply classify such pain as of "unknown" etiology. The whole problem is thereby bypassed. In one study, from an ambulatory-care clinic for internal medicine, the etiology of chest pain as the main complaint was regarded as organic disease in 11 percent, psychologic in 6 percent, and *unknown* in 83 percent.[2] Obviously, only the patients who were clearly nervous or hyperventilating were diagnosed as "psychologic." In another study, from an adult "drop-in" clinic, which included many more acute cases, the etiology was attributed to ischemic heart disease in 11 percent, possibly 17 percent; other disease, mostly acute respiratory infections, in 24 percent; chest-wall pain in 17 percent; *unknown* in 42 percent.[3] Some of the "unknowns" may have been esophageal disorders, unrecognized because of the absence of heartburn or other associated symptoms. It will be seen, however, from the data reviewed here, that many of the "unknowns" in both studies actually had emotionally induced "atypical" pain.

The "unknown" category, and what it might represent, is strangely omitted from the conventional textbook differential diagnosis of episodic chest pain. Instead, it includes many rare (biliary tract disease, cervical disk) and dubious (mitral prolapse) causes, whereas psychogenic chest pain other than "hyperventilation" is disregarded altogether.[4] This typifies the view of many physicians. The ubiquity of psychogenic chest pain is not appreciated unless the clinician is open to the diagnosis and familiar with the problem. In one study of 430 patients considered to have psychogenic regional pain, pain in the chest and arm was second only to pain in the head and neck as the most common site.[5] Psychogenic chest pain is most often unrecognized when it is the sole symptom of distress, as it was with Irene F. (Ch. 11), who had no obvious hyperventilation, anxiety, or depression.

Actually, psychogenic chest pain is a common condition. This should not be surprising. The chest is central to the emotional expression of both crying and laughter. Most people experience "tightness" in the chest during anger or fear. Many other basic observations may prove convincing to physicians who are reluctant to recognize psychogenic chest pain as a clinical reality.

Clearly, chest pain is an integral component of the common symptom cluster of anxiety: three of four anxious patients have chest pain.[6, 7] Of those in whom the diagnostic focus is hyperventilation syndrome, half or more have chest pain.[8, 9] When chest pain predominates, as it often does, and the nervous tension is not recognized, patients are often referred for treadmill EKGs or coronary arteriograms. As would be expected from the data just cited, the referred patients with normal tests have far more anxiety, panic attacks, depression, and/or psychosocial difficulties than those with frank disease, if systematically investigated. [10–17]

The failure to recognize psychogenic chest pain obviously precludes an investigation of its personal source. If the diagnosis is anxiety, panic disorder, or hyperventilation syndrome, but the management is strictly biomedical, the emotional basis is again bypassed. All this is indeed unfortunate, for if the specific underlying disturbing personal situation is not recognized, and the patient can find no way to make the necessary changes, as with Evelyn C. (Ch. 1), healing is not likely to occur.

Many chest pains, of course, are transient and minor, and the visit is prompted only by the patient's concern that the pain might indicate serious disease. Five percent of 1,410 adults (not patients) in a British neighborhood survey had noted chest pain during the brief period of two weeks before the interview.[14] Ten percent of the healthy population used as controls in another study reported episodes of chest pain.[7] Such pains can be caused, for example, by pectoral-muscle strain, as in driving a car many hours under trying conditions, or by the brief emotional tension of giving a speech. But persistent, distinctly disturbing pain, if it fits the ensuing description of psychogenic pain, is most likely indicative of major emotional distress.

We will focus here on the differential diagnosis of the three common types of persistent chest pain. Not discussed are problems of acute chest pain, chronic disease of the lungs and pleura, pulmonary hypertension, or other types of heart disease such as cardiomyopathy. Most of these chronic diseases can be ruled out by history, physical exam, chest X-ray, and EKG. In regard to the occasional unusual causes of chronic chest pain, the reader is referred to a more detailed analysis.[15]

First, Is the Pain Anginal or Psychogenic?

The "typical" anginal pain of coronary disease can usually be distinguished from the characteristically "atypical" pain of anxiety, designated here as psychogenic chest pain. Esophageal motility disorders and/or microvascular angina, as components of the emotional response, will be discussed later.

Chronic, stable angina pectoris is a transient, predictable, pressure-like feeling, mild to moderately severe, in a clearly demarcated central area, more often substernal than precordial, with repetitive radiation to specific areas. It is induced primarily by exertion, and disappears completely in a few minutes by standing still. It appears more readily after meals or when cold. It is rarely associated with shortness of breath, palpitation, fatigue, nervous tension, or other symptoms. The patient provides an objective description of the pain, including its onset and course. The chest is not tender. The physician feels secure about the evaluation.

In contrast, psychogenic pain:

· is persistent but unpredictable.
· often varies in quality (pressure-like but also sharp, shooting, jabbing, sore, aching, gnawing, twisting, burning, or of mixed character).
· varies in duration from a few seconds to hours or days, often at rest.
· bears no constant relation to exertion. With exercise the pain may appear soon, late, afterwards, or not at all; if it occurs, it rarely compels cessation of effort, and it may disappear as the exercise continues.
· varies in location, distribution (small areas or widespread), and radiation.
· is more often precordial than substernal, and the chest is commonly tender.
· is often severe, though varying in intensity.
· is less likely to be relieved by nitroglycerin. This has no value as a diagnostic test, however, because one-half of all patients with chest pain and normal coronary arteriograms report relief, [16–19] and nitroglycerin can relieve the pain of esophageal spasm, or microvascular angina.

· is often associated with shortness of breath, palpitation, fatigue, or other psy-chosomatic and emotional symptoms.
· compared to angina, the pain is more likely to be disabling, to dominate the patient's attention, and not to improve on treatment.

Patients with psychogenic pain, unlike patients with angina:

· often appear tense, have a history of other nervous disorders, and are more likely to request analgesics or tranquilizers.
· have difficulty describing the symptoms, their duration, and their onset. The descriptions seem anecdotal, tangential, evasive. The physician feels strangely insecure about the diagnosis and describes the pain as "atypical."

Second, Regardless of the Kind of Pain, Does the Patient Have Coronary Artery Disease?

Cardiologists classify chest pain as *definite angina*, *probable angina* (if the pain has most of the features of definite angina but is atypical in some respects), or *nonischemic* (such as the psychogenic pain described above). Within these three groups, the percent of patients with coronary artery disease, defined as the presence of >70 percent luminal narrowing of at least one coronary vessel on coronary arteriography, was found to be as follows:[20]

Diagnosis	Sex	Number
Definite angina pectoris	male	89
	female	62
Probable angina pectoris	male	70
	female	40
Nonischemic pain	male	22
	female	5

Thus the description of pain is a general guide to the presence or absence of coronary disease, but some patients with typical angina do not have the disease on arteriography, and some patients with "nonischemic" pain do have disease. A borderline abnormal resting EKG or exercise test (1 mm. ST depression) adds little to the diagnostic accuracy in patients with definite angina; in the other two categories, false positive tests abound.

The diagnostic problem is complicated further by pain at rest, which oc-curs in unstable angina and can be induced by coronary artery spasm. Large-vessel spasm is the principal cause of variant or Prinzmetal's angina (often nocturnal) and can be a factor in the pain of patients with occlusive disease. In these conditions, however, the pain, though usually more intense and prolonged, is similar in quality and location to that of classic effort-induced angina. How can these problems be resolved?

Nonischemic ("nonangina") chest pain. A negative exercise EKG generally suffices to confirm the absence of coronary disease.[21] If the exercise EKG is positive, then other studies are necessary. Further evidence that recurrent chest pain is not caused by coronary disease or spasm is provided by ambulatory electrocardiographic monitoring that shows no abnormalities when pain is present. If these tests are inconclusive, a negative thallium perfusion scan serves to rule out coronary disease. If positive, a coronary arteriogram is indicated.

Probable (but not definite) angina. A negative exercise EKG is insufficient to rule out ischemic disease. Negative ambulatory electrocardiographic monitoring that coincides with pain episodes may settle the question. If not, the negative exercise EKG combined with a negative thallium perfusion scan reduces the likelihood of coronary disease to less than 5 percent.[21] In regard to the remaining possibility of ischemic disease in the 5 percent with negative noninvasive tests, or in patients with *nonischemic pain* who have a positive exercise test and a negative thallium scan, one must first review every detail of the clinical data, the age and sex of the patient, the risk factors, the probability of alternative diagnoses, and the degree of positivity of the tests before proceeding to invasive tests. Depending on the circumstances, the cardiologist may recommend coronary arteriography with or without ergonovine to induce coronary artery spasm, or other special tests, to establish or rule out coronary disease. Arteriography is of course customary in patients with "definite" angina.

These studies will serve to rule out coronary disease in most patients with nonischemic pain, many patients with "probable" angina, and some patients with "definite angina." Be cautious, however, about the diagnosis of coronary disease in women: in the study cited above only 5 percent of those with nonischemic pain, and 46 percent with definite and probable angina, actually had the disease.[20] Summarizing the literature, Diamond and Forrester provide an elegant analysis of the probability of coronary disease in relation to type of pain, age, sex, risk factors, and noninvasive tests.[22] The probability, for example, varies from 1 percent in women, age 30–39, with nonanginal pain to 94 percent in men, age 60–69, with typical angina.

Third, If Not Coronary Disease, What Does Cause Persistent, Recurrent Chest Pain?

This question has been studied intensively, both biologically and psychiatrically, in patients who had been referred for arteriograms that were then found to be negative. Referrals are made for atypical as well as anginal pain. Thus the observations summarized here include both types of patients:

Psychogenic pain. At one time the problem of chest pain with negative arteriograms was classified simply as "anginal syndrome with normal coronary arteriography," an "important clinical entity . . . the cause . . . unknown."[23] This concept was indeed misleading. Even those who coined the term reported that 56 percent of these patients had "pain not predominantly related to exertion," and 80 percent had pain at rest.[18] Others have defined the pain more precisely as nonischemic in three-fourths of such patients.[9, 17, 24, 25] Finally, the striking prevalence of psychiatric disorders in patients with negative arteriograms,[9, 24–27] especially with atypical chest pain,[28, 29] is now well established. Thus the pain in most patients with negative arteriograms is not typically anginal, nor is the cause unknown. Many patients with the "syndrome" have psychogenic chest pain, as previously described.

Esophageal pain. Most characteristic is the "heartburn" of acid reflux, which is felt centrally from the upper epigastrium to the mid- or high-substernal region. It can be induced by meals, especially when followed by recumbency, bending, or stooping over, and it is usually relieved by antacids. It is often associated with sour eructations, regurgitation, or dysphagia. A symptom complex of this type points directly to the esophagus and would rarely be confused with "angina," nor would such patients be referred for arteriograms.

Esophageal pain can, however, resemble the centrally located "pressure" of angina, even with the same sites of radiation, and it can occur in the absence of other esophageal symptoms. About half of the patients with chest pain and negative arteriograms are found to have some type of esophageal dysfunction, either a motility disturbance or a problem of acid reflux, or both, if studied with manometry, 24-hour pH monitoring of the distal esophagus, acid infusion, and other provocative tests.[30–35] Perhaps most of these patients would be those with angina-like pain rather than the atypical pain most characteristic of emotional disturbance, but the kind of pain is not described in most studies.

Whereas acid reflux is a mechanical problem of an incompetent lower-esophageal sphincter, many esophageal motility disorders, especially the nutcracker type and allied dysfunctions, are commonly associated with emotional distress or can be provoked thereby.[35–37] This accounts for a considerable overlap in the esophageal and psychiatric analyses of chest-pain patients with normal arteriograms.

We see, then, that the somatic expressions of emotional distress can appear either as the angina-like pain of an esophageal contractile disorder or as the variable, diffuse, more characteristic pain of anxiety, or both. The clinical picture will vary according to the patient's proclivity for either type of stress reaction.

If coronary disease has been excluded and the patient's pain is typically "atypical," especially if there are other observations indicative of a nervous state, I believe the clinician should seek directly to determine the nature of the stress or emotional disturbance. If, however, the pain is central, always more or less the same, and something like angina, esophageal dysfunction would be the next consideration, particularly acid reflux, which is fairly common. In studies of pain sufficiently anginal to merit arteriography, which however proved to be negative, the same pain appeared during acid-infusion tests in 7 to 20 percent of the patients,[30] or during actual acid reflux detected by 24-hour pH monitoring in about 25 percent.[31] Special testing, however, may not be necessary. First, the history should be reviewed for any collateral esophageal symptoms or factors that could either reduce esophageal sphincter competence or cause gastric hyperacidity and distention. These would include eating too much too fast (especially fats), alcohol, smoking, coffee, restlessness, and nervous tension. Reflux, if that is the problem, may well respond to amelioration of these elements plus a therapeutic trial of H_2 antagonists or omeprazole and the other aspects of anti-reflux therapy. If there is no response, a GI series and referral to a gastroenterologist for special testing should be considered; reflux, with or without esophagitis, may be identified even though the therapeutic trial was negative. If, on the other hand, the pain is identified as a functional esophageal motility disorder, this may well have an emotional basis [35–37] that should then be explored if not considered previously. Attending to the source of distress may well be effective, whereas the available biotherapies for motility disorders are of limited value.

Microvascular angina (MVA): Impaired vasodilator response of the coronary microcirculation. Several investigators have demonstrated that abnormal lactate production indicative of myocardial ischemia can be induced by the unusual stress of atrial pacing in many chest-pain patients with normal arteriograms.[38] The usual pain of these patients is described by different observers as typical angina,[39] like angina but atypical in some respects,[40] or both.[41] Studies of coronary blood flow and vascular resistance in response to pacing, often with superimposed vasoactive drugs, show the physiological mechanism to be a persistent vasoconstriction of the coronary microcirculation (impaired vasodilator response) to increased demand.[38, 39, 42] This is not due to small-vessel disease.[39, 43, 44] Left ventricular dysfunction can often be demonstrated by radionuclide studies,[45] but the life expectancy of these patients is thought to be normal.

The appearance of the patient's usual pain during the study correlates statistically with the impaired response, but some patients develop pain during a normal study, and others have an impaired response but no pain.[38, 40] Thus, it is not clear how well the ischemia induced by pacing correlates with the patient's discomfort during the far less demanding stresses of daily life.

Similar studies have not been performed in patients who have not had coronary arteriograms. Thus the prevalence of the impaired response in random subjects with or without chest pain is not known. It might well be found in anxiety states, though chest pain is not the dominant symptom, as suggested by the following data.

First of all, the impaired response can be induced in from one-third to three-fourths of the chest-pain patients with normal arteriograms, [38, 41, 46] indicating here too, if only by the numbers, a substantial overlap with the esophageal and psychiatric disorders noted in other analyses of such patients. Patients with MVA do indeed also have esophageal motility disorders.[47, 48] Most telling is the remarkable prevalence of anxiety (73 percent) or a history of major depression (53 percent) in MVA when specifically investigated.[49] This is particularly striking because the patients so studied have chest pain predominantly; patients whose pain is more clearly psychogenic are not usually referred for invasive studies in the first place. And many MVA subjects are also found to have a similar vasoconstriction in the peripheral circulation,[50] or the same kinds of airway responses [51] noted in hyperventilation syndrome.[52] Clearly, the constriction of the cardiac microcirculation is but one aspect of a generalized systemic response.

The data, in accord with the many psychological studies of chest-pain patients cited previously, suggest strongly that MVA is a psychophysiologic phenomenon, a functional disorder. Like other functional syndromes, it may be induced by other factors, but emotional distress appears to predominate. In any event, the response as elucidated to date, or its recognition in individual patients, does not in any way preclude an emotional source.

Psychogenic Chest Pain and the Chest-Wall Syndrome

The major biologic expressions of anxiety fall into four categories: hyperventilation syndrome, adrenergic discharge, GI reactivity, and muscle tension generally. Microvascular angina perhaps fits the second category; esophageal contractility, the third. One or the other, or both, may account for the angina-like components of the pain. The more diffuse and variable aspects of psychogenic pain perhaps fit best the fourth type of psychophysiologic reaction: intercostal muscle tension is suggested by chest-wall tenderness, just as local tenderness characterizes fibromyalgia and other muscle-tension syndromes throughout the body.

Is there also an idiopathic "chest-wall syndrome" unrelated to nervous tension, trauma, or coronary artery disease, as so often described?[53, 54] Sometimes this is called costochondritis or Tietze's syndrome. Costochondritis is indeed a dubious entity (Ch. 6). "Tietze's," as defined, is restricted to costochondral swellings, [55, 56] which are rare. The diagnosis of chest-wall syndrome, if based on eliciting tenderness at the costochondral junctions or other areas of the chest wall, is clearly untenable, because the same tenderness is often found in psychogenic chest pain. Furthermore, patients with "chest-wall syndrome" are often described as depressed or anxious; emotional stress brings on the attacks; hyperventilation is common.[57] It is not likely that the pain is the cause of the anxiety; the anxiety is the cause of the pain. Patients can certainly have localized pain and tenderness due to unrecognized chest contusion or muscular strain. But if the pain is more diffuse, distinctly persistent and disturbing, I believe the "syndrome" is more likely to be psychogenic than "idiopathic."

Chronic Chest Pain: An Overview

A meticulous history is essential, looking just as carefully for the salient features of psychogenic chest pain, panic, or anxiety as for those of angina pectoris and the collateral symptoms of esophageal dysfunction. If the general history, physical exam, lab review, and chest X-ray are otherwise negative, the problem involves three overriding questions.

First, could the patient have coronary or other major cardiac disease? Regardless of the history, this must be excluded.

Second, if not that, could the patient have a problem of acid reflux or esophageal disease other than a motility disorder? This should also be excluded.

Third, could the pain have an emotional basis? If the pain is characteristically atypical, as in emotional disturbances, even though there are no other symptoms of anxiety or panic whatsoever, this question should be considered from the very beginning. Such pain is common, and it usually *is* psychogenic. If, on the other hand, the pain is not atypical but simulates angina, then its possibly emotional basis should be considered as soon as coronary disease, frank disease of the esophagus, and acid reflux have been ruled out. How far the workup should be extended to detect esophageal motility disorders or MVA is questionable. The same biotherapies (nitrates, calcium channel, and adrenergic receptor blocking agents), used in both conditions, are not very effective in either. Thus diagnosis does not yet lead to a specific therapy. And both conditions most often have an emotional basis.

We see, then, that the physiological mechanism of emotionally induced chest pain may be chest-wall muscular tension, an esophageal contractile disorder, microvascular angina, or any combination thereof. Therefore, it could be argued that what is most important is not so much its somatic biology but rather its emotional source and what can be done about that.

The same principle applies also to a psychobiological interpretation. It has been argued that perhaps half the patients with chest pain and negative arteriograms have panic disorder.[58] Does it help to identify such patients in this way? Yes, it certainly shows that they have psychogenic chest pain. Can the panic disorder be treated? Yes, but whereas *psychiatric* patients with panic disorder, many with agoraphobia, respond favorably to several classes of psychoactive medication,[59] the response of *medical* patients where chest pain is the predominant symptom is less impressive.[60] Nevertheless, such therapy might have provided Evelyn with some relief. If psychoactive drugs were the sole approach, however, she would have been left with her unrecognized, unresolved marriage problem, and her general distress would have persisted; and Irene, who had equally psychogenic chest pain but no panic or other recognizable psychiatric disorder to treat, would have gotten nowhere with a strictly psychobiological approach.

The many studies that have demonstrated the prevalence of psychiatric disorders in patients with negative arteriograms, especially those with atypical pain, have served well to switch the prevailing medical focus from "unexplained" to "psychiatric." Unfortunately, however, such studies rarely include any mention of an attempt to elicit or work through the patient's underlying personal problem. Only in two recent papers did I find the psychiatric categorization extended to include its personal source.[61, 62] But such an approach, at least a willingness to proceed in that direction, should be more universal. As emphasized before, the recognition of anxiety, panic, or depression should open, not terminate, the quest for understanding. Sometimes the patients are simply categorized as "hypochondriacal" [25] or "chronically neurotic and socially maladjusted."[63] This may be true: Evelyn was "neurotic and socially maladjusted," but this cleared readily when she learned to express her needs and emotions.

It has been noted that the chest pain persists in at least half, sometimes most, of the patients with negative arteriograms.[17–19, 25, 63–67] The investigators often express surprise that the patients, disabled by pain, fail to improve when advised not to worry about the disease that doesn't cause the pain. But obviously the pain will persist if the illness is not clearly identified for what it is, and its personal source attended to. How can patients be expected to respond favorably to a simplistic "reassurance" that their suffering, which can be intense, far more protracted than true angina, is just "nothing to worry about"?

A major difficulty here has been the lack of an acceptable name, such as tension headache or dyspepsia, for emotionally induced chest pain. As noted before, I use the term *chest tension syndrome*. The mechanism of the pain is now known to be some combination of muscular tension, esophageal spasm, and/or microvascular angina. The precise mechanism could be determined by more extensive and invasive procedures, but, because all of these conditions are usually induced by stress of some kind, it is of first importance to explore what that might be. In one study of panic disorder, for example, precipitating stressful life events could be identified in most patients, especially in association with symptoms of recent onset.[68]

I did look for sources in 25 consecutive patients I examined in the medical clinic for distinctly "atypical" pain, as described previously. The psychosocial survey was sometimes brief, sometimes extensive, but enough data were disclosed to provide a positive, though tentative, identification of the underlying stress in 18 of the 25 patients (unpublished data). This was explained to the 18 as at least one likely source of the pain (as with Evelyn and Irene, though they were not part of this series), and they were encouraged to move toward a more effective resolution, and told that the distress could be expected to improve accordingly. Admittedly, this kind of analysis, which fits more or less into the clinic time schedule, was much too brief and superficial. If it had been acceptable to the patients, it would have been more helpful to make referrals for a more intensive psychotherapeutic approach. Nevertheless, though not treated with psychoactive or other medications, 15 were well or improved, two were the same, and only one was worse when interviewed again within two years. Clearly, it is helpful to many patients if we listen carefully to their story, so as to elicit, if possible, the emotional source of the pain.

Chronic Abdominal Pain

The common painless disturbances of GI function do not usually constitute a diagnostic problem. Abdominal pain as the dominant symptom is far more perturbing. Such patients often undergo repeated workups without a positive diagnosis, and, therefore, no concerted plan for resolution.

Surveys of nonpatient populations provide a perspective: 11 percent of all children [69] and 20 percent of all adults [70] suffer from frequent bouts of abdominal pain. Conversely, most children [71] or adults [72] with pain, when referred to diagnostic centers after a negative preliminary workup, are not found to have specific disease on more intensive investigation. Stress or emotional disturbances, however, if investigated systematically, are found to be a major factor in most of the children, [73] as well as the adults.[72]

Most of these patients have the physiological pain of spasm, distension, hypermotility, gastric hyperacidity, and other dysfunctions of the gut, usually classified either as functional dyspepsia or as irritable-bowel syndrome (IBS). Some patients have somatoform pain disorder as defined in the preceding chapter (Mario L.). Some clinicians distinguish the somatoform from the irritable-bowel syndromes [72, 74]; others classify all functional abdominal pain syndromes as IBS.[75] Regardless of the mechanism of pain formation, the clinicians most concerned about such problems invariably emphasize the importance of a biopsychosocial approach.[75–80]

In two recent studies, patients with IBS were found to have more evidence of psychologic distress than did random subjects with similar GI symptoms who had never consulted a doctor.[81, 82] "Stress," however, which is not always interpreted as "distress," may well be a significant factor in both groups, but the nonpatients "have higher coping capabilities, experience illness as less disruptive to life, and tend to exhibit less psychologic denial than patients."[81] Stoeckle noted long ago that the patient's decision to seek medical aid is often based more on the extent of psychologic distress than on medical factors alone, even with organic disease.[83]

In this brief section we will focus on the persistent *pain* syndromes, which generally take one of two forms, sometimes both: the epigastric or dyspeptic syndromes, and the more generalized or lower-abdominal pains with or without diarrhea and/or constipation that comprise the irritable-bowel syndromes. Esophageal pain was summarized in the preceding section. Psychogenic anorexia and weight loss are common attributes of depression and other nervous states. The functional problems of painless diarrhea or constipation, "burbulence" or "gas," psychogenic vomiting, globus "hystericus," and proctalgia fugax are not discussed here; the reader is referred to Thompson's text, a warm and wise model for clinical care.[77]

The gut is second only to the head as the most frequent site of functional disturbances. Eighteen percent of the subjects in a neighborhood survey noted "indigestion" during the brief period of two weeks preceding an interview.[84] This is not surprising. Activity of the gut continuously reflects the balance of the vegetative and emergency functions of the autonomic nervous system. Stress of any kind readily activates the adrenergic system that overrides the parasympathetic state necessary for normal gastrointestinal functions.

Unlike psychogenic chest pain, in which emotional tension is usually the central issue, functional bowel syndromes have many other causes. These include eating too much or too fast, tobacco, alcohol, habitual use of laxatives or enemas, and irregular eating or bowel habits. Irritable-bowel syndromes may be related in part to low-residue diets and corrected by dietary fiber, but the fiber hypothesis remains controversial.[85] Dysentery can precipitate IBS that may persist long after the infectious agent is eliminated.[75] Many drugs affect the GI tract: salicylates and other nonsteroidal anti-inflammatory agents, corticosteroids, magnesium hydroxide containing antacids, certain antibiotics, beta blockers, and narcotics.

Some investigators regard food intolerance as a major cause of IBS.[86] Though specific food sensitivities can occasionally precipitate vomiting, diarrhea or constipation, and abdominal pain, most clinicians do not regard such sensitivity as a common factor in the usual persistent IBS.[87] Patients often inappropriately attribute symptoms to foods in a vain attempt to identify and remove the cause. If, however, the history and a food diary do suggest an adverse food reaction, appropriate elimination diets and food challenge can verify the diagnosis.[87, 88] Milk sensitivity is not uncommon in infants and children. When adults develop symptoms resembling IBS after ingesting milk products, they probably have lactase deficiency syndrome. Celiac sprue is a food-sensitivity disease induced by gluten, but it presents as a problem of steatorrhea or malabsorption, not with abdominal pain.

Epigastric Pain

Dyspepsia and ulcer. Recurrent epigastric "peptic" distress, variously described as a burning or gnawing pain, a discomfort or fullness, is a common symptom. In patients with peptic syndromes of sufficient severity to be referred for endoscopy, about 40 percent have a peptic ulcer.[89] Most of the other patients have functional dyspepsia. In primary practice, where the more common peptic syndromes are seen, the ratio of non-ulcer dyspepsia to ulcer is undoubtedly much higher.[90] In non-ulcer dyspepsia, the presence or absence of gastritis or duodenitis, endoscopically or histologically, appears to bear little relation to the symptoms or outcome.[89, 91] Whereas gastric infection with Helicobacter pylori appears to be a material factor in peptic ulcer disease, its relation to non-ulcer dyspepsia, especially in the absence of gastritis, is questionable; in dyspeptic patients who do have H. pylori infection, the long-term value of antibacterial therapy has not yet been established.[92]

Compared to ulcer pain, the epigastric distress of non-ulcer dyspepsia is more likely to be diffuse and associated with "gas," belching, and other symptoms of "indigestion." It is usually induced by eating, refractory to treatment, and absent at night. In contrast, ulcer pain (duodenal, especially) is usually a more specific, localized epigastric pain that appears on a relatively empty stomach, with few other digestive symptoms. It is more likely to be relieved by antacids, milk, or other foods, and it commonly reappears during the night. Nevertheless, the symptoms of ulcer and dyspepsia, which are often regarded as two poles of the same disturbance, can resemble each other. A GI series, or, if negative, especially in patients with intractable symptoms, an endoscopy, which can demonstrate an ulcer in an additional 20 percent ± of patients so studied, is necessary to establish the diagnosis.

The etiology of peptic ulcer, including excessive acid-peptic gastric secretion, diminished tissue resistance, and Helicobacter infection, is regarded as predominantly "organic," though collateral factors, such as stress, inadequate rest and relaxation, emotional disturbances, smoking, alcohol, and excessive coffee play a significant role in some patients. On the other hand, dyspepsia—

though the pathophysiology and resulting distress can be as disturbing to the patient as those of peptic ulcer—appears to be a more typically functional disorder in which the personal factors predominate. A positive diagnosis— what it is, not just what it is not (Ch. 3)—is essential. It is not known why patients with dyspepsia, unlike those with peptic ulcer or with the heartburn of esophageal reflux, respond so poorly to antacids or H_2 receptor blocking agents.[91] For this reason, however, amelioration of the underlying personal stresses may constitute the only effective plan for healing.

Hiatus hernia. One-third of asymptomatic adults have a hiatus hernia. Therefore, one-third of all barium meals, whether for strictly epigastric distress or for the substernal heartburn of esophageal reflux, will disclose a coincidental hiatus hernia. The distress of dyspepsia should not be attributed to the hernia, as this usually diverts attention from the personal factors that really precipitate the symptoms. Most hiatus hernias are asymptomatic (Ch. 6).

Biliary colic. Though usually located in or about the right upper quadrant, the colic is occasionally central, appearing only in the midepigastrium or periumbilical area. Such attacks of moderate to severe steady pain, which reappear unpredictably and last for hours or more, differ from dyspepsia both in quality and regularity. If there is a reasonable possibility of biliary-tract disease, an ultrasound study or oral cholecystography should be performed. Cholelithiasis, however, is not a cause of the typical dyspeptic syndrome (Ch. 6).

Cancer. Another problem is that of more or less *continuous* epigastric or central abdominal pain persisting for a month or more. If the usual laboratory tests are negative, and disease of the gastrointestinal and biliary tracts has been ruled out, the differential may fall between carcinoma of the body of the pancreas and somatoform pain disorder. This question can often be settled by a careful analysis of the illness and its setting and/or a CAT scan to survey the whole abdomen and retroperitoneal space as well as the pancreas for malignant and other disease.[93] A pancreatic carcinoma, however, may not be seen on either CT or MRI. Chronic pancreatitis is another possibility, but would usually be suspected because of the underlying alcoholism or previously diagnosed acute episodes.[94]

Irritable-Bowel Syndrome

Other than peptic syndromes, IBS is the most common cause of recurrent episodes of abdominal pain that persist for months or years with no physical or laboratory evidence of disease, especially when associated with irregularities of bowel movement, more than three movements daily, or alternating constipation and diarrhea.[95] If the patient notes distension, relief of pain with bowel movements, looser and more frequent movements with the onset of pain, mucus in the stools, and a sensation of incomplete evacuation, the diagnosis is even more positive.[96–98] If pain predominates, and most of these symptoms have recurred for two years or more, a more meticulous workup is unlikely to reveal any specific disease, although lactase deficiency should be ruled out in any illness resembling IBS.

A more difficult diagnostic problem arises when the pain of IBS occurs with minimal or no disturbance of bowel function. The pain can be right- or left-sided, or generalized through the lower quadrants or the whole abdomen, or it may appear at several different sites, and it can be colicky or steady and persistent.[75] If the pain is strictly continuous over an extended time period in the absence of bowel symptoms, it may well be somatoform; most longstanding functional bowel pain is intermittent and physiological.

We see that a positive diagnosis of IBS is strongly suggested by long-standing pain plus bowel irregularities. Nevertheless, the symptoms may closely simulate those of organic disease, and the diagnosis is in part one of exclusion. There are three problems here:

First, the workup may have to be fairly extensive. The symptoms of partial bowel obstruction, either in the colon by carcinoma, in the terminal ileum by Crohn's disease, or rarely in the small bowel, can be restricted to intermittent cramping sensations that persist for a year or more, sometimes several years, without blood in the stools, bowel irregularity, or other symptoms. Therefore, an air contrast barium enema and sigmoidoscopy, if not colonoscopy, and often a GI series with small-bowel study, are necessary. The terminal ileum should be visualized one way or the other. IBS pain from the hepatic flexure or transverse colon can occur mostly in the right upper quadrant, periumbilical, or epigastric areas; if so, cholelithiasis must be ruled out. IBS pain in the lower quadrants in women may simulate that of pelvic disease or the psychogenic pelvic pain syndrome described later in this chapter. Urinary-tract calculi, obstruction, or infection, manifested only as abdominal pain with repeatedly negative urinalyses, is highly unlikely, but an IV pyelogram may occasionally be indicated. Alcoholism, as the cause of hepatitis, pancreatitis, or simply gastrointestinal dysfunction, is another consideration. Functional bowel syndromes rarely appear for the first time in the elderly; abdominal pain is then most likely due to organic disease. Systemic disease such as porphyria, vasculitis, and tabes dorsalis are very rare causes of recurrent abdominal pain. In persistent GI syndromes in which diarrhea or steatorrhea, rather than pain, is the dominant symptom, the differential includes ulcerative and infectious colitis, malabsorption syndromes, Whipple's disease, and others.

My purpose here is not a detailed discussion of differential diagnosis but rather to recommend that whatever workup is indicated be completed so that the clinician can initiate a positive and, therefore, constructive evaluation of whatever needs to be corrected—either disease, if present, or the personal factors that lead to the bowel reactivity of IBS.

Second, as with hiatus hernia, one-third of all healthy asymptomatic adults over 40 have diverticuli in the colon. Therefore, *diverticulosis* will be found in one-third of all barium enemas in this age group. Symptoms of IBS are just as prevalent in those with normal studies and no diverticuli as they are in those with uncomplicated diverticulosis.[99] Like the appendix, diverticuli cause symptoms only *when* inflamed or otherwise complicated, and this can only be determined by the finding of local tenderness, fever, leukocytosis, or other abnormal signs during or after an attack. Too often what is really IBS is attributed inappropriately to "diverticular disease" (Ch. 6).

The final hazard here is begging the question. The workup is negative, but the physician, still concerned about disease, and reluctant to diagnose a "functional" disorder, continues to study the patient or shifts to symptomatic therapy without providing a positive diagnosis. The emotional background, which constitutes the basis of what is really an irritable-bowel syndrome, is not explored.

Chronic, Persistent Pelvic Pain

Chronic pelvic pain in women, unremitting for months or years, is usually psychogenic (Chs. 1, 6, and 12). The discussion here is restricted to the problem of diagnosis.

Pelvic pain that is clearly caused by pelvic disease is often acute or subacute, or if chronic, restricted to the week or so of menstruation, or associated with an obvious cause of pain. In contrast, psychogenic pelvic pain is a chronic problem that persists, often daily, much of the time, if not continuously. It is often accentuated with menses but should not be viewed as dysmenorrhea because it persists between periods and soon reappears if it abates transiently at the end of menstruation. It ranges from mild fullness, heaviness, or aching to severe, intractable pain. It is usually located in the lower abdominal quadrants (unilateral, central, or generalized) or deeper in the pelvis and pelvic floor, often including the lower back or sacrococcygeal area. It is sometimes referred to the bladder, vagina, or rectum with other complaints of dysfunction of these organs (endometriosis can cause similar symptoms). Sometimes it also involves the trunk more widely, the thighs, or more remote areas. The pain is often accentuated by prolonged standing, fatigue, or intercourse. Regardless of the severity of the complaint, the patient may or may not be tender and guarded on pelvic exam or appear to be having severe pain. There may be no obvious nervous tension, but a careful history usually reveals other psychosomatic and emotional symptoms.

When pelvic pain is of recent onset, organic disease is the primary concern. When the pain is chronic, major disease must obviously be ruled out, but the pain should not be attributed to painless lesions. Ovarian cysts, for example, regardless of size, rarely cause pain unless complicated by torsion and ischemia, rupture or bleeding, the pelvic incarceration of a large tumor, malignant invasion, or other unusual events. Similarly, uterine fibroids, though they may cause bleeding or dysmenorrhea, rarely cause chronic pain.

The overriding consideration here is that the kind of relentless pain described above is quite characteristic of psychogenic pain, and organic disease is not likely to be the cause. This holds true whether the patient is found to have (1) no pelvic disease, (2) pelvic disease that is usually painless, or (3) pelvic disease that, though it may cause dysmenorrhea or other symptoms from time to time, could hardly be expected to cause this kind of prolonged, steady pain. Such lesions include chronic cervicitis, cystorectocele, adhesions from old inactive inflammatory disease or other causes, mild to moderate endometriosis, and uterine adenomyosis, retroversion, or prolapse (Ch. 6). In these conditions, the *disease* is organic, and medical or surgical treatment may well be appropriate, but the *illness* (persistent pain) is often emotional.

Psychogenic pain often disappears after surgery. This may be due to several factors: (1) suggestion; (2) the intrinsic benefits of hysterectomy (Ch. 6); (3) the legitimation of illness by an organic diagnosis when conversion forces are involved; or (4) the apparent disability of postoperative convalescence, which, in these patients, may persist for a year or more, filling the same psychosocial needs that were previously achieved by the somatoform pain syndrome. Excision of asymptomatic organs, however, is a risky placebo. In a Mayo Clinic study, half of the women with pelvic pain had pelvic surgery; 41 percent of these patients still had pain four years later, though the pathology in question had been excised.[100]

Patients with psychogenic pain often give a history of extended periods of pelvic distress punctuated by surgical intervention following which the pain reappears sooner (Janet F., Ch. 1) or later (Rosetta C., Ch. 14) at the same or adjoining sites, or other psychosomatic symptoms take their place. The patient describes the past history by the names of the diseases and operations only, not mentioning the symptoms or their chronicity, and minimizing the pain if asked about it. The present symptoms are viewed as an unrelated, different, more severe illness. The physician is readily enticed into the patient's point of view. If surgery cured the previous disease, it will again. Women with psychogenic pelvic complaints give a history of previous pelvic surgery far more often than do other women.[101] In one comparative study, such patients had undergone seven times more gynecologic procedures than had healthy controls.[102] A history of previous pelvic surgery, including appendectomy, should immediately alert the physician to the possibility of psychogenic pain unless the previous pathology reports were those of a distinctly painful disease process (Ch. 14).

On the basis of the data provided in Chapter 12, psychogenic pelvic pain, unlike functional bowel disorders, is predominantly somatoform. It may, however, include psychophysiological components of the irritable-bowel syndrome (colon spasm in the right or left lower quadrant), muscular backache, vaginismus, or other forms of muscle tension, and it is superimposed on the physiological distress of primary or secondary dysmenorrhea. Pelvic vascular congestion was once thought to be a factor,[103] but few patients were found to have evidence for this on clinical exam,[104] laparoscopy, [105] culdoscopy, or laparotomy.[106] Severe pelvic pain need not have a nociceptive pathway.

The diagnosis of psychogenic pelvic pain is readily suggested by the way the pain is described, its chronicity, the whole medical history, the patient's "gestalt," and the negative physical and laboratory exams. The physician, however, must be aware of the very existence of such an entity, its nature, and its frequency, and assume the responsibility to establish the diagnosis. If not, all of the above will be overlooked.

For some responsive patients in whom all evidence points to a psychogenic pelvic-pain syndrome, laparoscopy need be recommended only if psychological assessment and treatment prove ineffective.[107] For many patients, however, laparoscopy, or at least ultrasound scanning of the pelvis, is necessary, for both the doctor and the patient. Laparoscopy can disclose pathology missed on pelvic exam or rule out pathology otherwise suspected. The usual laboratory screening tests for systemic, pelvic, and urinary-tract disease are also necessary. Occasionally, GI contrast studies, spine X-rays, or an intravenous pyelogram is indicated if any symptoms suggest disease of these systems.

Because the doctor's belief system about symptoms and disease often leads either to the organic or psychological opposite pole of the diagnostic spectrum, as we have seen again and again, the core problem here lies in interpreting the significance of abnormalities found at laparoscopy or laparotomy. Liston et al., reporting on laparoscopy in 134 patients with chronic pelvic pain, found no abnormalities in 76 percent, adhesions in 16 percent, and endometriosis or other lesions in 8 percent, but considered the latter two findings coincidental to the pain. They conclude: "If a clinical diagnosis cannot be reached, laparoscopy seldom provides one. It may be useful, however . . . where firm reassurance is the best form of therapy."[108] Castelnuovo-Tedesco and Krout, reporting on culdoscopy or laparotomy combined with a clinical and intensive psychological evaluation of 40 women with chronic abdominal pain, reached the same conclusion. Though disease such as a pelvic abscess was occasionally found to have clearly explained the illness, most pel-vic abnormalities, noted in 63 percent of the patients in this study, were deemed not to be the cause of the pain: "Chronic pelvic pain, even in the presence of definite organic pathology, is 'more' than pelvic disease. It is a complex psychosomatic entity . . . involving . . . the emotional status and total functioning of the patient."[106]

In contrast, note the conclusion of Lundberg et al. about the laparoscopic findings on 95 women with chronic pain: "55 had pathologic processes dem-onstrated in the reproductive organs, and in 52 it was felt to be the etiology of the pain."[105] This represents an all too common medical point of view. The assumption that *any* lesion discovered is the cause of the pain is, of course, the medical side of the polysurgery problem. In 29 of Lundberg's 52 patients, the pain was attributed to "adhesions" or "PID-chronic." Liston, however, concluded that adhesions had nothing to do with the pain, because he had found that one-third of all women studied only for infertility had the same findings, though they were completely free of pain.[108] (We referred to these data about adhesions earlier, in Ch. 6.)

On the basis of these data, laparoscopy, if indicated, should be performed with this understanding: (1) a negative study is a positive step toward the cor-rect diagnosis; (2) positive findings should be questioned as the cause of long-standing relentless pain unless the relationship is clear and obvious.

When the pelvic examination is negative, and disease seems unlikely, there is a tendency in practice to temporize without providing a definitive evalua-tion. This may be unwise. If emotional factors are significant, the patient must grapple with these problems sooner or later. A psychotherapeutic approach may or may not be successful, but it cannot begin until both patient and doc-tor are convinced that significant disease has been excluded. If the doctor or an allied therapist is willing to understand and work with the patient, both medically and psychosocially, and the patient will accept a multidisciplinary approach, most patients will improve, and some will become completely free of pain.[109–114]

Low Back Pain

Backache is indeed ubiquitous: 65–85 percent of adults over 45 have ex-perienced significant low back symptoms.[115–117] In any one attack, even with sciatica, there is a high rate of spontaneous recovery; 70–90 percent will improve in four weeks whether treated with "specific," symptomatic, or no therapy.[118, 119] The pain, however, will recur in most patients [120] and persist chronically in many.

In the medical model we prefer to think in terms of precise diagnosis.

Probably in less than 20 percent of backaches, however, whether acute, chronic, or recurrent, can a specific diagnosis be established that satisfactorily explains the whole illness.[119, 121] Of all common symptoms, backache is the one best described as "an illness in search of a disease."[122]

In acute or subacute backaches, it is often difficult to identify either the precipitating situation or the particular back derangement. Nevertheless, a specific injury has presumably occurred: tension, stretch, or tearing of back muscles, tendons, ligaments, fascia, or other soft tissues. This may occur with or without damage or degeneration, past or present, to intervertebral disks, articular facets, or other sensitive spinal structures. Long-term or frequently recurrent chronic backache, however, may be far more complex, involving occupational, social, and psychological issues as well as disk injury and the many postural, lifting, and other mechanical forces that strain the back structures generally.

Even when a structural defect that *could* cause backache is demonstrated, it is often difficult to know how much of a role it plays in the individual patient. For example, lumbosacral intervertebral disk abnormalities on magnetic resonance imaging were noted in 54 percent (bulge, 44 percent; herniation, 10 percent) of *asymptomatic* young women in one study.[123] In a similar survey of CAT scans in *asymptomatic* volunteers of both sexes, a herniated nucleus pulposus was noted in 10 percent of subjects under 40; 27 percent over 40.[124] Therefore, unless the location of the herniation is consistent with that of the patient's sciatica or neurological deficit, it may have nothing to do with the backache. When it does, surgical correction does not always provide substantial relief.

Thus, the recovery from chronic or recurrent backache often has little to do with specific diagnosis or therapy. Successful management boils down to a long-range collaboration, a joint enterprise designed to discover, evaluate, and revise the many possible factors that do underlie the symptoms and *can* be changed, with a program of appropriate exercises and rehabilitation. In short, we need to shift our focus from disease to the illness itself. Before this can be done, however, three preliminary steps are important:

First, Do Not Focus on the Wrong Disease

The sure way to a diagnosis that has little or nothing to do with the illness is to secure X-rays of the lumbosacral spine, then to attribute the pain to whatever lesions are found. Many comparative studies have demonstrated that the prevalence of most common spinal abnormalities on X-ray is no higher in patients with backache than it is in asymptomatic controls.[116, 117, 120, 125–131] The most common abnormalities to which backache is attributed erroneously are single disk narrowing and/or osteoarthritis, either osteophytes (bony spurs) of the vertebral bodies or degenerative changes in the articular facets (apophyseal joints). Such signs of degeneration correlate only with age, and are virtually universal in older people, even in those who have never suffered backache. Other abnormalities that are just as common in asymptomatic subjects are sacralization of L5 or lumbarization of S1 (symmetric or otherwise), disk calcification, Schmorl nodes, spina bifida occulta, and mild to moderate scoliosis. Of questionable or borderline significance (the abnormality is found more often in patients with backache than in controls in some comparative studies, but not in others) are spondylolysis (defects of the pars interarticularis of the vertebral arch in the region of the articular facets), retrolisthesis, and severe lumbar scoliosis or lordosis. Positive correlations of spinal abnormalities with backache are found for multiple disk narrowing, spondylolisthesis, lumbar osteochondrosis, congenital/traumatic kyphosis, and, of course, recent fractures. As with herniated disks in asymptomatic subjects,[123, 124] this does not mean that the positive correlations can necessarily identify the cause of a backache. In the Horal study, for example, disk degeneration was noted in 46 percent of the probands and 32 percent of the controls.[120] The correlation suggests only that for no clear reason, the abnormality causes pain in some subjects but not in others, or that it enhances the subject's vulnerability to other stresses which, combined with the defect, cause the pain.

Second, Is There a Neurologic Deficit?

If so, surgery is indicated for intractable pain or persistent recurrences, progressively worsening neurologic deficit, or cauda equina syndrome. A satisfactory outcome can be expected if the sciatic pain is more severe than the back pain, the neurologic exam demonstrates a specific root syndrome, the straight leg raising tests are positive, and a demonstrable defect (on myelography, CT, or MRI) [132] corroborates the neurologic exam.[133] A good result can be impaired by a background of psychological instability and psychosomatic symptoms, or by the secondary gains often associated with industrial or vehicular accidents.

The occurrence of sciatica in 17–28 percent of all adults, [115, 119] or 38 percent of men over 35, [134] with back syndromes suggests that disk disease or other causes of spinal stenosis or nerve-root compression are the most common underlying *spinal* source of low back pain. But few patients meet the criteria for surgery. Although there are no published data to indicate how often surgery would be effective in a population of patients with chronic backache in primary practice, it would probably be much less than 10 percent.

Third, Be Sure That the Illness Is Not Caused by Specific Disease Other than Structural Defects of the Spine

In brief, these fall into two categories. First are the diseases of the spine, including infection (osteomyelitis, tuberculosis, etc.), malignancy, ankylosing spondylitis and other forms of inflammatory arthritis, Paget's disease, and osteoporosis with compression fractures. Osteoporosis, unless complicated by compression, is rarely the main cause of backache. Second is visceral or systemic disease such as bacterial endocarditis, disease of the genitourinary systems, aortic aneurysm, or, rarely, gastrointestinal disease (posterior penetrating ulcer, for example).

Evidence of such diseases will nearly always be found on some aspect of a complete history and physical exam, routine lab including CBC, sed rate, UA, chemistry screening, and X-rays of the lumbosacral spine, all of which are essential in the study of chronic backache. Of special concern are any data, past or present, for systemic disease, cancer, tuberculosis, trauma or recent surgery, corticosteroid use, and drug or alcohol abuse. The general physical exam includes, of course, a careful neurological survey and examination of the back for the usual signs of impairment, also a rectal in both sexes, and a pelvic exam in women.

If all these laboratory examinations, and others that may be indicated for special symptoms, are negative, revealing no evidence of systemic, visceral, or spinal disease other than structural defects of the spine, bone scintigraphy is not necessary; the test would rarely provide the only evidence of cancer, infection, or other disease.[135–137]

In a random survey of a nonpatient adult population, ankylosing spondylitis was found in less than 1 percent of the subjects with back pain,[138] and it is highly unlikely that the disease will be missed on the first X-ray of the spine in likely suspects only to appear on subsequent studies.[139]

The incidence of these diseases as the cause of backache varies with the series studied. In one series of referred patients, age 50 or older, the incidence of any disease other than structural spinal defects as the cause of backache was 15 percent (mostly malignancy and osteoporosis).[135] A survey of younger patients with chronic backache would show a much lower incidence.

Low Back Pain: An Overview

Thus chronic backache is often a truly personal illness, as defined throughout this book, caused by many kinds of stress, perhaps mainly mechanical but also psychosocial, that *can* be corrected. The patient indeed needs a guide who is familiar with evaluating all aspects of the problem. What is usually most important is not what the therapist does to the patient in the form of prescription drugs, diathermy, ultrasound, manipulation, acupuncture, corset support, etc., but what patients learn to do for themselves. McKenzie puts it straight in his advice to patients: "The main point of this book is that the management of your back is *your responsibility*," [140]—a difficult concept for many patients as well as for the physician trained in a converse perspective.

Most medical texts focus on *what doctors can do* biomedically for the conditions that cause backache. If this is how we think clinically, we may get mired in an endless procession of ineffective anti-inflammatory, psychoactive, analgesic, and, finally, narcotic drugs, or feel pushed to inappropriate laminectomy. What patients can do for themselves is better described in portrayals of backache, both diagnostically and therapeutically, as a multifaceted personal illness. Such descriptions are written either for doctors [141, 142] or for patients [140, 143–145]; that of McKenzie is particularly brief and readable. In a collaborative program, such as has always characterized the work of physical and rehabilitation therapists, we can work with our patients to correct the actual sources of the problem.

The most common problems involve faulty postures and actions while standing, walking, working, bending, lifting, carrying, sitting, or lying. The basic fault is often a somewhat stooped forward position, or inadequate lumbar lordosis. Sometimes it is the opposite: excessive swayback. Associated problems include inappropriate support in chairs, car seats, or beds; inadequate physical conditioning and loss of flexibility that can be improved by exercise programs; unnecessary muscular tension during many activities with insufficient periods for rest, relaxation, or stretching maneuvers. We must also consider, when appropriate, the nervous/muscular tension of psychosocial disturbances, and the somatoform problems that evolve around issues of secondary gain.

The mechanical factors probably predominate in most patients, especially in those who remain active with intermittent pain and positive signs of back impairment (Richard D., Ch. 12). In others, psychosocial factors may be paramount, especially when the pain is unremitting, the disability prolonged, and the examination negative. Mechanical and psychosocial problems are both common; it is not surprising how often they interact in such a disturbing symptom. "The greatest handicap a low back pain physician can have is lack of interest in and awareness of the psychosocial environment of the patient," as the neurosurgeon Finneson puts it so well in his balanced view of the whole problem.[146] That nervous/muscular tension is a common factor in backache is evident from patient histories replete with other musculo-ligamentous-arthralgic syndromes over the years. Sarno emphasizes nervous tension as the dominant factor in chronic backache, but I find this component, though important, to be far less universal than his book implies.[147]

All healers, doctors included, prefer therapeutic programs, whatever they are, that can be applied across-the-board for a specific symptom or disease. This often fails to work for chronic backache. An educational and collaborative program for healing must be individualized to serve the unique needs of each patient.

Chronic Fatigue

In a Danish neighborhood survey of 40-year-old subjects, 41 percent of the women respondents and 25 percent of the men "felt tired."[148] In studies of medical practice in which all patients, regardless of the reason for the current visit, were asked if fatigue was a recent and major problem, 37 percent of those aged 17–50 replied affirmatively in one survey,[149] as did 24 percent of all adults in another study.[150] The ubiquity of fatigue, and the experience of most people who feel unduly tired from time to time, suggest strongly that the feeling (tired, weak, lack of energy, listless, low vitality), if not an indication of a real need for rest after a period of stress, is far more often a basic expression of the down side of the human condition (with zest and exuberance the expressions of the positive side) than it is a symptom of disease. This is borne out in all studies of fatigue as a medical complaint, from Allan's early studies [151, 152] to the recent survey of Kroenke et al.[150] In both reports the symptom was deemed to be psychogenic in most patients, on the basis of positive interview [151, 152] or psychometric data.[150] Known disease sufficient to be the main cause of *chronic* fatigue was found in ≤ 20 percent of the tired patients.

There is no question that chronic fatigue states usually have an emotional basis. The data to be summarized in this section clearly support this concept. It is now argued that a subset of fatigue, defined as "chronic fatigue syndrome" (CFS), may be due to a viral infection and/or a related immune response. Whether this proves to characterize some patients or not, it is obviously not the cause in most subjects with the same complaint. And in those who do have the infection, if such can be demonstrated, emotional factors are likely to be of major significance. Let us first consider here the problem of psychogenic fatigue. Later we will turn to the controversy about CFS.

"Lack of energy," whether the experience is physical, mental, or both, is characteristic of both anxiety and depression, especially the latter. Depression, as described in DSM-III-R: "A decrease in energy level is almost invariably present, and is experienced as sustained fatigue even in the absence of physical exertion. The smallest task may seem difficult or impossible to accomplish."[153] If the patient is focused more on feeling "down" than feeling "tired," the diagnosis is depression; if focused more on feeling "tired" than feeling "down," the diagnosis is a fatigue syndrome.

The problem for the clinician is the many patients who do not appear to be emotionally disturbed and simply feel tired. Patients who find it difficult to perceive, accept, or communicate affective distress [154] often describe the disturbance in the vernacular of fatigue. Such patients, however, may well be anxious, depressed, or suffering from other psychological disorders, but such problems will be revealed only by a structured inquiry like the Diagnostic Interview Schedule,[155] or perhaps by the self-rating scales (Ch. 14), which are rarely used in practice.

On the other hand, assessment of the symptoms of nervous disorders, so clearly defined in DSM, may be negative, and, too, the underlying psychodynamics are not often readily identified or verified. Nevertheless, I find, on the strength of many observations, that the process, in some patients, represents latent dismay about a life situation, though there is no overt problem. The subject feels OK about him/herself, successful, accomplished, neither anxious nor depressed. At some level, however, perhaps mostly unconscious, this person's ongoing educational goals, occupation, marriage, or other situation, though involving no stress as conventionally conceived, no longer seems right or satisfying. Yet change appears to be impossible, or it would be devastating to all concerned. The status quo is destined to prevail. This general problem is discussed in greater detail in Ch. 17. In such patients, if the interviews or assessment scales are directed only to questions of psychiatric disorders or obvious stress, the existential source of the fatigue will not be revealed. These are indeed difficult problems, but if, in psychotherapy, the patient can find some way to recognize and work through the situation more effectively, the illness may abate.

When patients complain that they are too tired to do anything, there is usually something missing in their lives. Some patients, however, feel tired because they *are* actually exhausted, and the emotional component may be minimal. A young mother of three children, for example, feels fulfilled with her loving husband and with her family, which has developed as planned, but she is exhausted from too much to do, too little rest or sleep, too little help, and no respite. Here the complaint takes a different form. It is not: "I can't seem to do much of anything." Instead, it is: "I ought not to feel tired no matter how much I do." Fatigue, of course, is the body's normal response to excessive physical or mental exertion, whether "stressful" or not, and such patients must learn to recognize and respond to their physiological limits.

Because fatigue is such a fundamental expression of distress, it may be the only or major symptom, or it may be one symptom of many in any functional syndrome or psychiatric disorder. It is most commonly associated with diffuse myalgia or weakness, headaches, and sleep disturbances.

Establishing the Diagnosis of Psychogenic Fatigue

The experienced practitioner, concerned about the possibility of disease, yet comfortable about recognizing psychogenic fatigue and exploring its source with patients, learns to distinguish the latter quickly, with considerable accuracy. A more extensive workup than is necessary can usually be avoided.[150–152, 156–161] The initial appraisal is based on a characteristic description of the symptoms in conjunction with an otherwise negative history and physical examination. Patients with frank debilitating disease, even disabling neuromuscular disorders, are usually active, doing as much as they can. They describe the difficulties of specific tasks but rarely complain that they are tired most of the time, lacking the energy to get started with what they want to do.

Fatigue can, of course, be one symptom of almost any major chronic disease: infectious, malignant, cardiac, pulmonary, renal, hepatic, hematological, endocrine, neurological, neuromuscular, rheumatoid arthritis or collagen vascular disease, or the drugs used in treatment. A general examination and appropriate workup are essential. Nevertheless, fatigue is rarely the first, the only, or the dominant symptom of any disease, especially in patients with no specific signs or symptoms.

A commonsense approach is helpful. The history should include personal factors, other than emotional distress, that may contribute to the tired feeling:

- sedentary life style, poor physical conditioning; or its opposite, the exhaustion of unusual stress.
- the malnutrition of reducing or other faulty diets, incipient anorexia nervosa or bulimia, laxative abuse.
- inadequate or restless sleep, or clinical sleep disorders.
- alcohol and psychoactive drugs, especially sedatives, hypnotics, tranquilizers, phenothiazines, antihistamines, narcotics, or the stimulus/fatigue dependency cycle induced by street drugs, smoking, or caffeinism.

Patients use the terms *fatigue* and *weakness* interchangeably. What is really meant? The "tired" patient is not weak; muscular strength as tested is normal or only slightly reduced. If the patient is unable to perform specific activities, repetitively or otherwise, or has significant weakness, generally or locally, disease is more likely. If the weakness involves specific muscle groups (limbs, ocular, bulbar), the differential would focus on diseases of the neuromuscular unit: neurological disease, myasthenia gravis, the muscular dystrophies, polymyositis, etc.

For chronic fatigue, with no demonstrable weakness or other signs or symptoms of disease, the workup (including chest X-ray) earlier suggested, plus electrolytes, is enough to pick up evidence for most of the diseases that might simulate psychogenic fatigue. A temperature curve could be added if there is a question of fever. Tests for adrenal or pituitary function are rarely indicated unless there is some clinical reason to suspect Addison's disease, Cushing's syndrome, or panhypopituitarism. The latter is rare but could be overlooked on the history, P.E., and lab survey. Special tests for polymyositis or other disease of muscle, rheumatoid arthritis or collagen vascular disease, Lyme disease, or HIV infection are not customary unless there is a specific indication. Chronic fatigue is rarely the *only* symptom present for any disease suggested by a positive test when the patient has no other clinical evidence for that disease.

As with pelvic pain or backache, the clinician may jump to the conclusion that any disease found on the workup explains the symptom, although the fatigue and the disease may well be coincidental. In one survey, for example, fatigue was attributed to hypertension in 15 of 300 tired patients in whom it was discovered,[158] although it is generally well known that fatigue is not a symptom of uncomplicated hypertension.[162] Or the symptom is attributed to mild hypothyroidism, although this is rarely if ever the cause of a pervasive, debilitating fatigue state (Ch. 6). Hypertension and hypothyroidism should be treated, of course, but if the vitality of the patient is the goal of treatment, another kind of understanding is usually necessary.

"Chronic Fatigue Syndrome"

The hypothesis of chronic Epstein-Barr virus (EBV) infection as a case of chronic fatigue became untenable for many reasons.[163] In particular, the range of EBV antibody titers in asymptomatic subjects was found to be comparable to that in tired patients.[149, 164] Nevertheless, because of the possibility that some kind of viral infection or immune response could be a factor at least in some patients with chronic fatigue, the CDC (Centers for Disease Control) proposed a subset for investigative purposes known as Chronic Fatigue Syndrome (CFS).[165] The definition is weighted toward the possible coexistence of a respiratory viral infection. The major criteria are (1) debilitating fatigue for at least six months and (2) no evidence of any organic disease or drug use known to cause fatigue, or of psychiatric disease, past or present. The minor criteria include other symptoms and signs (described later). There are several insurmountable problems with the concept and definition of the "syndrome."

The exclusion of a psychiatric disorder. As noted, this can only be done by a structured interview. In one study of 200 consecutive adult patients with chronic fatigue, 60 fit the CDC definition when a conventional psychiatric history was used to rule out a psychiatric disorder.[155] If, however, the more precise Diagnostic Interview Schedule was applied to all the patients, the 60 with CFS could not be distinguished psychologically from the 140 fatigued patients who did not otherwise fit the definition. The two groups had the same frequency of current psychiatric disorders (78 percent vs 82 percent), an active mood disorder (73 percent vs 77 percent), or preexisting psychiatric disorders (42 percent vs 43 percent). And the patients identified as CFS were even more likely to have had many other symptoms characteristic of functional disorders, often lifelong. If, then, the Diagnostic Interview Schedule had been used instead of a more conventional psychiatric history to rule out psychiatric disorder, only about 12 (6 percent) of the 200 tired patients would have matched CDC criteria for CFS. Thus the cause is not "unknown." It is psychogenic in most patients.

In a comparable study of 28 patients diagnosed as having CFS on the basis of standard criteria, and referred to the NIH for acyclovir therapy, 75 percent were found to have psychiatric disorders when the Diagnostic Interview Schedule was applied.[166] Of great significance, the disorders more often preceded the appearance of fatigue than followed it.

The symptoms and signs. Of the 11 symptoms specified in the CDC definition, six are characteristic of functional syndromes generally: weakness, myalgia, headaches, arthralgia, irritability and other psychologic complaints, and sleep disturbances. A seventh symptom, fatigue after minor exercise, adds nothing to the definition because it characterizes all "tired" patients.

The other four symptoms (low-grade fever, sore throat, painful cervical or axillary lymph nodes, sudden onset) and the three physical signs (low-grade fever, nonexudative pharyngitis, palpable or tender lymph nodes) are indeed those of viral infections. To fit the definition, however, the patient need not have the physical signs, which are themselves elusive. In any event, the symptoms are intermittent, and all these occurrences are common in the population at large. Patients who are not in any way "tired" often ask, "Why do I get 'colds' [or 'the flu'] all the time?" In short, even in patients with chronic fatigue, such findings can be presumed to be due to intercurrent coincidental infections. There is no way to know that they are specific indicators of CFS.

The functional nature of the syndrome. No distinct, clinically manifest evidence of chronic organic disease has been reported in any patient even after many years of fatigue. Impaired cognition, coordination, and other "soft" neurological symptoms have been attributed to "myalgic encephalomyelitis," as CFS is designated in British Commonwealth countries, but persistent CNS inflammation or damage has not been demonstrated, and the difficulties described are common in disturbed patients generally. In many ways, the syndrome cannot be distinguished from fibromyalgia.[167] Mental fatigue and fatigability characterize both CFS and major depression, but not myasthenia gravis, myopathies, or other frank diseases of the neuromuscular system, unless there is an associated psychiatric disorder.[168]

Severe infections such as mononucleosis,[163] influenza, or other acute infectious diseases can certainly cause asthenia in otherwise healthy patients for one, occasionally two, rarely three months, but, when all clinical evidence of disease is gone, most patients get on with their activities anyway. The weakness rarely evolves into a major complaint. The debilitating fatigue of CFS is said to represent a different kind of disorder altogether, but usually there is no well-documented acute illness at the onset.

Clearly, the CDC concept of CFS is fraught with difficulties, and very few patients with chronic fatigue fit the criteria stated. Nevertheless, let us allow the definition as a reasonable basis for further investigation of a possibly organic etiology. Positive findings have been reported, but they have not been replicated. At present there is no consensus.

In spite of the as yet unsubstantiated and controversial evidence for a viral or immune basis to the "syndrome," let us assume that it does indeed constitute a significant etiologic factor in some patients, either as the agent that initiated the process or as a continuing problem in the course of the illness. Is not the overriding question, however, not whether there is or is not a viral infection or immune dysfunction, but what is it about some patients that makes the illness so disabling? In any study there are likely to be control subjects with the same disease but no symptoms. In short, should not the clinical focus be redirected from the disease to the patient and the illness?

There are, after all, remarkable differences in response to any condition, depending on the previous or concurrent psychosocial state of the patient (Ch. 1). Consider the elegant prospective study of Imboden et al.[169] Six hundred healthy, employed individuals were given a battery of psychological tests *prior* to an epidemic of influenza. Of those who contracted the disease, about half recovered quickly. The others continued to complain of subjective symptoms for more than three weeks, though there were no longer objective signs of disease. The acute illness was clinically identical in both groups. The delayed recovery occurred in those who had previously responded to the psychological tests in patterns characteristic of depression-prone patients! The evidence supports the view that the preexisting emotional disturbance was the main cause of the persistent symptoms, not the virus per se. Eventually, "the patient regards himself as the victim of a chronic, enduring infection and is enabled defensively to avoid emotional problems."[170]

All physicians are familiar with this pattern. One patient with acute infectious mononucleosis insists on going skiing while still febrile with a palpable spleen, whereas another patient is still disabled long after all evidence of the disease has disappeared. One patient with severe, active, widespread rheumatoid arthritis manages a full-time job with considerable physical activity, whereas another patient with minimal disease feels incapacitated. In these situations, every physician would quickly see that the disability had little to do with the disease. But those who defend the disease theory of "chronic fatigue syndrome" argue that all patients are the same: the disease causes the fatigue, and, if depression is present, the disease causes that too; they deny or minimize the emotional factors.

There being no effective treatment for the infection,[155, 171] will not the focus on CFS as a "disease," a positive antibody titer, or other findings of dubious relevance, center the patient's concerns on the relatively hopeless aspects of the problem? The diagnosis will, of course, be immensely satisfying to patients who cannot or do not want to view the problem in any other way. But no healing will ensue. In spite of this, the patient often interprets the introduction of the possibility of psychological factors as an attempt to trivialize and "psychologize" a disease that the doctor neither accepts nor understands.

There is, of course, no question about the suffering and anguish of incapacitating fatigue. There is no question about the pain and suffering of the many patients with other functional syndromes described in this book. Those who are willing to explore the problem in terms of their life situations may get well. Those who are not so willing may not recover. A psychosocial stance about the illness, if it is pursued carefully and compassionately, and if some basic understanding can be achieved, is a distinctly positive and hopeful approach. Yet the psychotherapeutic approach is not easy. It is demanding, a real challenge. It takes courage. In no way can it be viewed as "trivializing" what is clearly a devastating state. On the other hand, the disease focus can be a dead end. But this is a difficult point of view for many patients.

Perhaps it could be explained that the illness, though perhaps initiated by a "virus," has now gone on too long, subtle blocks to recovery have developed, a reactive depression has evolved, and the patient now needs to get into a more active program of rehabilitation. Or, an infection, if there was one, readily results in an illness more severe or persistent than usual if it occurs at a time of any uncertainties or concerns about one's life situation; to get well the patient may now need to explore this aspect of the problem. Viewed either way, psychotherapy may well be helpful.

Psychogenic components are nearly always significant in chronic debilitating fatigue with no clear evidence of organic disease. The "chronic fatigue syndrome" was defined mainly for heuristic and investigational purposes. It was not proposed as a substitute for careful evaluation of the patient, psychologically and otherwise. Chronic fatigue should not be diagnosed as an incurable viral infection or disease of unknown etiology. This is an easy way out of a difficult problem, but it is not fair to the patient. It is a demanding task for patients to look realistically at life situations that underlie the symptom, but that is their best hope for getting well.

Aching All Over

Pain in widespread areas of the body (nonarticular rheumatism, fibromyalgia), often with specific tender points, persisting for three to six months or many years, with no evidence of disease, is a common functional symptom. Disease is ruled out by a negative physical exam (except for the tender points and other signs of muscular tension) and by the laboratory survey, as recommended previously. Determining the sedimentation rate is particularly important, because polymyalgia rheumatica can closely resemble the nondisease myalgic state. A serum creatine kinase is usually added for evidence of muscular disease. Other tests may include rheumatoid factor, antinuclear antibodies, a Schirmer test for Sjögren's syndrome, and, if backache is a feature, lumbosacral spine X-rays. If any of these four tests are positive in a patient who has a diffuse pain syndrome but no specific signs of rheumatoid arthritis, lupus erythematosis, Sjögren's syndrome, or ankylosing spondylitis, the patient probably has a functional myalgia unrelated to the incipient or early disease state indicated by the positive test. Such tests, however, alert the physician to all possibilities in the evolving clinical picture.

Lyme Disease

About 80 percent of patients with untreated Lyme disease will experience rheumatic evidence of the disease:[172]

1. Intermittent short episodes of localized joint, periarticular, or musculoskeletal pain with no objective abnormalities, or
2. Intermittent transient attacks of frankly inflammatory arthritis of one or a very few joints at a time, most commonly in the knees, or
3. Both syndromes.

The rheumatic episodes occur more often during the course of the disease than do the neurologic, cardiac, or other cutaneous manifestations.[172, 173] Such episodes can appear shortly after erythema migrans (the initial lesion) and recur for six to eight years, but their frequency and duration diminish steadily after three years.[172]

The typical picture of fibromyalgia is not characteristic of Lyme disease. The two conditions can usually be distinguished readily. Whereas fibromyalgic pain is diffuse and persistent, month after month, the arthralgic/myalgic episodes of Lyme disease generally affect but one or two sites at a time, lasting only a few hours to days in a given location, though the pain may migrate to other sites. Episodes are often separated by months of remission. Symmetrical trigger points are not usually found. Nevertheless, such attacks and/or the migrating pains of Lyme radiculitis or polyneuropathy, often associated with paresthesias if not more definite sensory loss, also with complaints of weakness and fatigue, can be more persistent.[174–176] In this way they can indeed resemble the functional myalgic/fatigue syndromes. And many patients with Lyme disease cannot recall the history of a tick bite or erythema migrans, nor have they had other manifestations of the disease.

Overriding such concerns is the epidemiology: fibromyalgia is common, Lyme disease, rare, except in particular endemic areas. If, however, there is any question about the diagnosis, an enzyme-linked immunosorbent assay (ELISA) for immunoglobulin G specific antibodies is indicated. The levels are usually elevated within six to eight weeks after onset and remain elevated indefinitely in untreated patients with continued infection.[177] A negative test rules this out. In an equivocal case, a positive test should be validated by a Western blot assay to identify false-positive ELISA tests, which, especially at low titers, can be caused by several autoimmune, infectious, and other diseases, and are often found when large numbers of serologic tests are requested in areas with little Lyme disease. Positive results of both assays provide strong diagnostic support for Lyme disease. The disease is unlikely, however, in patients with a positive ELISA but a negative Western blot assay; in one study of such patients, 91 percent had evidence of another condition, organic or psychiatric, to account for their clinical manifestations.[178]

It was noted in the long-term study cited above, describing the course of untreated infection after erythema migrans, that 20 percent of the patients remain asymptomatic for years.[172] Other serologic surveys of small endemic communities show that from one-third to almost one-half of those with positive tests are asymptomatic.[179, 180] In a similar survey of 964 random subjects in a Swiss community, only two of the 21 with very high Ig G titers had symptoms of Lyme disease.[181] Thus, even in patients who have the disease, atypical symptoms may be due to something else altogether.

Of 100 patients examined in a Lyme disease center, for example, 25 had fibromyalgia but were referred mainly because they had been found to be seropositive.[182] The ELISA titers were not reported, however, nor were the results verified by Western blot. Because there was no clinical response to antibiotic therapy in any of the fibromyalgia patients, the serology was presumably false positive in most cases, or, in some, the fibromyalgia could have developed coincidental to an asymptomatic Borrelia infection. Unless ELISA and Western blot are both distinctly positive in untreated patients, widespread persistent myalgia, fatigue, and other symptoms characteristic of functional syndromes, present for longer than three months, in the absence of inflammatory arthritis, any signs of neuropathy, or other objective signs of disease, are probably not due to Lyme disease.

The many aspects of this whole problem are discussed in the recent reviews of Steere [183] and Rahn and Malawista.[184]

The Nature of Fibromyalgia

The usual symptom complex, or "syndrome," has been delineated in many ways by rheumatologists.[185–190] Fortunately, the old term, *fibrositis*, a misnomer because no inflammatory process was ever confirmed,[191] has been replaced by the descriptive term *fibromyalgia*.[192] It is useful to have a name for every functional syndrome, for communicating both with patients and with other doctors. "Fibromyalgia" is a good name for the kind of diffuse pain described here.

Naming can be a problem, however, as we have seen. As the definition is restricted (for heuristic, descriptive, investigational, and communicative purposes) to subsets of the symptom complex—here, the subset of diffuse pain with a designated number of specific tender points and other biological concomitants—its meaning shifts accordingly to indicate a certain pathophysiologic insight.[193] Finally, the name, as used by an organically focused clinician to indicate a biological entity, perhaps even a "disease of unknown etiology," serves as a substitute for understanding the person with a functional disorder. This was not the intent of the major investigators who defined fibromyalgia; they were well aware of its usual psychogenic background. The transformation of emphasis takes place in practice, nonetheless.

Fibromyalgia is recognized by the diffuse pain and the diagnostic tender points, usually associated with fatigue, morning stiffness, and disturbed sleep. The association with fatigue is striking. In a recent series of 50 patients diagnosed as primary fibromyalgia in an academic rheumatology practice, 48 complained of fatigue, and 33 were never free of it.[194] Note that fatigue is a cardinal symptom of fibromyalgia,[190] just as myalgia is a major criterion for chronic fatigue syndrome.[195] Thus patients who complain primarily of fatigue are often diagnosed as "CFS," and the myalgia is listed as a secondary symptom, whereas patients who complain primarily of pain are referred to rheumatologists, who diagnose "fibromyalgia" and list the fatigue as a secondary symptom. Moreover, patients diagnosed as fibromyalgia cannot be distinguished from those diagnosed as CFS by most of the other ten symptom criteria for CFS.[194] Fibromyalgia is also frequently associated with headaches, irritable-bowel syndrome, anxiety and stress, and vague neurovascular symptoms such as coldness, mottled skin color, and paresthesias.

These data speak for themselves. It is clear that fibromyalgia is indeed a functional syndrome, often inseparable from other functional syndromes. Therefore, the source lies somewhere in the personal life of the patient. It is not an enigmatic "disease," nor is it as specific a syndrome as has been implied in rheumatology. It is enigmatic only in the sense that it may be difficult to sort out the many psychosocial and physical elements that are relevant, as in most functional or psychiatric disorders. Let us explore the problem from two points of view.

The Physical Basis: What Causes the Pain and Tenderness?

Though the mechanism is not clear, the process is basically physiologic, though somatoform features readily creep into the ultimate clinical picture. The physiologic basis of the pain is indicated by its variability in intensity and distribution, its incitement by many kinds of disturbance (climatic, sleep, psychic and physical stress, etc.), its interrelationships with other psychophysiologic symptoms, and the tender points.

Most likely, the pain is related to muscle tension, the physiologic readiness for action of so many emotional reactions. Patients often "relax poorly during examination, with spasmodic, inappropriate muscle contractions interrupting active and passive motion."[196] Many patients note cramps and tremors.[197] Usually, muscle tension cannot be demonstrated by EMG in fibromyalgia patients at rest,[198, 199] though it *can* be demonstrated, in contrast to controls, by specific maneuvers.[197, 200–202] Some patients are much improved in EMG-biofeedback training.[203] The most striking observations were those of Holmes and Wolff, who demonstrated widespread muscle tension induced by interviews that engendered the underlying emotions in 75 subjects with backache.[204] Unfortunately, such observations, directed to the core of the problem, have not been repeated, nor have they been made in patients with fibromyalgia.

Are the designated tender points specific? Yes, more or less; they are found much less often in other conditions.[205] Thus, the tender points constitute a marker for the psychophysiology of fibromyalgia, just as respiratory alkalosis constitutes a marker for hyperventilation syndrome. But if the diagnosis of fibromyalgia is restricted to patients with a certain number of tender points, as it is,[192] then how do we designate the many patients with diffuse pain but no tender points (or too few to fit the definition), or with tender points but very little if any diffuse pain? [206] The clinician must address the problem of all patients with diffuse pain, regardless of the tender point count.

Some patients appear to be prone to fibromyalgia. This means only that they are more likely to respond to a variety of stresses with diffuse muscle tension than they are with headaches or some other reaction. The process can be initiated by physical as well as psychosocial stress. This is particularly true for the fibromuscular system, which is so subject to the wear and tear of daily life. Thus, an unusual diffusion of pain can follow in the wake of back, neck, or shoulder strain, tendinitis, bursitis, or other localized myofascial pain syndromes. The pain of "fibromyalgia" is usually diffuse, predominantly truncal but also involving the extremities. Vulnerable patients, however, often give a history of multiple pain episodes at different sites, unusually prolonged and complicated, though each was diagnosed by the conventional medical name for pain at that site. Diffuse myalgia can also complicate the otherwise localized pain of rheumatoid arthritis or other diseases. It is then known as secondary fibromyalgia.

Many patients "ache all over" as the major symptom of physiologic fatigue induced by overextended physical or mental exertion. Smythe describes a "fibrositic" personality: patients who "set high standards and are as demanding of themselves as of others. They are caring, honest, tidy, moral, industrious . . . effective in their chosen field of activity."[196] Such patients drive themselves, find it difficult to recognize their limits, and cannot understand why they ache all over (or get migraine or some other symptom) when they are so well and have so much to do. In this situation the myalgia can be regarded as the physical expression of exhaustion; the patients are not anxious or depressed, nor do they feel emotionally disturbed in any other way. There are, of course, many other patients whose myalgia is caused more directly by nervous tension.

Regardless of the source of myalgia, a series of vicious circles are established. Muscular tension causes pain. Pain causes muscular tension, nature's protective device to contain the injury. The increased tension in turn causes more pain, and so on, with nervous tension bound to the whole process as both cause and effect.

Meanwhile the patient suffers from the nonrestorative, alpha-delta, non-REM sleep disorder found in most patients with fibromyalgia,[187] and also in many other conditions in which sleep studies have been done.[207–209] When it occurs, or is induced in healthy subjects, it usually results in the very symptoms that characterize fibromyalgia. Moldofsky: "This disturbance in sleep physiology could have been triggered in our patients by their traumatic or emotionally disturbing situations. The subsequent fatigue, irritability, depression, anxiety, and musculoskeletal aching and stiffness would become incorporated in a vicious, self-perpetuating, nonrestorative sleep cycle."[187]

The complex physical basis of fibromyalgia is complicated further by the superimposition of somatoform factors. The syndrome often evolves, for example, after a minor automobile or industrial accident, and does not abate until the litigation is settled. Or it evolves in a setting of insoluble domestic or other difficulties. The secondary gains are apparent. The constancy and strange distribution of the pain in somatoform regional pain disorders (see Diane B. and Rosetta C. in Ch. 14) usually serves to distinguish somatoform pain from the physiologic pain of fibromyalgia. But when pain is "all over" and similarly constant, rather than variable, as is usual in fibromyalgia, it may be difficult to separate the two aspects of the syndrome. Of the 400 consecutive patients in my clinic survey, 31 (8 percent) had diffuse pain syndromes without disease. In 20 of these 31 patients, the somatoform aspects of the illness appeared to outweigh the physiological. In eight of the 20, there were so many other symptoms that the illness fit the definition of somatization disorder, but the diffuse myalgia, viewed apart from the other symptoms, would be diagnosed as fibromyalgia. The findings in this survey are not representative of primary practice, but they do indicate how difficult it can be in some patients to separate the somatoform from the physiological elements of what is usually called fibromyalgia.

The Psychosocial Basis

The psychosocial basis for fibromyalgia has been emphasized by virtually all of its major investigators, as well as by those who have explored this particular question at greater depth.[185, 186, 210–212] The kinds of underlying personal problems are manifold. In the subgroup characterized as "fibrositic" personality,[196] and in many other situations, excessive stress or overexertion, if not an emotional disturbance, simply exceeds what is comfortably tolerable. In other patients the emotional basis will become apparent only by a careful exploration of the setting of the illness in relation to the patient's personality and life situation as a whole.

In the modern era of DSM categories and biological psychiatry, there appears to be more interest in "diagnosis" than in understanding persons. Thus, a rash of recent papers have reported studies of fibromyalgia patients with rating scales designed to disclose anxiety, depression, other psychiatric disorders, or personality variants. As described above, however, many patients are not hypochondriacal, depressed, or hysterical (as measured on MMPI scales), nor do they fit any DSM category, except for "psychological factors affecting physical condition" that are not disclosed by the scales used. Thus many patients will be "normal" when tested in this way. Nevertheless, most of these studies do disclose a higher prevalence of measurable psychiatric or personality disorders in the patients than in the controls.[213–216] In the only study that failed to show such correlations, the subjects were nonpatients discovered by questionnaire.[217] As discussed previously, this does not rule out causative personal factors in these subjects; it means only that they accept the symptoms as intrinsic to their life situation. When the emotional or physical distress exceeds their tolerance, they are likely to seek medical attention.

Chronic Recurrent Headaches

By the age of 13, from two-thirds to four-fifths of all children experience headaches.[218, 219] The ubiquity of headaches in adult life was noted previously (Ch. 4), as was the frequency (95 percent) of "tension headaches" and/ or migraine as the diagnosis for the chronic recurrent headaches of patients examined in headache clinics. Because chronic headaches, unlike many other common symptoms, are predominantly functional syndromes of one type or the other, or both, physicians in primary care are familiar with the problem, and the diagnosis is rarely enigmatic or controversial. The headache types, and the differential diagnosis in relation to the many organic pathologies that cause headaches, are well described in standard textbooks, and will not be repeated here.

The Type of Headache

Because specific biotherapy can be effective both in preventing and in treating migraine, it is important to recognize the classic, common, and other forms it takes. Nevertheless, migraine as the main type of headache is noted in fewer than 15 percent of children with headaches, [218, 219] and, of adults in treatment for headache, less than 30 percent [220–221] Most headaches, both in children and adults, are of nonmigrainous or mixed type.

Many recent studies cast doubt on the vascular constriction/dilatation hypothesis as the sole mechanism of migraine, [222] also on muscular contraction as the main characteristic of what is usually called "tension" headache.[223] These dysfunctions are often mixed in either type, and other electrophysiologic and neurotransmitter mechanisms have been proposed. Thus most chronic headaches can be viewed as the result of several mechanisms that combine to cause the pain but defy precise classification.[224, 225]

The headaches of anxiety and depression are not unique; they presumably result from the same physiological disturbances that can be precipitated by any kind of personal distress. Headaches are not often somatoform, but this can be suspected by the constancy and other aspects of a headache in conjunction with the function it serves for the patient. Most headaches are physiological disturbances that serve no such function.

Precipitating Factors

Migraine attacks can sometimes be precipitated by, or related in part to, menstruation, oral contraception, alcohol, exercise, vasoactive drugs, mountain sickness, tyramine-containing foods or wine, other kinds of reactions to certain foods such as chocolate, and, rarely, milk or wheat allergy.

Most common and most important, however, both in migraine and in nonmigrainous or mixed-type headaches, is the background of stress of some kind. This may simply be the fatigue of prolonged mental and/or physical exertion with inadequate rest, sleep, or recreation but no particular emotional distress. Or it may be an emotional disturbance in the absence of any fatigue from overdoing, or perhaps both kinds of stress are combined. The emotional disturbance may involve a crisis, or it may be related to a long-term state of anxiety, depression, or other forms of nervous tension. The immediate source of distress could be interpersonal conflict, a grief reaction, an existential quandary, or any of the problem areas outlined in Chapter 17.

"Perfectionistic" personality characteristics have been ascribed to migraine, but most headaches are of mixed type, and, even at the poles of this spectrum, I do not believe that there is a "migraine personality" not found with "tension headaches," nor any kind of "tension" not found in migraine. The nature of most psychophysiologic reactions is determined more by the patient's biological proclivity for that type of response than by the nature of the stress that induced it.

Migraine attacks can appear without any apparent provocation whatsoever, either immediately prior to the attacks or in the preceding week or two. This does not mean, however, that a problem situation of some kind is not a factor in many or most of the patient's headaches. The "stress" may be a steady state but subtle: a bit too much pressure at work, a half-hour too little sleep, two glasses of wine at supper instead of one. All this seems perfectly normal. But if the patient's propensity for migraine is sufficiently reactive, it may be enough. And, though the mechanism is unknown, the headache often does not evolve until the biological forces that are activated in response to stress are released, as on a Sunday morning.

A superb discussion of the clinician's approach to the personal situations that result in headache is that of Adler, Adler, and Packard.[226] In this book, Chapter 8, "Evaluating the Psychological Factors in Headache," is recommended as a model for the interview of patients with any functional disorder.

Organic Disease

If the patient's repetitive headaches began in childhood or early life and appear again and again in a characteristic pattern of migraine, muscle-contraction, or mixed-type headache without evidence of disease, the diagnosis is usually clear. Although the physician may feel compelled to order special procedures to rule out intracranial disease, such a workup is not really indicated or necessary.[227, 228] A meticulous history and physical is indicated, of course, with special attention to the neurologic exam (including the optic disks and cranial nerves) and to the possibility of systemic disease or disease of the neck, ears, eyes, nose, and paranasal sinuses. My personal experience, however, is that disease of these structures rarely simulates the more diffuse pain of migraine or mixed headaches. Sinus pain is rare in the absence of a respiratory-tract infection or allergic rhinitis. I have seen two such patients, however, with attacks of frontal sinus pain simulating migraine, one with a deviated septum, the other with a vasomotor response to cold wind exposure.

When intracranial disease is suspected, an MRI is the procedure of choice.[229] Skull X-rays and EEG are no longer regarded as components of the workup for chronic headache in the absence of special indications such as trauma or the question of a convulsive state. An MRI will pick up most aneurysms and arteriovenous malformations, and cerebral angiography would rarely be necessary. The use of lumbar puncture in acute or subacute headaches to detect meningitis, encephalitis, or subarachnoid hemorrhage is well established but would rarely apply to the investigation of chronic recurrent headaches without a specific indication.

In chronic headache, intracranial or systemic disease should be suspected in the following circumstances:

1. Headaches of recent onset are more or less continuous and become increasingly severe, at any age. Most ominous would be their initial appearance after the age of 35. Or, the long-term pattern of recurrent headaches has recently changed to one of greater intensity and frequency. A constant, unremitting headache is always of concern, though it may be found to be an unusually severe mixed-type headache, or somatoform.

2. A sudden, severe, and unusual headache occurs during the course of chronic headaches. This may well turn out to be a particularly severe migraine attack, but the diagnostic considerations should include onset of organic disease.

3. The headaches have begun to appear with exertion, to awaken the patient at night, or to be induced by coughing, bending over, straining, lifting, or sex. Such symptoms, though quite common in migraine, may also indicate increased intracranial pressure. Unilateral headaches that *always* occur on the same side should also be investigated, though this too can occur in migraine.

4. Any other indication of organic disease is noted. Of particular importance: even minimal optic edema, hemorrhages, or exudates; any signs or symptoms of neurological disease or history of a possible convulsive epi-

sode; a history of cancer or trauma; abnormal vital signs, especially fever, hypertension, or wide pulse pressure; any question of neck stiffness; the patient is drowsy, confused, looks ill, suffers a memory loss or other deterioration in intellectual functioning; or the headaches are associated with persistent or episodic but distinct personality change.

Temporal arteritis should be considered in every elderly person who develops headaches, regardless of their site, quality, severity, or time pattern.[230] The sedimentation rate is characteristically elevated.

Transient visual field defects and, rarely, vertigo, unilateral sensory or motor deficits including hemiparesis and paresthesias, speech disturbance, or cranial nerve impairment can precede or accompany the headache of migraine. Patients with such phenomena, except those with the characteristic transient visual scotomata, should be studied, especially if the dysfunction persists.

Nervous Tension

Adrenergic discharge, hyperventilation syndrome, muscular tension and tremor, headaches, functional GI distress, easy fatigability, insomnia, and/or apprehension and irritability are the common physiologic expressions of emotional distress that anyone can experience if sufficiently disturbed. When multiple symptoms of this kind appear concurrently, they are readily recognized as expressions of nervous tension. Obviously, the physician must consider the differential diagnosis of nervous states, reviewed briefly in this section, but the characteristic picture of multisymptomatic anxiety is rarely mimicked by organic states.

Drug Effects

An exception to the above generalization is the effect of drugs. The use and abuse of, or dependency on, psychoactive agents, alcohol, nicotine, and caffeine, most commonly, or amphetamines, cocaine, and other stimulants or psychedelics, can result in nervous states. And withdrawal, especially from alcohol, barbiturates, benzodiazapines, or opiates, usually results in profound disturbances. Nervous tension may, of course, be the cause as well as the result of the use, as with alcohol, smoking, and coffee dependencies. The patient is caught in a vicious circle. From 20 to 30 percent of American adults, for example, consume more than an intoxicating daily dose of caffeine (500 mg), in coffee, tea, colas, cocoa, and/or certain over-the-counter medications.[231] This may be at least one factor in a nervous state. And certain prescribed medications,[232] particularly prednisone at high doses,[233, 234] can cause mental disturbances.

A careful query about alcohol (as outlined previously), smoking, caffeine, street drugs, and all medications, whether prescribed or over-the-counter, is essential.

Endocrine/Metabolic Disorders

The possibility of such disorders should be considered in any anxious or depressed patient. The history, physical examination, overall picture of the illness, and the laboratory screen recommended in the introduction to this chapter, including T4 and TSH, plus electrolytes, would provide the necessary data to rule out most of the more common conditions.

In my experience, however, endocrine diseases are not often confused with nervous disorders. The clinician must keep in mind that almost half of the patients with new illnesses in primary care have an underlying nervous state of one kind or another.[235] When such patients are found to have en-docrine disease, the correlation is often coincidental.

Thyrotoxicosis is readily distinguished from anxiety by physical exam and laboratory confirmation. Even in the absence of a palpable thyroid or early prominence of the eyes, the patient's warmth, particularly of the hands, as opposed to the usually cool vasoconstriction of anxiety, may suggest the di-agnosis. Subjects with mild hypothyroidism detected by surveys of TSH are generally asymptomatic.[236] If a patient with "fatigue" is found to have mild hypothyroidism, recall that about one-third of adult patients, regardless of the chief complaint, also feel tired; the fatigue is probably not caused by the thy-roid deficiency. Patients with *overt myxedema* may be slow, methodical, lack-ing animation, but they rarely complain of fatigue, though they will confirm a low energy level if asked about it. And rarely do they feel or act depressed, though the TSH should be checked in any depressed patient.

Hypoparathyroidism, though rare, can cause muscular and abdominal cramps, irritability, anxiety, and other personality and mental disturbances. Hyperparathyroidism is a dubious cause of fatigue or nervous tension. In any event, either condition would be indicated by the abnormal calcium level on the screening panel.

Adrenal cortical disease would require special testing. *Cushing's syndrome*, which is occasionally associated with mental symptoms ranging from mood lability to psychosis, would usually be evident from the characteristic physical signs and symptoms. *Addison's disease*, though rare, should be considered in the differential diagnosis of weakness and fatigue. Its presence would often be suggested by pigmentation (not always present), hypotension, a small heart, asthenia, and/or electrolyte abnormalities.

I have encountered one healthy-appearing normotensive woman whose paroxysmal symptoms at times of stress resembled those of panic attacks, though without the usual fear or apprehension.[237] She proved to have a *pheochromocytoma*, but her blood pressure was normal on several consecutive visits, and hypertension was not noted until she got to an emergency room during an attack. The urinary VMA, however, was elevated at all times. Though it is not customary practice, pheochromocytoma, though rare, should be ruled out in what appear to be anxiety states, especially discrete panic attacks, unless it can be ascertained that the blood pressure is consistently normal while symptoms are active.

Premenstrual tension syndrome is usually diagnosed when nervous and other symptoms appear only during the late luteal or premenstrual phase of the cycle. The interactions of endocrine fluctuations and emotional stress that may come to bear at this time are controversial, and presumably vary from subject to subject. A comprehensive approach, embracing both the physical and psychological factors that may play a role, is appropriate, as with any illness.

Many endocrine diseases are described as simulating nervous states. Such assumptions are often untenable. It is said, for example, that autoimmune thyroiditis is characterized by sudden fluctuations in circulating thyroid hormones that upset the patient's emotional balance, causing overwhelming anxiety coupled with significant depression, or that hyperparathyroidism is associated with severe anxiety in most cases.[238] But a review of the data cited show that such conclusions were not substantiated, the mental disorders described were obviously coincidental,[239] or the report represented a typical example of ascertainment bias.[240] This occurs if the clinical focus is an endocrine disorder, from which the few patients with mental symptoms are segregated and reported, or if the focus is a mental disorder, from which the few patients with an endocrine disorder are segregated and reported. The clinician should be careful to avoid inappropriate correlations of this kind whenever an endocrine disorder, or any other disease, is associated with nervous symptoms which, though common everywhere, rarely characterize the disease detected.

Actually, studies of subjects with autoimmune thyroiditis detected by screening surveys of a nonpatient population show that most are asymptomatic, and their thyroid function is generally stable from year to year, though clinical hypothyroidism evolves slowly at a rate of about 5 percent a year in women who initially had elevated concentrations of both TSH and thyroid antibodies.[241] In another study, specific thyroid antibodies were found in 16 percent of elderly women without clinical evidence of thyroid disease.[242] And, in a random necropsy series, focal thyroiditis was present in 19 percent of the males and 45 percent of the females.[243] Asymptomatic disease is the rule, not the exception.

Similarly, most patients with hyperparathyroidism, detected by screening surveys of clinic patients, are asymptomatic, even with calcium concentrations > 12 mg%.[244] Other observers have suggested, however, that when the non-specific fatigue and nervous irritability of patients appears alleviated by excision of the parathyroid adenoma, such symptoms must, therefore, have been related to the hypercalcemia.[245] Such an inference, however, is tenuous unless substantiated by long-term follow-up. One keeps in mind that nervous symptoms not only are common but often abate when, like psychogenic pelvic pain, they are diagnosed and treated as though caused by disease. When the magic of naming wears off, the symptoms often reappear.

Frontal and Temporal Lobe Lesions, and Temporal Lobe Epilepsy

In primary care, patients with the complex partial seizures originating from the limbic temporal lobe area, or with the psychiatric manifestations of frontal and temporal lobe lesions, or both, are rare. And the bizarre symptoms rarely simulate the usual spectrum of anxiety or depressive reactions. I have encountered just two patients. The interested reader is referred to the excellent descriptions in the texts of Benson and Blumer.[246]

Nevertheless, the clinician should be aware that unusual, often episodic, changes of personality or behavior, intensified or fixed emotional responses, apathy or indifference to life events or sexuality, memory impairment, or psychotic ideation can constitute the only symptoms of such conditions, in the absence of more obvious neurologic deficits, intracranial disease, or a convulsive episode.

Temporal lobe epilepsy is characterized by the sudden arrest of ongoing activities associated with a stereotyped sequence of strange psychic experiences and/or behavior lasting seconds to a minute and a half. The episode may include focal motor, somatosensory, autonomic, or mental phenomena, or hallucinatory visual, auditory, olfactory, or gustatory sensations. The passive experience is unrelated to the environment, and the patient is out of contact during the episode. The patient may recall some aspect of a very brief aura but is amnesic for the central behavioral, muscular, and autonomic ictal events and the postictal confusion, which persists for about two to ten minutes. Therefore, the patient may or may not be aware of, or report, some kind of a lapse in consciousness. If there is any question about this, an observer should be interviewed, and EEG, MRI, and neurological consultation considered.

The Hyperdynamic Beta-Adrenergic Circulatory State

The adrenergic discharge has been described in this way, as though it were a primary fault of the autonomic nervous system or its receptors,[247] though there are no data to suggest a premorbid abnormality. In no way is this a problem for differential diagnosis. The terminology provides nothing but a physiological description of the adrenergic expressions of anxiety. Mary S. (Ch. 3) had such a hyperdynamic circulatory state, or, if viewed psychiatrically instead of biologically, it would be classed as panic disorder; from either point of view, however, the condition was the result, not the cause, of her personal distress.

The Problem of the Isolated Symptom

Now let us turn to the main problem in the diagnosis of nervous disorders: the patient who does not feel nervous or depressed and complains of only one or two physical symptoms that resemble those caused by disease.

If, for example, a nervous-appearing patient complains of many typically nervous symptoms—heart pounds, can't breathe, dizzy, no energy, etc.—the possibility of a nervous state is obvious, and it is not necessary to think through the theoretically possible differential diagnosis of each individual symptom. But if the "pounding" of the heart, perhaps irregular though the patient is not sure, is the sole symptom, and the current exam is negative, the sinus tachycardia of emotion cannot be distinguished from premature beats or a pathological arrhythmia from the history alone. A Holter monitor or other studies may well be necessary, and a precise diagnosis is essential. I have seen many patients whose isolated complaint and denial of nervous tension suggested a paroxysmal tachyarrhythmia, and, sure enough, when this was finally demonstrated, specific treatment could be applied. In other patients with the same complaint, however, healing was possible only when the symptom was identified as the sinus tachycardia of adrenergic discharge and its source elicited—in one man, for example, a sexually frustrating problem with his wife. Once again, until you know what is really going on, you don't know what to do.

Let us briefly review here the cardinal physiological expressions of nervous tension (anxiety and/or depression), any one of which may appear to be the sole or dominant symptom:

heart pounds	no energy, tired all the time
can't breathe	feels tense and trembles
dizzy	no appetite, weight loss
faint	upset stomach, nausea
numbness or tingling	insomnia, or sleepy all the time
chest pain	restless, irritable, keyed up, on edge
aches and pains	can't think clearly, concentrate

As we saw in a study cited previously,[248] an organic basis for most of these symptoms can be established in only about one of six patients. Nevertheless, when the symptom is the only expression of distress, the possibility of disease must be considered, in each case. The differential diagnosis for each symptom is beyond the scope of this discussion. If, however, the clinician considers the possibility of a functional disorder as the history unfolds, in conjunction with whatever workup is deemed necessary, the true nature of the illness can usually be recognized readily, as with Joseph's dizziness (Ch. 1). These kinds of questions should run through the clinician's mind:

1. Is the chief complaint really the only symptom? Are there perhaps other symptoms, though less prominent, that suggest a nervous disorder?
2. Does the patient appear to be tense, distracted, withdrawn, tangential, disturbed in some way, though denying feelings of emotional distress? Is the symptom described as you would expect it to be if caused by a coincidental disease process in an emotionally healthy person?
3. Could the symptoms be associated in some way, though not precisely in time and place, with any kind of stressful situations or events?

If neither the diagnosis nor the personal background of the illness is clear, and the physician does not use a health-history questionnaire that includes a mood category, it may be helpful at some point to have the patient complete a standardized inventory of the emotional states that characterize depression and anxiety, as will be described in Chapter 14.

Problem Drinking

About 13 percent of all U.S. adults have experienced alcohol abuse or dependence at some time in their lives; 3 percent suffer such problems at any one time, or 5 percent during a period of six months.[249] Because problem drinking causes, accentuates, or interlocks with so many clinical disorders in both the subjects and their families, the incidence of problem drinking will be found greater in patient populations than in the public at large. In surveys of adults in primary care, it is reported that from 19 to 36 percent meet criteria for a past alcohol abuse or dependence disorder, and from 5 to 12 percent are so afflicted at any one time.[250–253]

We are trained to recognize alcoholism as the cause of alcoholic disease: syndromes of chronic use, intoxication, and withdrawal; alcoholic disease of the liver, pancreas, and central and peripheral nervous systems; cardiomyopathy; and fetal alcohol syndrome.

What is more likely to be overlooked is alcohol as a major factor in, if not the cause of, many functional, behavioral, and psychiatric disorders, not just in the subject who drinks, but often in the spouse or children who appear as "identified patients" in the troubled family. Also overlooked may be alcohol as the main problem in accidents, sexual and physical abuse, and hypertension, or as aggravating the severity of illnesses caused by diseases other than those more directly related to alcohol. It is imperative to recognize alcohol overuse as a barrier to recovery in any condition. Treating the physical or emotional symptoms of anxiety or depression, for example, with psychoactive drugs, or even with psychotherapeutic interviews, will accomplish little or nothing if alcohol dependency persists and is not recognized as the patient's established route of escape. To make matters worse, the patient may infer that if the alcohol is not talked about, it cannot be such a problem. Or the patient believes that the first order of business is the medical or psychotherapeutic resolution of ongoing physical or emotional problems, rather than the alcohol dependency per se.

Over and above all these considerations is the personal and familial devastation that goes on and on, though it does not surface as clinical complaints. Clearly, this is an overwhelming problem for all concerned, and a major problem for medical practice.

Clark and McIntyre have delineated the essence of the disease in an exceptionally informative and compassionate discussion [254] that should be read by every health professional. The core problem is an imperceptible evolution, often over years, with less and less healthy drinking patterns increasingly associated with ever greater loss of control. Defensive strategies and psychological blocks, some conscious, some unconscious, limit the person's capacity to perceive what has happened. It is difficult for physicians, counselors, and family members to understand how complete and impenetrable these blocks can be. Therefore, both diagnosis and an effective therapeutic liaison can be difficult.

Recovery, of course, begins with a recognition and affirmation of the alcohol problem. Fortunately, several techniques for screening interviews, validated in careful studies, have been developed in recent years, and they are far more effective than asking patients how much they drink.[253–255] As I read the current literature, I am appalled to reflect on the generally inadequate training for this problem that characterized medical education in the past, thus my own difficulties and those of many colleagues in recognizing alcohol dependence, especially in the absence of an associated alcoholic-disease condition. We did not know how to address the problem. If we did know, there were few effective treatment programs available for referral.

The brief discussion here is restricted to the CAGE screening test.[256] Regretfully, I have had no personal experience with this approach. The commentary is mainly that of Clark:[254] "Every patient should be asked if he drinks; if the answer is yes, one should proceed to the CAGE questions. *Do not* next inquire about pattern and amount of drinking, because this question provokes defensiveness, minimization, and lying, and augments the sense of guilt and shame." The CAGE questions:

Have you ever felt the need to .... Cut down on drinking
Have you ever felt .... Annoyed by criticisms of your drinking?
Have you ever had .... Guilty feelings about drinking?
Have you ever taken a morning .... Eye opener?

This approach opens the discussion. Positive responses lead to a more com-prehensive alcohol interview, as described in the article. Note that "How much do you drink?" implies an accusation of direct responsibility, whereas the CAGE questions lead into a disease-model approach. The implication is that many people drink. Some slide into trouble. Could this have happened? If so, perhaps we could explore the problem together? In other words, the CAGE questions, which assess the major issues, are less likely to trigger defen-siveness or evoke shame and low esteem. Even if the answers are negative, the questions may turn the problem drinker's attention to the core problem. Fo-cusing on the patient and his/her experience (Is this a problem for you?), rather than on alcohol and the act of drinking, fosters a partnership rather than an adversarial relationship.

This kind of interview sets the stage for the allied question: Do you use marijuana? Cocaine, amphetamines, or any other street drugs? If yes: Have you ever felt, or has anyone else ever felt, that this could be a problem for you?

Finally, because an addictive problem in one person may be the source of any number of nervous or behavioral disorders in the family constellation, any disturbed person should be asked about the other family members. Are there any concerns or adverse effects of their drinking patterns, drug use, or other behaviors?

Pseudoseizures

Somatoform pain disorders are by far the most common kind of "con-version" in medical practice today. Anesthesias, found unexpectedly on physi-cal exam, though not a complaint of the patient, are also common, but other conversions simulating neurological disease, such as pseudoseizures, paraly-ses, weakness, aphonia, coordination disturbances, and blindness, are rare. Because we are unfamiliar and often uncomfortable with such conditions, the correct diagnosis may be too long deferred, or an erroneous organic diagnosis may be established instead. Nevertheless, if at least the possibility of a conver-sion is considered, the nature of the illness can soon become apparent. The symptoms are unusual for the disease suspected, and, conversely, there is no clear disease basis for the symptoms, nor do they fit into any recognized ana-tomic or physiologic pattern. Then, if the setting of the illness is explored, it may be possible to perceive its function for the patient.

I will focus here on pseudoseizures, because they are often misdiagnosed as epilepsy. From 22 to 23 percent of the patients referred to epilepsy centers for confirmation and further characterization of seizure type do not have epilepsy.[257, 258] In Mattson's study, 40 percent of the nonepileptic attacks were pseudoseizures; the others were identified as problems of syncope, drug toxicity, and other psychiatric disorders, including hyperventilation syndrome, sleep disorders, movement disorders, and, occasionally, severe vascular headaches with confusion and erratic behavior. The differential diagnosis of syncope [259] and other disturbances of consciousness, with or without twitching or other limited motor components,[260, 261] is beyond the scope of this discussion. "Hysterical" seizures or pseudoseizures, however, most often mimic a frank convulsive episode, but they can usually be distinguished from epilepsy.

Though the pseudoseizure may superficially resemble a neurogenic convulsion, it does not "ring true" to an experienced observer. The patient, though detached and uncommunicative in an altered, dissociated state, does not appear to be strictly unconscious. Postural control in the sitting position may be maintained in spite of the twitching. Hyperventilation may be present, but breathing is not impaired by a spastic oropharynx. Some patients will moan or even talk during the attack, and some attacks can be terminated by suggestion. A grand mal convulsion usually evolves in a sterotypic tonic-clonic sequence lasting less than five minutes, not usually more than once a day, with a characteristic obtundation after each attack. Pseudoseizures rarely begin with a purely tonic phase. The jerky movements are often random, bizarre, sometimes pseudopurposive, and do not evolve in a pattern consistent with an expanding cerebral focus. The attacks often vary in length or pattern, sometimes lasting 10 to 15 minutes or longer, and recur, perhaps several times in a day. Even then there is little or no postepisodic drowsiness or confusion. Tongue biting, incontinence, and injury are unusual but do occur rarely. Pseudoseizures characteristically occur when the patient is awake, usually indoors, at home, in the presence of others, and often under special circumstances of stress. They will also occur during the medical examination, especially when the doctor's confirmation of a convulsive disorder or disability is expected, or its effect is to distract the doctor from the pursuit of the emotional source of other symptoms. The EEG is normal during the seizure and also between attacks, unless the pseudoseizures have followed in the wake of true epilepsy, which is not at all unusual.

If there is any question about the diagnosis, and there often is, especially if the seizures are not seen, the patient should be referred for consultation. If appropriate, extended EEG monitoring can be done simultaneously with videotape recording of the patient.[257, 262–265] This can often distinguish pseudoseizures from epilepsy or, if the latter, the type of seizure.

Clearly, it is of critical importance to make the correct diagnosis as soon as possible. Unfortunately, partly because we are poorly trained to recognize and work with "hysterical" seizures, and partly because these patients will accept a diagnosis of epilepsy far more readily than will true epileptics, patients sometimes go on for years on anticonvulsants without relief. Their illnesses are further complicated by the side effects of medication, and by the many life difficulties attendant to having "epilepsy." Of the 388 patients referred to one epilepsy unit, 34 had pseudoseizures; recognition of the true character of the attacks led to a positive approach to the core problem and improvement in 25.[257] Effective, empathic, psychotherapeutic management of this trying problem for both adults and children is well described in the two excellent texts cited above.[260, 261]

As a general internist, seeing many patients with functional disorders, I realize how difficult it may be to classify the symptoms in medical terminology. Is the myalgia the primary problem; the fatigue, secondary? Perhaps, but was it not the reverse with this patient six months ago? And what about the headaches? Does it make sense to diagnose tension headaches, a fatigue syndrome, and fibromyalgia in the same patient? Does it matter whether the symptoms are physiological or somatoform? Is not the nervous state now so obvious that the main diagnosis should be anxiety or depression, and the physical symptoms secondary?

Or should I just try to get to know this person and see what the real problem is?

Person-Centered Care

CHAPTER 14

Collaboration Begins:
The Medical History

*The medical history is a record of medical data and a study of the pa-
tient's illness experience. The latter should include (1) the symptoms—
all the symptoms, just as they are—and (2) those aspects of the patient's
personal situation that bear directly on the illness. We fail to elicit these
two cardinal features of the subjective database, however, if we question
patients from a premature and exclusive focus on disease. Doing so, our
diagnoses are often erroneous, and we are unable to formulate a comprehensive clinical judgment about the whole illness. The purpose of this
chapter is to suggest how history-taking can lead to the discovery of the
true nature of a clinical problem, whatever it may be.*

∾ "When someone is seeking," said Siddhartha, "it happens quite easily that
he only sees the thing that he is seeking . . . because he has a goal, because he
is obsessed with his goal. Seeking means: to have a goal; but finding means: to
be free, to be receptive."[1] This quotation from Hermann Hesse's *Siddhartha*
describes all too well the conventional medical history. The physician *seeks* to
identify the disease. That is the goal. Each disease has characteristic symptoms.
So the patient is questioned to see what disease the symptoms represent. Such
questioning often characterizes the entire history, from its very beginning.
Sometimes the same goal is pursued steadfastly for years. The goal is eventually achieved: the diseases are ruled "in" or "out."

Listening

In this kind of history-taking we hear the answers to our questions, but we are not listening. The questions are tuned to disease, not to the person, not even to the illness as it is. For many patients, therefore, we fail to *find* what is there. We do not understand the illness, and we err in our diagnosis. This can happen whenever we process the symptoms as indicators of disease, without listening carefully to the patient's concerns, or to the description of the whole illness in the patient's own words. "Finding means: to be free, to be receptive." *Seeking* instead of *finding*, as described by Siddhartha, is not what our best clinicians teach about history-taking.[2–13] It is, nevertheless, what actually happens in practice much too often:

> *Resident*: What's troubling you?
> *Patient*: I have this pain in my stomach (indicating with his hands the entire abdomen).
> *Resident*: Where is it?
> *Patient*: Pretty much all over.
> *Resident*: Is it here (pointing to the patient's epigastrium)?
> *Patient*: Yes, I feel pain there.
> *Resident*: When do you get it?
> *Patient*: A lot of the time.
> *Resident*: Before meals?
> *Patient*: Yes, before meals, but I get it any old time.

In this videotaped interview of a resident physician with a new patient, note that the doctor is not listening. He begins to structure the history with his second question, "Where is it?" The question may be open-ended in regard to location, but it cuts off the patient's own description. Henceforth, the patient will only answer questions. He will not be expected to participate in the interview in any other way. A better approach at this juncture would be to wait until the patient continues, or a simple encouragement such as "Tell me more about it." Instead, the doctor goes on to ask increasingly "closed-end" questions. At the end of the examination he diagnoses probable peptic ulcer disease and orders a GI series.

In this kind of interrogation the doctor cannot perceive that the patient, if not interrupted, is describing the typical symptoms of what he actually has, a functional bowel disorder. But that is not what the doctor wants to hear. He would prefer the patient to have a peptic ulcer, a straightforward organic disease he knows how to treat. Though he regards himself as objective and scientific, he manipulates the data to fit his concept of disease, but is not aware that he does so. He does not discover a pattern; he generates one. He cannot see that he has structured the history to fit the patient to the medical model, rather than the other way around. He makes little effort to know the person or the illness well enough to see how medical care, combined with his personal understanding of the whole problem, can be individualized to fit the needs of this particular patient.

The GI series was negative. Had it not been for a videotape review and interaction with his consultant, this doctor might then have diagnosed peptic disease anyway, or ordered more tests and X-rays.

Perhaps this is too flagrant an example of poor history-taking, but I don't think so. Major disease is our primary concern. Specific information is essential, and specific questions are sometimes the quickest way to get it. So that is what we do. Openness to what is there varies from doctor to doctor, but when pressed for time we all stop listening and start questioning soon after the patient begins to talk.

Ideally, patients should be encouraged to describe their illnesses and concerns fully, in their own words, before any questions are asked. Then, when more specific information is necessary, the transition from the most open-ended questions (What was the pain like? How did you feel?) to the more specific (Was it sharp or dull? Were you sad?) should be carefully graded so that the interviewer does not unwittingly shape and thereby misconstrue the answers.

The major purpose of our examination is to discover the true nature of a clinical problem, whatever it may be. To do this the clinician must listen carefully, be open to all possibilities, from the very beginning of the history, and elicit the symptoms, all of the symptoms, exactly as they are, without shaping them one way or the other. Although exceptions do occur, most illnesses have characteristic symptoms. When symptoms are vague, the chronology indefinite, the patient unable to provide a clear description, this does not mean that the patient is a "poor historian." It means only that the "uncharacteristic" symptoms do not fit the usual descriptions of organic disease. Actually, the patient's difficulty in describing the symptoms is quite characteristic of functional illness. Most of the time the symptoms—the facts as well as their "tone" or quality (Part II of this volume, on Symptoms)—provide an excellent, though tentative, guide to the kind of illness, and, therefore, to the information needed.

Taking the medical history provides the doctor a pivotal opportunity to elicit the relevant personal as well as biomedical data. The history is *the way* to learn about the *patient* and the *illness*, while the physical, laboratory, X-ray, and other special examinations delineate the *disease*. As outlined previously, the emphasis varies according to the kind of illness. No physician has unlimited time. We must focus on the central issues. If what emerges from the *present illness* is a characteristic story of organic disease or injury, we first get the information necessary to identify the disease. Knowing the patient may or may not be important, but that comes later. If what emerges suggests a functional or psychiatric disorder, or any illness with a reasonable possibility of significant personal components, then we can direct our attention accordingly. We can be alert to any verbal or emotional clues, "listening with the third ear," as Reik [14] puts it, and pick up on each opportunity to learn more. Indications about the specific life situation or associated emotions may surface at any time. The strategic moment to respond is whenever they appear. The patient's need to share is often most poignant at the first encounter. If not encouraged, or if actively squelched, patients get ever more mired in their own repression.

The history is far more than a method of acquiring information. It is the physician's opportunity to be creative, sensitive, responsive. After years of practice, filing medical data into the categories of a routine history over and over again is boring, whereas an imaginative interview can have meaning for the patient and be a stimulating experience for the physician.

The history is the crucial first step that determines whether the care will evolve into an effective collaboration, or into a prescribing doctor/compliant patient relationship, or something between. If collaboration is to evolve, it begins with the history itself, as it becomes a learning experience for the patient. Viewed in this way, the management of an illness is not deferred until the examination and workup are completed. It begins when the doctor first greets the patient and continues through every step thereafter.

If the physician is competent, interested in the patient as a person, and in the illness as well as the disease, communicates clearly, listens carefully and consistently, asks open-ended questions indicative of a desire to understand, and responds to the patient's concerns and emotions, the patient is encouraged to share, and responds accordingly. The sharing should be mutual. The physician needs to explain the medical approach, the probable nature of the illness, the purpose of the workup, what can and cannot be done medically, what the patient can do, and other salient features of their interaction.

If, however, the doctor is half listening, not open to all possibilities, not responsive to the personal aspects of the illness, and persists in a disease-oriented interrogation, the history and the entire doctor-patient relationship is soon polarized if the patient has a personal illness. The doctor has an agenda of disease; the patient is concerned about his or her life and illness. There may be little connection between the concerns of these two individuals. Though patients may not realize that their doctor has retreated into the medical model, they too respond accordingly, revealing less and less, learning little about themselves in relation to the illness.

Eventually, we must share with the patient our understanding about what is wrong and what each of us can do about it. This leads to a division of responsibility. It may be the patient who must bring about whatever changes are necessary to be well. The patient cannot begin to do this, however, until these issues have been clarified. Patients are best prepared to accept our interpretations about the personal source of an illness when they have discovered this for themselves, during the natural flow of the interviews.

Interviews are either nourishing or polarizing. They move steadily along whatever grooves they are nudged into. If a polarity develops during the history, and the doctor persists in a strictly disease-oriented, symptom-suppressive approach, it will become more and more difficult to reverse this path when the patient founders in the medical model. If the doctor feels that it is mandatory to rule out every conceivable organic disease before even considering the possibility of a personal illness, little effort will be made during the history or early encounters to understand either the person or the illness. Then, when the workup is finally completed and negative, it is too late to do so. Either the patient is reassured about the absence of disease; or a probable nervous basis for the illness is suggested; or the patient is referred to a psychiatrist. All of these paths are doomed to failure. The patient has lost confidence, regards the switch in tactics as a "put-down," and usually goes on to another doctor to find the elusive disease. If a better understanding is to be achieved, it must begin in the first encounter, or very soon thereafter. In the most effective interactions the facts and feelings speak for themselves, the essential understanding evolves steadily, and the summation at the end of the first visit, or in subsequent interviews, is *not* a confrontation.

The purpose of this chapter is to describe aspects of history-taking that lead to more accurate diagnosis and a more effective collaboration, especially when a realistic appreciation of the human side of the illness is necessary. The basic biomedical data must, of course, be obtained, but as we will see, the facts are often perceived in ways that lead us astray. I assume that the reader is already familiar with the basic principles of medical history-taking, as so well described by Morgan and Engel,[8, 9] for example, and these are not reviewed here.

In this chapter I describe my own experience, expecting that the reader will pick and choose or adapt the ideas to complement her own style with different patients. I do not pretend that I am able to apply these concepts in every situation, or that all patients respond. (To simplify the writing here I will refer to doctors as "she," patients as "he," except where otherwise specified.)

Meeting the Patient

First I introduce myself to the patient by full name, make sure I know the patient's full name and the names and relationships of anyone else present, and exchange briefly whatever friendly remarks seem appropriate from whatever I know about this person.

A relative or friend sometimes accompanies the patient in the consultation room, expecting to be present during the interview. As much is to be learned from such relationships, I usually proceed without asking anyone to leave, but first I ask the patient if it is his wish that the other(s) be present. The patient customarily agrees because he is bound into the relationship, whether it is nourishing or not. When alone with the patient, usually during the physical exam, I make it clear that I intend to relate directly to him, that I am not an agent of the other person(s), nor will I share confidences without previous discussion. But I use the initial opportunity to observe these persons together to understand the nature of their relationship. I note who does the talking, who dominates, how they react to one another, and try, in general, to be as sensitive to the relationship as I am to the patient when I am alone with him. The presence of these people together in the interview is often the key to the diagnosis. With children, one uses considerable discretion in moving between a direct and open relationship to the child and the legitimate concerns of the family unit.

Before beginning the history, I seek to clarify the setting: the general purpose of the visit, whether for consultation or for continuing care, how the patient came to be here, whether referred by a friend or health professional, what other doctors are presently involved, and related matters.

I believe it is important to ascertain the patient's expectations of the visit. Similarly, the patient will need to know our overall plan and the goals for our interaction. There are often major discrepancies between these two sets of assumptions that may not surface until later. The sooner these differences can be clarified, the better will be the relationship (Ch. 15).

Opening the Medical History

I seek to start with an open attitude about whatever may concern the patient, to listen and learn from the beginning. I often open the history with a simple statement: "Please tell me now your main *concern*, what it is that has prompted you to see a doctor." Alternatively, particularly in patients with a known chronic illness, as when referred for diagnostic consultation, the statement may take this form: "I'd like you now to begin by telling me *how you are feeling*." Note that these are here-and-now statements, not questions, identifying me, right now, as concerned about you, a person, your concerns or ill feelings, whatever they are. The present tense emphasizes the immediacy of the relationship. The intent is to start and continue ("tell me more about it") with open-ended statements that invite the patient to participate by setting a tone for sharing. I seek to avoid a premature interrogation by which the patient might perceive me solely as a scientist processing information, or worse, as a prosecuting attorney questioning the indicted.

Concerns, or *feelings,* are terms that include subjective states without excluding objective data. The patient can respond with, "I've been short of breath for three weeks, and my ankles are swollen," "I've turned yellow," or "I feel miserable, I cry all the time, and I don't know what's the matter with me." In short, these terms allow the patient to respond with a whole range of concerns or emotions, as well as the usual symptoms and objective observations of disease. In obvious acute disease or injury, the doctor will move more directly into the problem itself, but when the diagnosis is not yet clear it is more revealing to begin as above.

In medicine we seek to elicit the *chief complaint.* In general usage, however, "complain" has a pejorative connotation that in a way puts the patient in a demeaning role as complainer. Patients are better viewed as persons who have *concerns* about their health and seek advice. One need not "complain" to enter the medical relationship. So *complaint* is a term perhaps best avoided. Similarly, the terms *symptoms* and *present illness,* implying disease to most people, may also invoke the medical model prematurely. However put, we need to get across that we really do seek to understand the ill person. Avoiding medical jargon in this way may appear to be stretching my point, but it is important to see how the conventional history-taking process can insidiously block us from hearing what we need to hear.

> *Cynthia S., 27, was referred for evaluation of chronic neck pain that had disabled her for two years. In her doctor's referral letter, the neurosurgical and orthopedic consultation reports, and the resident physician's medical history, the neck pain was described in detail: its quality, intensity, radiation, what made it worse, what helped, etc.; X-rays, a myelogram, and many other studies had been negative.*
>
> *Then, when I met the patient to confirm the findings, I stated simply that I would like her to begin by telling us how she was feeling. She proceeded to do just that: she felt sick and ached all over, she trembled and felt dizzy, she was worried and fretful, she couldn't hold still, couldn't sleep, etc. This vivid description of agitation went on without interruption for two or three minutes. Finally, I asked, "Was there not something about a pain in your neck?" and she replied, "Oh yes, right here."*

Obviously, the neck pain was but one of many symptoms—*feelings*—that any physician should recognize as an expression of emotional tension. The diagnosis was clear from her response to the more open-ended request. Somehow, this whole symptom complex had been lost during the previous examinations as the neck pain was singled out as the *chief complaint*, then identified as the *present illness*, the focus for investigation and treatment. This is a common problem in practice. Innumerable case histories could be cited to illustrate how the questions of a conventional history serve as pigeonholes for sorting data but provide no perspective of the whole problem. The *present illness*, therefore, often fails to reflect the actual expressions of the very illness it is supposed to describe.

The "how you are feeling" overture may facilitate a deeper understanding from the outset. The patient sometimes responds, not just by a better account of the symptoms, but by expressing the underlying emotions directly. One patient started with a matter-of-fact statement, "My hands are cold and blue," then suddenly burst into tears and told of the impasse in her marriage.

If the patient responds with, "Do you mean how am I feeling right now?" or "How have I been feeling since I've been sick?" I reply with, "Why don't you start with now, and then tell me about how it developed." In this way I may learn of the person's feeling *about* the illness as well as the symptoms per se. The "feeling" statement allows a greater flexibility from which the interview can flow along whatever path seems appropriate.

The Symptoms: How Does the Patient Feel Sick?

The medical purpose of the *present illness* is to delineate the symptoms. Asking about symptoms, however, often elicits a misleading objective response. *Feeling* calls for a subjective response; we need to know primarily *how* the patient feels sick. This is not as easy as it sounds. We must keep this problem in mind constantly, or we may prematurely objectify a symptom before understanding what the patient really feels. This happened, for example, to Joseph (Ch. 1), whose dizzy feeling was objectified to vertigo, faintness, or disequilibrium; the correct diagnosis was not revealed until just *how* Joseph felt sick was clarified. This is a particular problem when patients have already converted how they feel into nouns (objects) with ambiguous meanings: *indigestion, constipation, heartburn, palpitation, insomnia, blurred vision, impotence, bruising,* many others. *Pain,* because it is perceived and described so differently, is especially difficult. Just what has the patient experienced?

Even worse is when patients substitute diagnostic names for subjective data. The patient says "flu" or "arthritis" when the actual experience is "I feel weak, tired, and achy," or "I hurt in my joints." Even the common term "gas" is a diagnosis, not a symptom. Reduced to the latter, it usually means, "I feel distressed in my belly as though I were distended." This feeling leads to the syndrome of repetitive belching induced by unconscious air swallowing. If we fail to perceive that the patient uses a *diagnosis* to describe a *symptom* we may fall into the same diagnostic error, and, though antiflatulents are prescribed, the patient may not improve until the symptom and the aerophagia are explained.

Other diagnostic terms that patients use in this way are *allergy, virus, sinus,* the *menopause* or *change of life, disk, hormone imbalance.* Such terms are seductive. They could explain the symptom if not describe it. Letting the term pass, without asking patients what they mean, avoids a possible argument. Sad, when inappropriate, because the patient remains stuck with the diagnosis, and nothing can change. The problem is reinforced if an erroneous diagnosis has been established medically. Any diagnostic phrase is readily fixed in the patient's mind when it serves as a convenient medical explanation for functional symptoms.

I was the doctor in this exchange:

Doctor: Tell me how you feel.
Patient: I was found to have hypoglycemia three years ago when my blood sugar fell to 42 on a glucose tolerance test.
Doctor: Yes, but tell me your symptoms at that time.
Patient: Are you a psychiatrist or something?

Creative Listening

Creative listening [15] means giving undivided attention to whatever happens, from moment to moment, remaining alert to every clue, every opportunity to learn more, to respond sensitively, seeking clarification of what the patient is trying to say. Nothing should slip by unheard, unseen, not understood. I maintain direct eye contact and make no notes during the *present illness* or other poignant moments of the history, though I usually record data during the *past history* and *review of systems.* The interview moves with the momentum of the moment when the patient indicates, ever so tentatively, some inkling of an inner meaning to the symptoms. Tapping into this gently by acknowledging what just happened, one seeks to encourage the flow of the patient's own process of sharing. Listening carefully is important in any part of the history, but particularly so in eliciting the human side of the illness. If at the end of the interview the clinician's tentative diagnosis is that of a functional or psychiatric illness, but no evidence has emerged so far about its personal or emotional basis, a more directed interview may be necessary (Chs. 16, 17), but the personal data are far more explicit when they emerge spontaneously. That is the purpose of creative listening.

> *Diane B., 45, was an intelligent married woman with a responsible secretarial job. Two years previously she noted a dull ache in the left pelvis with menorrhagia, and was found to have an enlarged uterus. Hysterectomy and left salpingectomy were performed for uterine fibroids and a small tubal cyst. The ovaries were normal. Two months later, pain reappeared in the right lower abdomen and soon became continuous, radiating into the right back at the same level, across the groin into the right thigh anteriorly, and finally on down into the front of the right leg and foot. During this time she was examined by specialists in gynecology, internal medicine, orthopedics, and neurosurgery, and underwent many studies, including repeated GI series with small-bowel studies, barium enemas, IV pyelograms, and a gall bladder visualization that showed several stones. A cholecystectomy performed one year after the hysterectomy had no effect on the pain. At this operation the ovaries were again found to be normal, as was the rest of the abdomen and pelvis. Nine months later a right adnexal mass was noted on pelvic exam and confirmed by pelvic pneumogram, and the right ovary, with a serous follicle cyst 4 cms. in diameter, and the remaining pelvic organs were removed. The pain continued. Because of nervous tension and marital difficulties she was referred to a psychiatrist, who began working with her personal problems, but he too remained baffled about the pain and referred her to the diagnostic clinic. She was taking Valium, codeine, and other medications.*

First, I reviewed the referral letters and other data with the medical student who was working with me at that time. I expressed the opinion that this might be a somatoform pain disorder, the most likely diagnosis when a pain is severe, continuous, and widespread in a seemingly healthy person with extensive negative workups. The operations may or may not have been appropriate for their respective indications, but the diseases found are often asymptomatic and probably had little or nothing to do with this patient's pain; also, the abdomen was found at surgery to be otherwise negative.

An important aspect of creative listening, perhaps more important than the technique of listening, is the attitude of the listener. We were open to all possibilities. If this pain was caused by an undetected organic disease, it was our responsibility to find it, but, if it was of psychogenic origin, we would have to move along other lines. I advised the student that interviews with patients like this can be difficult, that resistance to any interpretation other than organic disease might be anticipated, especially after two years of technical medical interventions. Ideally, however, the interview would move forward, and we could find a way to help this person.

We started by asking Diane to describe how she felt. She had difficulty doing so. Though disturbed, she was bright, verbal, open, pleading, desperate to communicate, and not uncomfortable with us. But words were insufficient, her descriptions labored and tortuous. We were prepared to respond to any clues about her inner world, but not until a few minutes into the description of the symptoms did occasional tangential remarks about her marriage or job first appear. Fortunately, it was not necessary to bring these out by questioning. Whatever she said was acknowledged immediately—that is the critical component of listening creatively—and she was invited to say more about her marriage or job, that being on her mind at the moment. She slowly seemed more secure with us. After a few more such exchanges, in which, each time, we learned a little more about her personal situation, we said that we could not be sure such matters had much to do with the feelings in her body, but they had emerged spontaneously while she described how she felt, and they might be related. Perhaps because of the previous exchanges, this triggered an unexpected reversal of her mindset. She affirmed that her personal problems might well have a lot to do with her symptoms. This statement led quickly to another, and another, and her tale of anguish then came forth with all the emotion that might have been anticipated from the intensity of the pain.

In brief, the problem involved a conflict of values between Diane and her husband. She saw him as overbearing, but at the same time she was passive and allowed herself to slip into the role of victim. Verbal communication with him was difficult. All in all, the transformation of the communication of distress into the more eloquent nonverbal expression of pain was understandable.

At the end of this interaction she appeared calm and relieved. The physical exam was again negative. We concluded with a straightforward statement that we thought the symptoms were mostly related to psychological stress. We explained the necessity for the operations, and how the discomfort of the conditions for which they were performed, plus the operative pain, had sensitized the area and fixed her body expression of distress in the regions around her pelvis. We suggested that she would slowly feel well as she dealt with the emerging values in her life, was more explicit about her personal needs, and found ways to be responsible for herself rather than feeling victimized.

She returned to work in a week. Three months later her psychiatrist informed us that the pain had disappeared, and that she was working through the problems that she had not faced before. Although many factors other than the interview itself contributed to the successful outcome in this case, it illustrates how careful listening can release understanding when the patient is ready or, more important, when the listening can facilitate the readiness.

Indications of the inner meaning of the illness may occur any time: in the *chief complaint*, during any part of the history or physical exam, as the patient leaves and walks out the door, during later visits, or after many years of care. They may appear emotionally or as a frank statement about personal problems, or they may take more the form of an indirect clue.

In a taped interview, during the *review of systems*, a patient, who has so far described only physical symptoms and diseases, suddenly interjects: "Sometimes I think maybe my nervous tension is the cause of all my troubles." In this case the patient is giving the gift of a diagnosis to the doctor. Most doctors would respond immediately. The resident did not. He went right on with the system review.

More commonly, the spontaneous clues are subtle, little more than a superficially innocuous remark. Examples:

> *Patient A:* "When did the pain begin? Three months ago *when I moved to California.*" Doctor, responding to the clue: "Why the move to California?" Patient: "My husband was transferred to the Palo Alto office. *I didn't want to move.*"

> *Patient B, during the system review:* "The headaches were bad *in my teens—I missed a lot of school.*" Doctor, responding to the clue: "Why so bad in the teens?" The patient's extended answer indicated how headaches were both a response to stress and the means for avoiding a problem.

> *Patient C, during the exam of the male genitalia:* "*That's an important part of the exam, isn't it?*" Doctor, responding to clue: "Why did you ask—are you concerned about something?" Patient: "Sometimes I don't think I'm normal."

In each case the exchange led to an understanding of the real core of the illness. Even if the answer is negative, the interviewer has indicated a concern, and the patient may respond on a subsequent visit, "Remember when you asked me about _____? Well, the truth is that _____."

Listening is difficult. Communication is difficult. Both require concentration and patience. The physician is used to the process; the patient is not. So it is the physician's responsibility to facilitate the process of sharing. To do this, she has certain inherent advantages. She has a broad perspective about illness and human nature, drawn from her clinical and personal experience. She can intuitively be aware of what the patient is trying to say. She can identify with the patient and enter into his world as the patient experiences it, but simultaneously be objective about it. She cares about the patient but does not live with him.

Emotions and Nonverbal Clues

Doctors and patients are most comfortable talking with each other, and a verbal interview can result in a deep emotional understanding. Words, however, are often limited to the patient's cognitive constructs about how things ought to be, whereas the physical expression of emotion delineates more eloquently how the patient really feels (Ch. 11). We have all experienced in ourselves and others the extraordinary conflicts that can develop between these two ways of viewing situations. This is especially true for psychosomatic symptoms in which the emotion is suppressed and the symptom has taken its place. The interview in which the patient *talks about* the symptoms or even his personal situation may not reveal the intensity of the disappointment, grief, anger, fear, frustration, or whatever characterizes the emotional ground of the illness. Thus we can often learn more by "listening" for and responding to nonverbal clues than from talk.

When symptoms can be converted back to the primary emotions and personal situation from which they arose, both patient and doctor understand immediately what the illness is all about. It can then be approached realistically. The experiencing of emotions is often the first step of the healing process, and the experience itself, in a supportive environment, sometimes suffices to exorcise the symptoms. An emotional eruption, if it occurs, is the fruitful climax of an interview, and it is important for a successful outcome that it not be denied if it "wants to happen."

Daphne G., 53, single, variously employed, was a talkative, superficially sophisticated woman who came often to the clinic with different symptoms of nervous tension. I had examined her four years before for what I took to be physical symptoms related to a personal problem at that time. She disagreed with my interpretation but was relieved that my examination showed no disease. As I saw her from time to time with the staff, she was friendly but seemed to view my concern about the human side of illness with a certain cynical amusement.

On this visit she had a new symptom, an intractable headache that had lasted three months. The physical examination was negative. I explained again that there was probably some underlying nervous tension. There ensued an unrewarding interview exploring her life situation, about which she denied any problems. Finally, I suggested that sometimes the problem is something missing rather than something happening. At that she burst into tears, the first emotion I had seen her reveal in years of care. I sat quietly, saying nothing. She soon told of the death of her lover, the one person whom she had loved the most in all her life, after which the headaches started. She had not previously allowed herself to experience her grief or share it with anyone else. When the tears subsided, she said she did not want a tranquilizer or follow-up. I phoned her several months later and learned that the headaches had disappeared after the interview.

Recovery from a major loss usually takes a long time. It begins with the acknowledgment of the loss and the experience of the grief itself. Circumventing this by denial or repression may block the whole process.

An emotion need not be overt—tears or clenched fists. One becomes sensitive to the wide range of expression through tone of voice, facial expression, gesture, posture, gait, animation, breathing, body tension—the many indications we all look for in family and friends to learn how they really feel. The interviewer responds with discretion. Usually, it is better to acknowledge what is noticed, allowing patients to respond in kind, or not to respond, as they will.

If, for example, a subtle change occurs—the patient looks away, voice trails off, eyes appear moist—the simplest response is just to be there, quietly, or, if the patient begins to cry, simply to offer tissue wipes. Silence acknowledges your awareness, and invites the patient to share. If, however, the patient resumes talking as though nothing had happened, you might say, "I thought perhaps we had touched on something there that was important to you." If the patient does not respond to this, so be it, but if there is obvious resistance to strong emotion, this in itself will help to explain the illness.

There are innumerable ways to pick up on one's observations and initiate a process of sharing. "I'm concerned about how you are feeling right now." "I notice you have begun to tremble." "Could you stop for a moment and just be aware of the tension in your body?" "You seem very quiet—are you concerned about something?" I mean here only to suggest a few possible responses. Each physician uses her own intuitive sensibility.

I simply seek to open channels of sharing. I do not push an emotional expression on the patient. Nor do I block the process. Whatever the response, something is gained in the relationship, and nothing is lost. If the emotional state is deeply suppressed, nothing happens. If the patient is aware at some level but not ready, afraid, unwilling or unable to share for any reason, he simply stays where he is. It is rare for an emotion released to be so devastating that the patient is worse off for the experience. The patient's usual compensatory and defensive systems will continue to operate, and in these situations are usually sufficient to block the emergence of the emotions in the first place. By and large, there is far more suffering in isolation than in sharing. Most people experience the sharing as a great release of energy that had been stifled much too long. They do not feel devastated as they may have feared. They are both relieved and strengthened by the experience, which in retrospect is felt to have been valid and necessary.

We do need to respect the patient's defenses. There are patients whose life situations have been truly devastating. A precipitous emotional confrontation with a lost or wasted life, or guilt-ridden past, could be a painful, unproductive experience. The physician proceeds cautiously. Nevertheless, we are generally too fearful of emotions and too cautious in our approaches. Our unwillingness to elicit emotions is based on our training, our apprehension about emotions in ourselves and others, our feeling that emotions are somehow bad or wrong, and our compulsion as doctors either to avoid emotions, to suppress them with drugs, or to "cure" the patient of the whole problem. In this frame of mind we cannot see that the sharing itself is of first importance. What can be done about the problem comes later, and that is mostly for the patient to decide. We cannot see how often patients need desperately to share the realities of their lives, and that they may first become aware of this opportunity in the presence of a concerned and compassionate physician. Ideally, such sharing should occur readily in close human relationships, but it doesn't. The individual's needs in the medical relationship are uniquely poignant.

The Medical History in Perspective

The most precious attribute of any clinician is the capacity to formulate an independent, creative, clinical judgment accurately describing the unique problem of the patient. The history is often the crucial determinant—how it is obtained, put together, and interpreted. In referrals of diagnostic problems, a consultant will occasionally discover an unobserved physical sign, order a revealing laboratory test, or reinterpret medical data to establish a precise disease diagnosis. Most often, however, especially in psychosomatic disorders, but also to a great extent in organic disease, it is the basic *subjective* data that make the crucial difference. The same history can be recorded 20 times on the same patient with the same unresolved problem, until a new physician, unperturbed by the apparent complexity of the past, starts over *from the beginning*, seeks a fresh evaluation of the *symptoms*—how the patient actually feels—and approaches the entire problem with an unbiased mind, open to all possibilities. The history as a whole, even the symptoms per se, may be quite surprising, in no way resembling the previous formulations. The facts now speak for themselves, and the correct clinical judgment is obvious.

Rosetta C. was a married woman of 37 referred for evaluation of a continuous pain encircling the lower trunk, groin, and right lower extremity for two

> *years. The physical exam and all the usual lab and X-ray exams, including a myelogram and electromyograms, were negative. In the referral letters and resident's history, the present illness and workup were described in some detail. In the review of systems, certain other symptoms were noted, and, in the past history, medical data about her childhood illnesses, childbirths, and operations. The latter included appendectomy, age 15, uterine suspension and tubal ligation, age 23, after three pregnancies, and panhysterectomy, age 31.*

The format of this medical history is classical. Any variation would be most unusual. Medical facts are, of course, important, and this history did indeed cover the major events. But the most important element in a medical history is missing altogether: the *symptoms!* What were the symptoms that led to the three operations? So I asked.

> *Was the appendicitis acute or chronic?* Chronic, it hurt for almost two years. *What was found at the operation?* The doctor didn't say. *Did you ask?* No. *Why was your uterus suspended?* It hurt all the time after my third baby. *Did the pain recur after surgery?* Yes, it was especially bad for four years before they took out my uterus.

We can now view this case in a different perspective altogether. The present illness did not really begin two years ago—it began 24 years ago, when the pelvic pain first appeared, at age 13, two years before a probably normal appendix was removed. At various times, ten years altogether, it was present continuously. Knowing only these facts about the pain, even without any corresponding psychosocial data, or without linking the pain to the other symptoms (headaches, palpitation, muscular pains) that were buried in the *review of systems*, a diagnosis of psychogenic pain disorder is immediately suggested. When we later obtained the path report ("cystic endocervicitis," "small follicle cysts of the ovaries"), the operative report (no endometriosis or other lesions noted) and enough personal history to understand the psychodynamics of this illness, we were sure of the diagnosis. Historical evidence for previous psychosomatic disorders does not indicate necessarily that present symptoms are not due to a new and coincidental organic disease, but when the symptoms are similar and consistent, and there is no evidence to the contrary, the symptoms can often be understood best as a continuation of the same problem.

A more informative recording of the present illness in such a patient would read: "The patient gives a long history of pain in the region of her pelvis and lower abdomen. It first appeared at the age of 13 as a daily pain in the right lower quadrant. After two years, the appendix was removed. She then had three pregnancies between the ages of 17 and 21. A similar pain reappeared in the lower abdomen after the third birth and persisted for two years, when a uterine suspension and tubal ligation were performed. . . ."

In giving their medical histories, patients almost invariably divide their illnesses into discrete episodes, each with medical names, just as the doctors do. When asked about the kind of pain each time, patients may report "similar" or "different." If different, it often turns out, nevertheless, that each episode was an expression of the same problem, a psychogenic pain syndrome.

Note how the compartmentalization of the standard history blocks perspective. Several things go wrong.

The names of episodic diseases or operations are substituted for subjective data, by patients as well as physicians, and what may be the same illness all along, or symptoms in different systems but due to the same underlying personal situation, are arbitrarily split into separate problems. After all, is it not the diseases that count, not the symptoms? Once an illness is labeled, that's it. If there is no label, then the name of a procedure, or a treatment, suffices. How often do we record *hysterectomy* under *operations*, or *thyroid* under *drugs*, without asking why? The principle here is that we should always question any diagnosis, any procedure, any treatment, including our own, past or present. *What were the symptoms? On what data was the diagnosis based? Is it correct? Whether correct or not, in terms of a test or X-ray report, does the diagnosis adequately explain all the symptoms?* The diagnoses that particularly merit each physician's reconsideration in relation to the symptoms were summarized in Chapter 6. The patient may have a condition—*mitral valve prolapse*, for example—but what were the symptoms? If discomfort in the chest, was MVP really the cause of the pain?

Long-standing emotional stress can be expressed as symptoms in several different ways. It may reappear as the same or a similar symptom (Rosetta). It may appear as many symptoms simultaneously in different systems (Orvieta, Ch. 2; Cynthia, this chapter). Or it may appear as separate illnesses in different systems over many years.

When there are multiple symptoms, we often err when we view the symptoms as separate illnesses of different systems. Even though concurrent, they can still be split between the *present illness*, the *review of systems*, and other divisions of a traditional history, or they can be viewed as separate problems in a problem-oriented record. For example, John T., a patient with concurrent headaches, epigastric pain, and backache, was identified as having three problems, each of which was "SOAPed" (Subjective data, Objective data, Appraisal or Assessment, Plan) separately. The *Appraisal* for headaches was tension headaches vs migraine; that for the epigastric pain, rule out peptic ulcer, rule out gall bladder disease; that for the backache, lumbosacral muscular strain, possible disk syndrome. Each problem then had its own distinct diagnostic and therapeutic plan for resolution. There could, of course, be certain factors unique to each symptom. Posture at work, for example, could be one factor in the backache but not in the headaches. But these three problems will remain separate even after their respective diagnostic plans and therapeutic trials have been completed. Nothing will happen to change the clinical logic that divided the illness in the first place. In fact, the workup may serve to reinforce the division, especially if extraneous factors are disclosed, such as a hiatal hernia or congenital defect of the spine, both of which may be asymptomatic. Because of the division, the common denominator, fatigue and emotional stress, will not be recognized, nor will the fact that the tension headaches, the dyspepsia, and the muscular backache (the true subdiagnoses) are all functional expressions of the same problem. Even when the stress is noted, it may be recorded on this problem list as a fourth and still separate problem!

The errors here result from the reductionism inherent in medical-model thinking, not from the problem-oriented record format per se. When the clinician perceives the illness in its entirety, either at the beginning or later, the problems should be integrated. The *Appraisal* would be that of a multi-system functional illness related to stress. Under *Subjective data* the symptoms in the three systems, as well as the stress, could be described briefly. The *Plan* for this one overall problem would still include a GI series and X-rays of the spine to rule out a possible second or third problem. Most important, the major theme of the therapeutic plan would be what the patient can do about the life situation, for that is the core problem of the whole illness.

Thus, when the history reveals a long series of previous or concurrent illnesses, perhaps masquerading as disease, whether of one or several organ systems, we must consider that these may not be purely coincidental pathological events. A realistic clinical judgment is based on the history *as seen in perspective*, but there can be no perspective unless this question is introduced: *Could there be a common denominator to the components of the past and present medical history?*

Health-History Questionnaires

A properly devised form has distinct advantages for person-centered care. First of all, few doctors in practice have enough time to record even the basic medical data. Most of the published questionnaires [16] are far more comprehensive than doctors can be in the details of past and family medical history, review of systems, previous diagnostic tests and doctors attended, travel and immunizations, medications, allergies and sensitivities, and health habits (nutrition, exercise, sleep, rest, work and play, smoking, drinking, and street drugs). Many questionnaires include sections on affective disorders—the feelings, behaviors, concerns, and symptoms associated therewith—as well as the problems of sexuality, family interactions, social support, and stresses of modern life that give rise to the disturbances. In the usual medical history many of these questions are never asked, even when they bear directly on the patient's illness. In one study of this problem, the doctors had asked but one-fourth of just the basic medical database covered by the self-report.[17]

Special questionnaires are available for pediatrics, adolescents and young adults, obstetrics and gynecology, the medical specialties, occupational health, and the evaluation of stress, headaches, and other aspects of health, functional capacity, and disability.[18]

Some patients, wondering why the doctor appears to have singled them out in the interview to ask personal questions, especially in regard to the presence or absence of emotional disturbances, respond reluctantly, whereas they will complete a questionnaire readily, knowing that many patients receive the same form. Responding on their own time before the visit (or after, if necessary) opens the way to thoughtful answers, and the patient can even be invited to indicate areas of special concern. The questionnaire serves as an educational device as the patient becomes aware of the doctor's concerns about the personal and biological background of health and illness, especially when reviewed together during the visit. The patient is clearly involved in the health-care process.

Most important, in terms of the doctor's needs, the time required to obtain the database can then be better used for the more sensitive interactions suggested in this chapter. The information provided by most questionnaires can quickly focus the doctor's attention on problem areas. If symptoms in many systems are checked positive, for example, that alone should suggest the possibility of a common source. I found that one glance at the responses in the mood and general-health categories of one form used in our clinic [19] provided an immediate evaluation of whether the patient was emotionally disturbed or not, directing my attention then and there to the probable nature of the illness. Unfortunately, the clinic doctors who avoid the emotional aspects of medicine would not notice these responses, nor do they obtain the same data on their own, and their workups for nonexistent disease would become unnecessarily prolonged, and expensive.

For the purpose of detecting unrecognized emotional disturbances, self-report questionnaires may serve their most useful function in primary care. The disturbance may, of course, explain the present illness or be a major contributor to illness caused by disease. Even when the patient has more obviously emotional complaints, the magnitude of the disturbance may not be apparent. And it can be important to know that a patient is disturbed, though the presenting illness or injury is unrelated.

The General Health Questionnaire, as one example, was developed in England specifically as a "technique for the identification and assessment of non-psychotic psychiatric illness" in primary care.[20] Its efficacy has been demonstrated in various practice situations.[21–23] A questionnaire of this sort includes elements of depression, anxiety, social/behavioral concerns, and problems generally. It does not make a specific "diagnosis," but it distinctly calls the physician's attention to disturbances of importance to the patient.

In this country, depression, generally more difficult to detect than anxiety, has been the major focus of similar questionnaires. The Beck Depression Inventory (BDI),[24] the Zung Self-Rating Depression Scale,[25] and the Burns Depression Checklist,[26] were developed for this purpose. Here too, the value of the instrument (the BDI, particularly) has been demonstrated in primary care and recommended for general use.[27–29]

Useful probes for anxiety are the Zung Self-Rating Anxiety Scale [30] and the Burns Anxiety Inventory.[31] One of these could be combined with the BDI or the Burns Depression Checklist as a general survey for emotional disturbance. When anxiety and depression are interfused, as they often are, positive responses can be anticipated in both aspects of the survey. These checklists can be completed in just a few minutes. Because each question calls for a range of responses, from normal to slightly, moderately, or most affected, the patient does not feel singled out in any way. The queries are "user-friendly."

Because it is simply awkward in most medical histories to ask the kinds of questions that determine if a person is affectively disturbed, and how much so, and because the verbal format provides no opportunity for multiple-choice responses, the self-report forms are usually far more effective. If not already incorporated in a general-health-history questionnaire, they should be used more widely, especially when the illness is not fully explained as a typical disease type of problem.

The medical history is often the foundation of clinical judgment. To obtain the personal as well as medical data necessary for an accurate diagnosis and comprehensive appraisal of the whole illness, the physician must listen carefully, be open to all possibilities from the very beginning.

Each kind of illness tends to have characteristic symptoms. Thus the critical first step in the history is to determine just how the patient *feels*, to elicit all the symptoms without premature manipulation into medical pigeonholes.

We need to understand the life situation of any patient when this is the source of the illness. The personal data are most explicit when shared freely by the patient. We can facilitate the sharing by responding sensitively to the patient's verbal and emotional clues as they appear spontaneously during the history. A critical judgment about the illness may also hinge on a review of the entire medical history in perspective, looking for the common personal denominators that may underlie what previously appeared to be coincidental medical illnesses.

Clinical judgment ultimately depends on how all the data, subjective and objective, past and present, are assembled and integrated. The disease, the illness, and the person are all important. History-taking provides an exceptional opportunity to begin to understand all three.

CHAPTER 15

Misunderstandings and Hidden Issues

Patients often have unstated reasons for coming into care, or expectations of the encounter other than diagnosis and treatment. If such concerns are not elicited and resolved, the entire medical plan may be misdirected. The purpose of this chapter is to summarize some of the more common covert issues that underlie the visit.

∾ In most medical visits a patient feels ill and comes to learn what is wrong and what can be done to be well again. The doctor responds by categorizing the illness as a disease that can be diagnosed and treated. The basic format of this interaction is much the same in all healing systems, though what is thought to be wrong, and what is done about it, varies. In general, the patient comes with a symptom, and the healer responds with a specific regimen.

In medicine, however, unlike most other healing systems, patients often have reasons for coming into care, or expectations other than the diagnosis and therapeutic considerations of the doctor.[1] Nevertheless, because of the "rules of the game," patients almost invariably feel compelled to describe a symptom. That is what they are supposed to do. If there are alternative expectations, hopes, promptings, a hidden agenda of some kind, they rarely volunteer what it is. Meanwhile, the doctor, unaware of these covert concerns, naturally assumes that the patient suffers as described and expects something to be done about it.

In this way, patients describe symptoms in matter-of-fact statements, without offering a clue about their underlying concerns. Then they follow the doctor's lead, wherever that takes them. Once under way, the medical process can go far astray, and the void in communication can persist indefinitely. So, in addition to understanding just what the patient means by the chief complaint (Ch. 14), it may be critical to determine just what the patient wants, needs, worries about.[2] What prompted the visit? Why now? What does this person really hope will happen? Keep in mind that the patient's underlying concerns may be conscious, unconscious, or a little of both. In any case, they are often not clearly expressed.

Common Covert Issues

Is the Patient's Main Concern for Specific Treatment or for Understanding?

Understanding, here, should be taken to mean an explanation of what is wrong, what causes it, and what can be done about it. Medication is but one aspect of what can be done, and to many patients it may be the least important. Obviously, the relative importance of these concerns varies with the urgency of the disease or injury and many other factors. In medical care generally, however, doctors and patients often view this question quite differently, and this is a common source of misunderstanding and patient dissatisfaction.

The doctors, of course, want to be helpful, and symptomatic drugs, if that is all that can be done biomedically, do indeed relieve suffering. Patients know this, and the doctors tend to believe that patients expect, perhaps "demand," a prescription at almost every visit. But the doctors have their own covert agenda, and one component of that agenda may be an explicit message that the prescription is *the treatment* for the problem. Therefore, implicitly, the visit was appropriate because the problem is appropriate for medical treatment. The biomedical relationship is sanctified. Similarly, the healer/client relationship of any system is affirmed when the treatment peculiar to that system is applied. Thus there is a strong compulsion to treat.

This question has been surveyed objectively. In one study, four of five doctors in general practice estimated that patients expect prescriptions in more than four of five visits; 22 percent of the doctors thought that a prescription was expected at 99 percent of all visits.[3] In surveys of patients, however, only about half expect prescriptions.[4] More pertinent to this question was a survey of 100 outpatients, all with recurrent headache, and 50 physicians, which explored the question of what such patients most want when coming to a doctor.[5] Of the top three priorities, pain relief was listed by 96 percent of the doctors, 69 percent of the patients. How was this to be achieved? Medication was thought to be most important by 68 percent of the doctors but by only 20 percent of the patients. Because most patients (77 percent) named explanation of the illness as their dominant concern, the majority obviously hoped to participate in the healing process in some way other than taking drugs. In another study of a large prepaid group practice, it was found that the patients who did not receive prescriptions reported the most satisfaction with the visit as a whole, but particularly with the doctor's communications.[6] This does not mean, of course, that the prescription per se hindered patient satisfaction; it presumably did so by substituting for other, more meaningful, more communicative interactions.

Note also, from national household survey data, that of those adults who reported high levels of both life crisis and emotional distress, 65 percent of the women and 79 percent of the men had not used medically prescribed mood-changing drugs in the year preceding the interview.[7]

Many patients, of course, will be disappointed if they do not receive a prescription. Nevertheless, it can be seen that the perception of many doctors about the expectations of patients is often a projection. It may be related more to what they want to do than to what they know about their patients.[8]

To obviate such a mismatch, we need to keep in mind that patients, while describing their illness, will rarely volunteer that what they want most of all is to understand it. And when prescriptions are most of what they receive, they comply, but begrudgingly, that being the only path to healing they have been led to follow. If there is to be a more comprehensive understanding, it must be introduced by the doctor. Provided with such understanding, knowing that the medication proposed is for symptom relief only, many patients choose not to be medicated. *The understanding is the treatment.* The collaborative plan for getting well in any kind of personal illness is implicit in the understanding, and pharmacotherapy falls in place according to the responses and clinical situation of the individual patient.

Is Relief or Reassurance the Core Issue?

This question is allied to the first, but here the patient is concerned, not about feeling ill, but only about what a transient symptom may signify. Nevertheless, the symptom is the "complaint." The patient makes no mention of the underlying concerns that prompted the visit, nor will such concerns be elicited unless we ask. If we assume again that the patient expects relief, that being our customary role, a relatively minor complaint can sometimes be taken seriously, studied, and even treated when all the patient had hoped was to be reassured that "it" was not an impending stroke or heart attack, cancer, high blood pressure, etc. Medical articles in the lay press, or the diagnosis of a major disease in someone known to the patient with similar symptoms, give rise to such concerns.

Another common situation in our health-conscious culture is the patient's compulsion to "cover the bases" during a health evaluation. Thus the list of symptoms does not necessarily indicate disease, a nervous disorder, or hypochondriasis. The patient simply uses the opportunity of a checkup to mention everything that has been noticed in the recent past.

In the absence of disease it is wise to ask, "What are you concerned about? What are you afraid you might have? What do you think really causes this?" This can then be followed by an explanation of the many transient symptoms that result from the stresses, strains, and physiological variants of daily life.

Could the Symptom Be an Excuse to Get into Medical Care, When at a Deeper Level the Patient is More Disturbed in Other Ways?

As cited previously, Stoeckle found that significant psychic distress coincided with the present illness in 84 percent of the patients attending a general medical clinic, regardless of the diagnosis.[9] The distress often appeared to transform symptoms into complaints, and to precipitate the visit. The patients, for example, would not otherwise be concerned about the arthritis, varicose veins, bursitis, or whatever the chief complaint, if it were not for the more personal disturbance that has caused them to focus on a minor, perhaps chronic, condition. Or the patient feels a diffuse need for help, a doctor is someone to turn to, and, though not thinking it through in this way, the symptom appears as the ticket of admission. Or, though quite aware of the underlying distress, and hoping to be able to confide in the physician, the patient is too self-conscious to bring it up and feels compelled to start with a conventional complaint. In other words, personal stress, though not necessarily the cause of the symptoms, results in the decision to visit a doctor or, sometimes, to adopt the sick role.[10–13] Depression is the most common of these underlying feeling states.

In spite of the matter-of-fact complaint, the more important issues may appear as clues, or suddenly break forth in the interview. Or they are readily elicited if the doctor provides an opportunity such as, "You appear to be troubled in some way, perhaps not just by the arthritis. Could this be so?"

A comprehensive evaluation of the symptoms—not just in relation to the disorder under consideration, but also to the patient's circumstances, needs, and emotional state—is often helpful. Providing an opportunity to share the underlying problems may mean more to the patient than would sticking with the chief complaint. Otherwise, the medical regimen is likely to be more convoluted than is appropriate.

Is the Symptom the Problem, or Is the Problem an Arbitrary Standard of Normality Against Which the Symptom Is Compared?

Roger H., 46, was a happily married man complaining of impotence. Detailed questioning, however, revealed that his sexual life was generally more imaginative and vigorous than most, but that he had failed to achieve erection on a few occasions when he was unusually tired and distracted. Presumably, on these occasions, his mind was telling him what it thought he ought to be feeling, that is, sexy on Saturday night, a customary time for sexuality, whereas his body was expressing, or rather not expressing, what he was really feeling, that is, a need for rest and not being sexual on those few occasions. Actually, he was not at all impotent. The symptom was not the problem. The problem was an arbitrary standard that he should always perform in a certain way at certain times, no matter what. Perhaps he had simply not yet learned to accept gracefully just not feeling sexually inclined for whatever reason.

This "problem" was readily handled as a nonproblem by pointing out that there was, in fact, no "symptom" but merely a waning of sexuality in times of fatigue or stress. In fact, he merited a commendation, having never before noticed this in the preceding years of a rewarding sexual relationship!

The patient's misconception here is obvious. Few doctors would be misled by such a complaint. But we need to keep this kind of problem in mind in such conditions as functional constipation (bowels *ought to* move every day), insomnia (*ought to* sleep eight hours), obesity (*ought to* weigh 5 or 10 pounds less), even mild depression (*ought to* feel happy all the time). The hidden agenda is in part the patient's fixed ideas of normality. In the case of eating and weight, the concept of self focused on physical appearance is often what needs attention more than the weight itself.

The "*ought to*" problem appears most commonly in any syndrome caused by stress when, for example, people insist that they ought to be able to work 14 hours a day and sleep six, or whatever the stress demands upon self may be, and not have the headaches, GI disturbance, or whatever other symptoms occur. Here the symptom itself is indeed a problem, but the deeper problem is the patient's expectation—and, sometimes, that of the physician, as well—that there should be no symptoms regardless of the stress, and, therefore, it is the sole responsibility of the doctor to provide the cure.

I do not mean to imply here that we should not be concerned about the patient's concerns, or help medically in any reasonable way. But in these kinds of situations, an explanation of the range of normal physiology and the factors that affect it, or an exploration of the background that led to the patient's concerns, may be most important. Otherwise, the management, either by the patients themselves, their doctors, or both, can be much too manipulative. The solution to the "problem" should not be a bigger problem than the "symptom" itself is.

Are There Indications of Narcotic or Psychoactive Drug Dependence?

It is natural to assume that your new patient, who appears to provide a straightforward description of the present illness, expects to be examined, diagnosed, and treated appropriately. It is indeed disconcerting, especially after a painstaking examination and plan for workup, to discover that the patient's hidden agenda was mainly to get a prescription for a narcotic, hypnotic, or other drug now denied by previous physicians.

The problem here is not strictly that of the patient. The drugs, after all, *were prescribed medically,* and the psychological aspects of what was in many cases a psychosomatic pain disorder have perhaps never been explored. Such patients rarely regard themselves as drug-dependent, nor are they fully aware of how much and how often they use. They "need" the drug for relief and cannot appreciate how continued use can block a more effective healing process (Jean G., Ch. 5).

Confronted for the first time by a patient with chronic pain but no distinct disease, it is wise to ask immediately, shortly after the chief complaint: "What do you take to relieve the pain? How much do you take? Who prescribes it? Does the doctor plan to continue prescribing? What do you expect of me?"

I may be prepared to help a drug-dependent patient recover, but to do so, I will have to deal with the psychosocial factors in the illness, and the therapeutic plan will usually involve the withdrawal of narcotics. With new patients, such questions must be settled early in the encounter, or, with established patients, as soon as we realize we have overprescribed.

Secondary Gain

In a conversion or somatoform pain disorder, the symptom expresses a conflict, or in some way resolves a personal problem, more effectively than does direct confrontation. That is the hidden agenda. If someone suffers disease or injury, the illness can serve the same function if, for example, it provides a desirable but unexpected release from work, relief from personal stress, or monetary compensation. When this happens, the disability is readily accentuated or extended from what it would have been otherwise.

Whether the illness is a primary somatoform disorder, or a secondary gain is superimposed on another condition, the patients are focused on the pain or whatever the symptoms may be. They provide a straight and earnest story of the illness. They suffer, and implore the doctor for relief. The exceptional intensity, quality, or persistence of the symptoms, unusual for the disease or injury that has been sustained or is now suspected, is readily overlooked. Whether the function of the illness is more or less unconscious, as in primary somatoform disorder, or well known to the patient, as in one who deliberately seeks to manipulate the industrial-accident system, nothing is said about these issues. There is no mention of the hated job, or the various duties, behaviors, or demands to be evaded, no mention of the special attention that takes their place, no mention of the hoped-for compensation or impending litigation. Many patients do not even mention the disability. Only the symptoms are described.

Thus, the secondary-gain issues may not emerge until the doctor has long since become mired in fruitless workups and therapeutic trials. Or they may never emerge, even after years of care. Obviously, if the patient is to be well, the hidden agenda must be elicited and in some way resolved, the sooner the better. The general nature of somatoform disorders was the subject of Chapter 12. Here, we will consider briefly the secondary gains superimposed on overt disease or injury.

Mainly, the doctor should suspect the possibility of secondary issues whenever an illness appears to be unduly persistent or disruptive. In such situations, there are two sets of issues to consider. One is the patient's psychosocial situation. The illness may have occurred coincidentally at a time of personal distress, or the illness itself causes problems that are difficult to surmount. If so, the illness may be accentuated by the somatoform effects of secondary gains, or by the psychophysiological effects of unresolved emotional conflict, or both. The other set of issues is that of litigation, compensation, authorized disability, and allied questions. As with George B. (Ch. 2), both sets of problems may play a role in the illness.

First, to begin to solve the problem, it is usually necessary to know the person, the family, and the setting of the illness in the patient's life situation. What can be done about all this varies, of course, with the unique situation of each patient, the understanding achieved, and the feasibility of change. Of the three patients described in Chapter 1, for example, the problem of shoulder pain was resolved by a frank statement about the obvious secondary gains, the diagnosis of a superimposed somatoform reaction, a settlement based on that reaction and a change of jobs. The problem of post-mononucleosis fatigue was resolved by academic counseling and an adjustment of the student's class schedule, in conjunction with the dean. There appeared to be no way to effect a real change in the arthritis patient's dependent personality, but she became ambulatory in a rehabilitation program with the support of her husband. Clearly, healing depends on recognizing the sick role adopted by the patient. Perhaps the underlying problems can be resolved, as they were in the first two patients. If not, as in the third case, the physician, perceiving the realities that actually cause the illness, if not the disease, can adjust the collaborative plan accordingly.

Next, compensation or disability issues, if involved, must be elicited and resolved. Whenever any patient mentions an illness following an injury, for example, no matter how trivial the latter or unlikely the possibility of compensation, I have learned to ask immediately: "Is there litigation?" If you do not ask, you may not find out until after many visits and a major workup, even though the litigation is now the core of the whole problem. The compensation, of course, may be quite appropriate. The patient did suffer a whiplash injury, let us say, through the fault of another driver. But the persistence of pain for many months or a year (instead of the usual three to six weeks if the compensation is soon settled) may have more to do with the patient's expectations of a major monetary award, or adverse personal situation at the time of the accident, than with the original injury, which was not unusual in any way. I try to approach the personal issues as considerately as I can, explaining how readily muscular tension can complicate the original injury. But there inevitably comes a moment of truth when I must explain the limits of the injury and the difference between law and medicine: "Your lawyer's concern is your sickness; the worse it is and the longer it lasts, the better the settlement will be. My concern is your health. There has been no unusual injury here. You are expected to recover, but you are unlikely to do what you need to do to be well again until the settlement is behind you. I can't guarantee anything, but generally speaking, you will improve steadily from that point on."

Another covert issue is authorized disability for welfare or Social Security benefits, release from work, school, or military duties, or compensation in many ways other than accident litigation. Especially when the actual disability is not obviously disabling, the patient simply appears again and again with the same symptoms, never improving, hoping perhaps that the complaints will speak for themselves, but reluctant to ask outright for disability. Most doctors tend to focus more on symptoms than on functional impairment,[14] and the patient's concerns about the latter may be overlooked. In any unduly persistent illness, I have learned to ask directly: "Do you regard yourself as disabled?" A positive answer to this question may be the key to understanding an otherwise enigmatic diagnostic or therapeutic problem. In any event, the course of the illness, when this is a factor, will not change until this question is brought out and settled one way or the other.

An allied problem is the patient you have treated, let us say, for a respiratory infection or backache. You did not consider the person disabled, and this question never came up during the encounter. Then, a week or two later, you are confronted with a disability form. Again, the hidden agenda must be resolved as soon as it appears. Ideally, this question would have been introduced at the original visit, but the disability aspect often comes as a surprise, as can other underground issues in the medical encounter.

Alternate Belief Systems

Are the patient's health beliefs at variance with biomedical models? There are many such beliefs, far too many to be mentioned here. Examples would include the hex, or possession by spirits, of many cultures, or the Mexican-American concept of *susto*, or fright disease. Such beliefs may well block healing unless elicited and resolved in some way. Berlin and Fowkes provide a LEARN model [15] for the resolution of these issues in cross-cultural health care:

L   *Listen* with sympathy and understanding to the patient's perception of
    the problem.
E   *Explain* your perceptions of the problem.
A   *Acknowledge* and discuss the differences and similarities.
R   *Recommend* treatment.
N   *Negotiate* agreement.

Obviously, such a model can be useful in any differences between doctor and patient about what is wrong or what needs to be done about it. The model could well be applied to most of the misunderstandings outlined in this chapter.

CHAPTER 16

Collaboration Continues: First Talks About Personal Illness

How any illness is explained to the patient is a pivotal juncture for what happens thereafter. If the illness is deemed to be caused mainly by personal distress, it is described both in "medical" and "personal" terms. This discussion can be relatively straightforward in responsive patients, especially if the history has already disclosed the probable troubling situation, but in defensive patients it can be difficult. The purpose of this chapter is to consider ways to facilitate these communications.

᭤ When the patient has a clear-cut disease or injury, and the plan for healing is mainly the responsibility of the doctor, the diagnosis, workup, and treatment are easily explained. The patient needs to understand the nature of the illness, its cause, and what can be done about it, but the communications are straightforward. If, however, the patient appears to have a functional or psychiatric disorder, or any illness caused mainly by personal distress, clear communications about its nature may be more of a problem.

In terms of the *medical* interactions, the illness must be named, diagnosed, or characterized in some way, and the mechanism of symptom formation explained. How to do this is not always clear, as, for example, in psychogenic fatigue states and somatoform pain disorders.

In terms of the *personal* basis of the illness, it is not necessary to explore the background of every transient mild stress reaction, and such understanding may be deferred in the major depressive and anxiety disorders until relief is secured with pharmacotherapy. In most functional disorders and nervous states, however, especially when the illness is distinctly troubling, persistent, or recurrent, patient and physician must seek together to understand its source as well as they can. The personal phase of the interviews may well continue over many visits. Although most patients appreciate the opportunity to share their life situations in relation to the illness, others do not. And it may be difficult to understand the core of the problem even in the most responsive patients. Nevertheless, patients have a right to know what is wrong, and, as with any illness, if the source can be known and dealt with in some positive way, the better the outcome.

How to proceed with these interactions, when person-centered care is deemed appropriate, is the quest of this and the following chapter. The suggestions here are but one approach. Every doctor must find her/his own way of communicating with patients comfortably.

Integrating the Medical and Personal Phases

The initial history and physical often provide the clinician with enough data to be quite sure that some kind of psychosocial distress underlies the illness. If so, and time permitting, the interview at the end of the first visit provides an optimal opportunity both to name and explain the symptoms and to know this person a little better. The patient, not yet locked into the medical system, is generally open to whatever interactions the physician proposes. The clinician, however, often lacks the time, cannot be sure enough of the diagnosis to proceed, or for other reasons chooses to defer one or both phases of the interview until the workup is completed. Nevertheless, if there is a reasonable likelihood of a personal illness, this should be explained before the workup is begun: other diagnostic possibilities are to be investigated, but the special studies may well be negative, and a more extended personal interview later will be necessary to understand the problem.

How the medical and personal phases of the interviews are phrased, timed, and integrated will vary considerably, depending on the nature of the illness, the patient's responsiveness and medical sophistication, the physician's diagnostic confidence, communicative skills, receptiveness to personal illness, office schedule, and many other factors.

How such interviews are integrated with decisions about pharmacotherapy is still another important consideration: depending on the urgency of the distress, the doctor's judgment, and the patient's position on this question, medical treatment may be introduced at once, or deferred, or the interpersonal understanding may take its place.

In any event, regardless of how and when the workup, the therapy, and other aspects of the medical program are ordered, if the personal understanding is too long deferred, it is apt to vanish in the procedures of the medical model. It may take some time, of course, to understand the basis of a long-term nervous disorder. On the other hand, many patients have an obvious emotional disturbance of recent onset, expressed as anxiety or with physical symptoms, yet deny any problems. In this situation, the understanding should not be deferred. It is imperative to state clearly that the illness indicates emotional suppression of some kind, and to pursue a definitive resolution.

Opening the Interview

Let us consider several possible beginnings to a collaborative approach. This could be introduced on the first or second visit or as soon as the illness is recognized for what it is.

If, for example, in a typical functional illness, there is good reason to suspect the likely source of the problem, such as Joseph's grief and loneliness (Ch. 1), Orvieta's stress (Ch. 2), or Mary's recent marriage (Ch. 3), it may be well to begin there, stating the reason and hinging the interview on what is already known. In this way, especially with a responsive patient, the interview begins in the personal phase, which flows naturally from the medical history, and the medical phase follows. For example:

- You said that you have three small children. That could be quite a problem. Tell me how this is.
- You say these symptoms began shortly after your marriage (or, the pain seems to recur every time you return to the steel mill). Tell me more about the marriage (the job, the school situation, etc.), especially at that time.

What turns up may or may not be significant in terms of the illness. You have merely indicated that some kind of stress or nervous tension may be involved, and further understanding about this may be helpful. This is then followed by a general medical statement about the illness and its relation to the personal situation, such as was described in the text for the three patients cited above. Either the problems disclosed in the preliminary interview are related, or other issues need to be explored later. Other diagnostic concerns and the purpose of the workup are also explained. Collaborative care evolves over time. This is a beginning.

If, on the other hand, I have no clues about the source of what I nevertheless take to be a mainly personal illness, I would usually begin with a general medical description but soon move to include the personal aspects. For example:

- I can't be sure yet just how to categorize your stomach distress that recurs from time to time. What you have sounds most like what is called a dyspeptic syndrome, that is, an acid distension of the stomach, but sometimes it can be caused by an ulcer. You should have a GI series X-ray to be sure, but an ulcer has not been demonstrated previously, and is less likely. The study may well be negative. This kind of distress is quite common. It can be induced in part by [name any adverse health habits already disclosed] and other things. Often, it is related to some kind of stress or nervous tension.

This is then followed by an overture such as:

- Could this be part of the problem here? . . . Is there anything about the stresses in your life, job, marriage, or whatever you have to do from day to day, that you are concerned about?
- I may be able to understand this problem better if I could get a feel for the setting of this illness in your life situation. Would you tell me something about that, whatever may be important for you?
- I need to know more about you. Could you give me an overview—anything that you feel might be somehow related to this illness.
- [Or, time running out] Perhaps we could talk more about these things on the next visit when the lab and X-ray findings have been reported.

These are just openers, of course. At the beginning, you want mainly to provide patients an opportunity to tell their own story. "I'd like to know . . . ," or "Tell me more about. . . ." are gentle overtures. Most patients can appreciate the wisdom of paying attention to personal situations that may well be interconnected with the illness, either as causes or effects. Obviously, the physician hopes to sort this out. The patient is soon involved in the give-and-take of the interview. Open-ended questions, even if they touch only on the patient's daily life, may readily disclose, without asking, any number of conflictual, existential, or physically stressful problems. The tone of the interview is pitched to help patients feel secure that the emphasis is on symptoms, not as "mental disorder," but as responses to stress that anyone is likely to experience under similar circumstances.

An alternative way of opening the interview, especially with any functional disorder or disease that can be caused by multiple factors, such as chronic backache, headache, or hypertension, is to make a general statement about this issue, then review each factor systematically, if not already covered in the present illness. With chronic backache, for example, you might start with occupation, posture at work, modes of lifting, etc., then later introduce the questions of general physical or emotional stress. In this way, the patient can readily appreciate your comprehensive approach. You are not viewed as the kind of doctor who either finds a disease or thinks the patient is "crazy."

The preliminary overtures described above may not begin to reveal the main source of a personal illness, and a more directed, more extended interview may be necessary (Ch. 17). In any event, let us return next to the medical phase of the interview, which usually comes first.

Medical Explanations

A positive statement about the nature of a personal illness is essential, the sooner the better. Sometimes the diagnosis will not become evident until the workup has been completed and the physician has had enough time to come to know the patient, but a special effort should be made to formulate a definitive clinical judgment as soon as possible.

To be affirmative, the physician cannot be disappointed that no disease has been found, nor feel any consternation about confirming and explaining the nature of functional and psychiatric disturbances. She must be confident of the diagnosis, willing to express an opinion, and prepared to engage in a dialogue with the patient about any aspect of the situation. A positive approach is also built upon the physician's interest and her encouraging approach. The illness is a common expression of distress. It is fortunate for the patient that it is *not* due to disease. And the illness can be expected to resolve with better understanding, and with the healing plan to be developed.

Naming the Illness

A diagnostic name is important, especially for physical-symptom syndromes, whenever possible. This signifies that the condition is known. The concept of illness predicated thereby can be shared by doctor and patient, indicating a path for further investigation and treatment.

Some common symptoms have no medical names, and multiple-symptom complexes often fit no specific medical category. In DSM-III-R terminology they would be classified as *psychological factors affecting physical condition,* or as *adjustment disorder with anxious mood, with depressed mood, with mixed emotional features,* or *with physical complaints,* but such terms are not suitable for talking to patients on medical visits. If the dysphoria predominates, and the patient is aware of feeling anxious or depressed, the illness might well be described as an *anxiety state* or *depressive reaction.* In general, however, the "benign nervous states" (Ch. 17) and multiple-physical-symptom complexes so common in medical practice are better described simply as a nervous condition, a stress reaction, or in other familiar designations that clearly indicate the nature of the illness.

However characterized, a positive diagnostic statement as the cornerstone of collaboration proved effective in the many patients followed by Balint and the general practitioners with whom he worked.[1] In psychiatry this was whimsically designated by Torrey as the Principle of Rumpelstiltskin.[2] In the Grimm fairy tale the queen saved the baby by correctly naming the evil man who wanted to take it.

I learned this lesson years ago in the case of a patient with a functional bowel disorder. My meticulous examination and workup, careful explanation of the physiological disturbance, and consideration of possible underlying factors, came to naught. The patient was quite upset. So I arranged a consultation with a distinguished gastroenterologist who examined her briefly and then said to me in her presence, "Why this is a case of irritable-bowel syndrome." The whole atmosphere changed as she smiled, now secure and gratified. I realized then how I had failed to provide a name.

Thus, identifying the illness can be a very positive beginning. The elusive underlying causative factors are secondary considerations. Play doctor first, then psychologist.

What name should you use? The medical name is best, if there is one. Functional disturbances with generally accepted names include tension headache, migraine, hyperventilation syndrome, dyspepsia, irritable-bowel syndrome, and fibromyalgia. Descriptive names characterize anorexia nervosa, bulimia, and functional disturbances of sleep and sexuality. Psychoactive substance dependence or abuse are designated with the name of the particular agent.

If there is no customary name, a descriptive phrase combined with an explanation of the physiological disturbance is usually satisfactory. Muscle-tension syndromes, for example, are common in the back and elsewhere in the body and can be so described, and how various combinations of muscle tension, spasm, strain, or sprain are involved can be explained. Or, as suggested previously, psychogenic chest pain may be described as chest-tension syndrome to convey the concept of physiological pain, emotionally induced, or the pathophysiology may be categorized further, as summarized in Chapter 13.

Patients need to see clearly how the condition (though, from their point of view, not a "real disease") can cause such severe distress. Thus, it can be explained how cerebral vasodilatation, adrenergic discharge, hyperventilation, gastric hyperacidity and distension, bowel spasm and hypermotility, muscle tension and spasm, and other disturbances cause the distress of the corresponding disorders. It can also be explained how the physiological disturbances of depression and other nervous states result in dysfunctional sleep, appetite, sexuality, mental acuity, and energy levels.

I emphasize here that emotionally induced distress is often far more intense than similar symptoms caused by disease. The spasm of irritable-bowel syndrome can cause more pain than food poisoning or cancer. Fibromyalgia is often more disabling than rheumatoid arthritis. The pain of chest-tension syndrome is usually more severe and sustained than that of angina pectoris. And so on.

Psychogenic fatigue. This poses a major problem of communication. The concept of "chronic fatigue syndrome," indicative of a chronic viral infection or impairment of the immune system, is known by most patients. That is often the reason for the visit. The patients expect the infection to be identified and treated in some way. Actually, very few patients with chronic fatigue (6/135 in one study) fit the CDC definition. Recall (Ch. 13) that many suspected of CFS are found to have probable causative psychological/situational problems. Many patients and doctors are not aware of such data, however. And the patients, who do not feel disturbed except by the fatigue itself, are often unwilling to consider that their life situations or ways of viewing themselves or the situation, to which they are strongly committed, may have something to do with the way they feel. In this way, the term *chronic fatigue syndrome*, describing in words what the patients experience, has appropriated the concept of *psychogenic fatigue*, which, though common, known, and well described for many years, was never established, like so many other functional disturbances, with a medical or psychiatric name of its own. CFS, with its implications of organic disease (psychiatric "disease" having been excluded), is a very misleading concept.

Thus, when my final clinical judgment is one of psychogenic fatigue, as it often is, I can explain the symptom to my patients only as a common and characteristic expression of some kind of underlying personal predicament, though just what this may be is often not clear when first explored. I would then move, whenever possible, into the personal phase of the interview.

If necessary, I would clarify my position, confirming that I am aware of the CDC definition and its implications, and know there are many doctors and investigators who support the disease concept. Nevertheless, summarizing what I have learned about this patient so far, and citing the data and perspectives of Chapter 13, I would point out that I do not believe that such an infection is a material factor here, nor is this my point of view generally. If indeed a "virus" were identified, it would lead to no useful therapy. On the other hand, figuring out the psychological, social, or existential components of such an illness may well lead to a better understanding of what could be done to be well again.

Somatoform or psychogenic pain disorder. Obviously, it is unacceptable to most patients to have their pain characterized as somatoform, psychogenic, or hysterical, or a conversion reaction. To the patients this means that their experience of intense suffering is interpreted as "imaginary." Functional pain disorder would be a less threatening but still unconvincing descriptive phrase. And, unfortunately, there are no good medical names for most somatoform pain disorders. Moreover, if the patient is fixed on "the disease," it may be difficult to introduce the possibility of a nervous reaction of any kind as a factor in the pain. So how can we be straight with these patients?

It is possible. Most patients remain quite disturbed. The underlying personal problems persist. They suffer from both the pain and the emotional distress, and they are aware to some extent of the emotional source of the illness. Remember, too, that the patient's silent-observer self, who knows what is really going on, is also present at the interview (Ch. 12). Thus, if one proceeds cautiously, open to clues along the way, the patient may well be open to the personal phase of the interview, as well as an interpretation of the illness as an expression of nervous tension.

Usually, there are aspects of the pain that can be described to make plausible the diagnostic explanations to the patient. First, most somatoform pain disorders follow in the wake of disease or injury, or the painful physiological events of menstruation and childbirth. One might say, for example: "You have suffered a lot of pain here. When you have so much pain it usually sets up vulnerable pain circuits that are more reactive to stress than other areas of your body are. That's where you will feel the pain, rather than getting headaches or something else, as other people would." Note that this kind of explanation, which perhaps describes well the actual situation, circumvents the implications of the more precise psychiatric diagnosis. The pain is a kind of "reflex pain" that is common. You have seen it again and again. It is understandable. And the pain in such sensitized pain circuits, as in pelvic-pain disorders, for example, is characteristically more intense and sustained than is that of frank pelvic disease generally.

Second, it is often difficult to separate the psychophysiological from the somatoform aspects of a chronic pain disorder, and elements of disease are also sometimes present. To Janet F. (Ch. 1), for example, I would say: "I can't be sure of the precise nature of this pain. You say you have had some disturbance in your bowel function. Some of the pain may be caused by the colonic spasm of irritable-bowel syndrome. You could also have some reflex pelvic pain set up by the pelvic disease and menstrual cramps you have suffered. And there is likely to be a superimposed painful tension of the pelvic muscles. In any event, I am sure there is no active pelvic disease any longer, and it is now emotional distress that most likely triggers most of these reactions."

Or, to a patient whose chronic backache now appears to be complicated by more obvious psychophysiologic or somatoform features: "You suffered this painful back injury three years ago. That sets up a lot of muscle spasm, which is nature's way of protecting you from further injury. That too is painful. Probably most of the original injury has healed by now, but it has set up a kind of vicious circle in which the spasm hurts, and the pain itself causes more spasm. Any stress or nervous tension, whether from the disability itself or from other problems in your life, causes muscle tension all over your body, but it is only in your back, where you are most vulnerable, that you will feel the pain. We've got to look into all the things that may be keeping this muscle tension going, and see what can be done to get you well."

In general, I find it more acceptable to most patients, also more comfortable for me, to explain somatoform pain disorders in physiologic terminology, even though I know the mechanism may be for the most part "supra-physiologic." The goal is to get to the personal phase of the interview and work with the core issues, and this may be the most effective way to get there. In some situations, however, especially with conversions simulating neurologic disease, or when the patient's awareness of emotional distress has been wholly displaced by the physical symptoms, when the symptom is strictly symbolic and not superimposed in previous disease or injury, or when pressed for more precise explanations, it may be more effective to be explicit about its psychological function as the patient's way of dealing with an underlying problem.

Major psychiatric disorders. DSM-III-R terminology is often appropriate in communications with patients, especially to explain the need for psychopharmacology. If, for example, a patient has a long-standing panic disorder with agoraphobia, the source is obscure, and tricyclics are indicated, the illness is perhaps best described in psychiatric terms. In this situation, it would be explained how the symptomatic attacks, though they may have had an emotional basis at some point, often reappear without obvious provocation, and, because they engender such fear, tend to be self-perpetuating. On the other hand, though Mary S. (Ch. 3) also had a characteristic panic disorder, its source was readily ascertained, and drug therapy was unnecessary. In my interview with her the illness was better described simply as an expression of the underlying emotional distress. Identification as a psychopathological disorder would have been counterproductive. The descriptive phrases used to discuss a psychiatric condition should be adapted to the situation unique to each patient. To establish an effective relationship and get to the personal source, it may often be wise to avoid the official psychiatric nomenclature.

The Workup

To be affirmative about a functional disorder, the physician must be satisfied that the illness is not caused by disease. The patient must also know this and feel confident with the doctor's comprehensive analysis. Thus an appropriate workup is often essential.

In a collaborative approach, the clinician must plan, predict, and explain each step of the diagnostic and therapeutic process as well as this can be done. The workup is a crucial juncture. Its obvious purpose is to demonstrate disease, if indeed that is the cause of the illness. In the care of a probable functional disorder, it is equally important as the means necessary to resolve doubts about the diagnosis. Its purpose, positive or negative, is to resolve the problem and establish the diagnosis, whatever kind of illness it may be. If contrived instead to find any abnormality that could be installed as the diagnosis, inappropriate causation is likely to be ascribed. When that happens, the workup will have compounded the problem of the illness rather than solved it, though the clinician will not be aware that the process has miscarried.

Thus, how the workup is planned and explained depends on a preliminary clinical judgment in which the probabilities of the diagnostic possibilities are ranked. If a personal illness is most likely, it should appear at the top of the differential, with the disease rule-outs in a secondary list. Then the workup can be explained accordingly. If, on the other hand, the doctor fails to recognize the possibility of a functional disorder, or prefers not to think about it until the workup is completed, says nothing, and orders tests and X-rays with implications of organic disease, a dead end is likely. The illness may slip into any one of the paths of nonresolution described in Chapter 6.

If, however, the possibility of a functional disorder has been delineated from the start, the discourse about it continues naturally at the visit following the negative workup, or, if significant disease is demonstrated, this is readily explained. The purpose of the workup, after all, was to cover all possibilities. Whereas it is a simple matter to reverse a tentative diagnosis of a functional disorder to one of disease, when both possibilities were discussed before the workup was started, it can be quite difficult to reverse the diagnosis from disease to functional disorder if the latter possibility was never mentioned.

Abnormalities disclosed on the physical exam or workup often have little or nothing to do with the illness (Chs. 1, 4, 6, and 13). These should be described and, if appropriate, treated, but with a clear statement that what has turned up is common and rarely causes symptoms, and there is no indication that it is more than a coincidental or marginal finding in this case.

The Patient Parries

In spite of the inherent difficulties in explaining a functional illness to patients who are not aware of any stress in their lives and do not feel emotionally disturbed, the physician is not often confronted with a total rejection of this point of view—if, indeed, the approach has been comprehensive, and the doctor has developed a genuine interest and concern about this person and whatever the problem may be. Nevertheless, patient resistance is not uncommon, especially in a consulting practice to which the most refractory problems, especially those with entrenched secondary gains, are referred.

Resistance, after all, is understandable (Ch. 11). Repression and dissociation are powerful forces that evolve for very good reasons. The patient has found it impossible, or so it seemed, to recognize or deal more directly with the underlying problems; to do so now would appear to be personally devastating. It could undermine or destroy an important relationship. Or the patients may know about the problem but, focused on the physical distress and unaware of the suppressed emotions, they cannot believe that they could have so little ego strength, control, self-possession, whatever, that this situation somehow got the best of them.

Thus it is important to accept and respect the patient's defenses, to proceed gently but clearly. I don't pretend to be effective most of the time with patients who are strongly resistant to the whole concept of a nervous disorder. I don't like to push my point of view on unwilling patients, especially if the illness is a well-established way of life. It may be appropriate, whenever the patient's responses so indicate, to retreat to the medical model, reasserting the descriptive diagnosis, but not pursuing the personal phase of the interview at this time. On the other hand, the patient has a right to know my clinical judgment, and I prefer to be more explicit, especially with an illness of more recent onset, or when the patient has been referred as if to a "court of last appeal." So these contrary forces need to be balanced. Occasionally, I push my point of view too far too fast, and upset a patient unnecessarily. At other times I know that I have retreated prematurely and lost a real opportunity to change the course of the patient's illness.

Often the resistance is more of a front than a fixed position. So I hope that the patient may be aware at some level that we are on the right track, or may respond more positively later, if not now.

Let us consider here some common arguments of patients and how the physician, if confident of the diagnosis, might respond.

"I don't believe that's all it is. There must be something really wrong. Can't you get more tests to find out?" I reply that these pains [specify the symptoms, whatever they are] seem very strange to you, but the pains of [specify medical name of the functional disorder or other descriptive phrase] are not at all unusual. Doctors encounter this kind of condition far more often than they do the diseases [specify] that can sometimes cause similar symptoms. Actually, the way you feel is quite characteristic of this kind of illness, and I believe it to be the most useful way to view what you have. I don't see it as a diagnostic problem. The tests we have done rule out the possibility of other diseases very well, and I am pleased that they are negative. You would be in real trouble if you had [specify disease].

"Can you be sure about all this?" No, medical judgments are usually probabilities rather than certainties. But I believe there are enough data here to be fairly sure about the kind of illness you have, and that's a good place to begin looking further into the different kinds of things that may be affecting the way you feel. I plan to reevaluate the diagnosis and your whole condition periodically, but I don't expect to find something else wrong in the near future. If you would feel more secure, I'd like to arrange a consultation.

"How could I have so much pain [or whatever symptom] if there is nothing really wrong with me? Is that what you are saying? Is it in my head or something?" I say: There *is* something really wrong with you. You have a serious disturbance in the function of this part of your body. The pain is precisely as you describe it, just where you say it is. Is there not a lump in your throat when you hold back tears? Do you not feel your heart pound and your body tense when you slam on your brakes to keep from hitting a child crossing the street? The body's reactions to stressful situations are very real indeed. They persist, and they can be extremely disabling. The problem in medical conditions of this kind is that the concerns, worries, stresses, or needs, or whatever it is that causes your body to react this way, are not so obvious. This is a common problem. You must be aware that most of the pains, headaches, GI troubles, and many other nervous conditions that so many people suffer from are not caused by specific diseases. But if they can find ways to reduce the stress in their lives, get in better shape, generally speaking, or attend to whatever kinds of problems there may be, they get steadily better.

"The pains [or whatever symptom] come on at odd times when there is nothing happening. How could that be due to nervous tension?" My response: Your body has become sensitized to its own particular way of reacting to stress. In this kind of condition there are usually ongoing problems that don't change much from day to day, but because your body has been sensitized in this way the reactions can be provoked by many other factors, just by losing sleep or worrying about something else, for example. Or the body will react without any apparent provocation whatsoever. That is the way it usually is. If you felt the way you do only when you were angry or disappointed about something obvious, you would not be seeing a doctor to find out what was wrong.

"There is nothing in my life to be upset about. I'm not nervous. The only thing wrong with me is the pain [or whatever symptom]. If I didn't have the pain, I would be perfectly OK." All I can say is that I feel quite sure that what you have is this kind of illness. Often, the underlying problems are not at all obvious. Clearly, as you say, you are not aware of anything to be upset about. Nevertheless, in my experience with many patients who feel just as you do, something turns up, sooner or later, which, in retrospect, was the source of the distress. It is easy to suppress negative feelings about something, especially when everybody, including yourself, would be upset if you were to express yourself more freely. Or sometimes something happens that, though not in itself too unusual, triggers some old concerns that have lain dormant for years, perhaps since childhood. Or you may just be needing something that you're not getting. There are many different kinds of nervous or stress reactions. From what we have talked about so far, I have no idea what the problem here might be, but it may be helpful to talk more about these kinds of things at some other time, and perhaps your spouse should participate. I believe it is possible to reach a better understanding.

It should be understood, of course, that in medical practice generally (except in psychotherapy) and in most alternative healing systems, a directed quest for psychosocial understanding is more the exception than the rule. So there are many ways to proceed in other ways when the patient's opposition to the psychosocial aspects of a comprehensive approach become apparent.

Strategies that serve to bypass the personal source of illness were described in Chapter 6, but I believe it is essential neither to beg the diagnostic question nor to suggest a diagnosis that is not really the cause of the symptoms. The most acceptable practice is a diagnostic appraisal that accurately describes the symptoms in physiologic or psychiatric terminology, and the customary therapeutic plan of the biomedical model, usually with symptomatic or psychoactive drugs, especially at the beginning of care. To this may be added referral for other health-promotion measures and/or a stress-reduction program or other means of behavioral modification. Fortunately, partial symptomatic relief can be provided for many functional and psychiatric disorders. Often the therapy is effective mainly as a means of providing support, or as suggestion or placebo (as with Mario L., Ch. 12). Any positive approach is likely to be helpful, even though the psychosocial basis of the illness may be bypassed altogether. Later, the relative medical and psychosocial aspects of recovery can be adjusted in various ways according to the patient's particular situation, as discussed further in Ch. 18.

There are, however, illnesses that persist indefinitely until the moment of truth when the core problems are identified and a realistic plan for their resolution can begin. Some patients, however, as in a somatoform pain disorder, when finally confronted by the need to look at an emotional component to the illness, cannot do this and leave to find another doctor who is better able to identify the "disease."

There are many medical situations in which patient and doctor must come to grips with their divergent views of illness. If I am convinced, for example, that disability benefits are not warranted, that antibiotics are not indicated for what is a viral respiratory infection, or that recovery cannot be expected without identifying the emotional source of an illness, I feel that it is important to state my case, gently but clearly. If patients then decide to find a doctor who views illness as they do, or with whom they feel more comfortable for one reason or another, they should do so. Losing an occasional patient in this way is no proof you have failed.

CHAPTER 17

The Core of the Collaboration:
The Personal Interview

This chapter summarizes some of the more common sources of distress in adult life that often result in personal illness and suggests ways to explore these issues in one or two hour-long interviews.

The Directed Interview

Ideally, clues about the source of distress in a personal illness emerge during the medical history (Chs. 14, 15) or in response to the open-ended queries at the beginning of the interview (Ch. 16). It may turn out, however, that no troubling situation has been disclosed, yet your tentative judgment is that such distress may well be a major factor, and the illness is not likely to resolve until the source is determined. Thus, a more structured interview designed to begin this process is essential. Many busy physicians will be unable to find the time for such an interview. Referral is necessary. Nevertheless, it is helpful to appreciate the more common sources of distress. The physician may then be able to restrict the interview to those aspects that are likely to be most significant. There are several important considerations here.

The Patient/Doctor Relationship

The responsiveness of patients to an interview depends on the ambience of the relationship. The patient must view the doctor as medically competent. This should happen if there has been a careful history and physical examination, a discussion of the major diagnostic considerations, both functional and organic, and a pertinent workup to rule out disease. The patient must also feel that the interviewer is interested, caring, empathic, supportive, and open-minded, and listens carefully and responds accordingly—in general, is comfortable to be with. How to proceed with such an interview is beautifully described by Reiser and Schroder [1] for adult medicine, and by Green [2] for pediatrics. As described in Chapter 14, establishing an effective relationship with the patient and acquiring the medical data go hand in hand throughout the medical history, and the focus shifts from the person to the symptomatic problem or back again whenever appropriate. Clearly the doctor must be comfortable eliciting emotions and sharing human problems. If not, someone else should do the interview (Ch. 10).

A major barrier for physicians is our compulsion to fix everything, as we try to do when treating disease. We can, of course, treat the symptoms of personal illness, but we need to keep in mind that our major contribution is simply to help the patient become more aware of the underlying problem in relation to the illness. The very process of sharing the problem with the doctor can relieve the isolation of many patients. This in turn leads into a therapeutic alliance in which this person can begin to consider alternative approaches, plans, choices for a more effective adaptation or resolution. Eventually, this is the patient's responsibility, not ours. This is very much like sharing the problem of a spouse, or friends, or colleagues, who do not want to be told how they ought to solve a problem as much as they want your personal support while they consider their own options.

Some patients, such as those who have a rigid self-image and are dissociated from suppressed emotions, or those who have a distinct secondary gain from the illness, or are fixed on a specific organic diagnosis or medication, will resent the quest for understanding. Even with the most defensive patients, however, a reasonably productive interview may be possible. Resentment occurs most often when I have failed to provide an adequate explanation for the understanding I hope to achieve, or push ahead in an interview without first recognizing and acknowledging the patient's discomfort.

Cultural barriers may also block disclosure: customs may dictate that emotional or family problems are never divulged, or perhaps mentioned only within the family or to a spiritual guide or healer; or the patient simply cannot feel understood or accepted by an outsider with different values and background. The professional ambience of the doctor's office may be an obstacle in itself. The physician needs to be aware of these problems and, when appropriate, should reach out to help the patient feel comfortable. Possible difficulties in understanding each other could be acknowledged, for example, at the beginning of the history, and the doctor can affirm explicitly that he/she hopes clearly to understand the patient's concerns by checking back to be sure. The patient is also invited to clarify, elaborate, or correct at any time. If, later in the visit, it is necessary to state that nervous tension about something is a likely source of the distress, the doctor must nevertheless respect the patient's reticence about personal disclosure, and terminate the interview accordingly.

The Patient's Personal Situation

The kinds of situations that lead into the common functional disorders and emotional disturbances of medical practice are mainly the same kinds of problems we all commonly encounter. McWhinney summarized the main social factors: loss, conflict, change, maladjustment, stress, isolation, and failure.[3] Ireton and Cassata provide a concise psychological systems review that includes the patient's emotional status, life situation, personality patterns, and outlook on life.[4] Many clinicians have made this point. Osler, in a lecture to medical students: "To you, as the trusted family counselor, the father will come with his anxieties, the mother with her hidden grief, the daughter with her trials, and the son with his follies. Fully one-third of the work you do will be entered in other books than yours."[5] Kirsner, describing the emotional factors in functional bowel disorders: "In most instances, the disorder seems to originate in relation to the ordinary frustrations, anxieties and disappointments of life, rather than from serious psychiatric problems."[6] Allan and Kaufman surveyed nervous factors in 1,000 unselected patients attending the Lahey Clinic for general medical examination. Of the 406 patients with significant "neuropsychiatric" components to the illness, 80 percent were viewed as having "benign nervous states" due largely to external situations; 20 percent as "psychoneurosis" related more distinctly to intrinsic personality factors.[7]

Each person brings to the "ordinary frustrations, anxieties, and disappointments of life" his/her own unique approach to problem-solving, his/her own ego defense system or adaptational style.[8] In this sense, every personal illness is psychosocial; that is, it involves a person (the "intrinsic" component) and a situation (the "extrinsic" component). The observations cited above simply indicate that the personal problems that result in the functional disorders and "benign nervous states" of medical practice, or accentuate the illnesses caused by organic disease, can be viewed for the most part as responses to particular situations. Though intrinsic forces clearly determine the response, and may affect other areas of the patient's life, understanding begins by identifying the precipitating situation: the marital conflict, a state of exhaustion from inordinate stress, a grief reaction, the effects of adverse health habits, an existential dilemma, whatever it may be. That is the appropriate goal of the interview in primary care. What the patient can personally do to change the situation, or whether the intrinsic factors need to be understood in greater depth and modified accordingly (the province of psychotherapy), are secondary considerations.

My point here may better be clarified by reviewing five patients, each with a marital problem. In each case, the interview revealed the situation in which the emotional disturbance arose. In each case, either the problem had not been previously recognized or it had been brushed aside with too little attention. Ruth B. and her husband (Ch. 1) were able to improve their relationship simply by talking it over together more openly and honestly. Mary S. (Ch. 3) needed only a better understanding of her sexuality and some birth-control advice. Evelyn C. (Ch. 11) had to alter her adaptational approach to the marriage, but she was fortunate enough to discover how to do this in an early interview, and her husband was receptive to the "new" Evelyn. Diane B. (Ch. 13) had to make similar changes, but this required several months of intensive psychotherapy. Janet F. (Ch. 1) found her situation untenable, and the marriage ended in divorce.

In each case, emotional distress was expressed as an illness with physical symptoms: somatoform pain disorder, panic disorder, or chest-tension syndrome. The key point: until the illness was correctly diagnosed, and its source identified, neither the illness nor the marital problem could be resolved.

The frailties of the human condition are manifold. I do not pretend to be comprehensive in this brief survey of distressful situations. I will focus mainly on certain situations or ways of viewing them that I believe should receive more attention than they customarily do. A psychotherapist would find this account woefully lacking in psychodynamics, but in primary care a simple survey of the more common situations that patients must resolve one way or another often provides the crucial insight to the inner core of the illness.

The Flow of the Directed Interview

One's assessment of the patient's situation flows naturally from the overtures described in the previous three chapters. You have already told the patient that it may be helpful to understand the illness in relation to the patient's life situation, and you would like to know more about that. "So I'd like to talk with you about the kinds of situations that are important for most people, if I may." The patient willing, I proceed to explore whatever areas I feel most likely to be significant, continuing with "Tell me something about . . ." statements rather than with direct questions. I often ask first for a detailed description of the patient's daily life. Virtually everyone can talk comfortably about this, and the account may reveal the problem, as it did with Joseph H. (Ch. 1) and Orvieta T. (Ch. 2).

As with any conversation, there is no simple way to describe the flow of an interview. It is a series of responses, one to the other, and it changes its course continuously, depending on what evolves. Each patient, and, therefore, each interview is unique. Each doctor has her/his own general style, but the tone of the queries, the phrases used, and their sequence will vary according to the doctor's sense of the patient's rapport at each moment.

It is often possible to get to the core problem quickly, simply by following up on the basic data from the social history (Ruth B., Ch. 1; Mary S., Ch. 3). In other patients, it may be necessary to explore several possible problem areas before getting to the main issue. Jean G. (Ch. 5) is a good example. I first considered here that perhaps the problem might lie in the marriage. This soon proved to be her strongest asset, so I asked about several other possibly troubling situations—stress, conflict, loss or disappointment—but found no apparent disturbances. I did not feel that this was a problem of contained emotions about any one of these situations, but, of course, one can never be sure about this. I had not yet asked about her daily routine, because I usually introduce this question when I believe the patient has too many stressful demands rather than too little to do. It was this question, however, posed much later in the interview, that finally disclosed what I took to be the main issue, an existential problem of meaning and joy in daily life.

When a problem is disclosed, how do you know it to be the source of the symptoms? It may be self-evident (Joseph H., Ch. 1; Ann F., Ch. 5). It is obvious if the patient breaks forth in tears or anger (Janet F., Ch. 1; Evelyn C., Ch. 11). It may be plausible, but clarity will evolve only after time. Sometimes the patient attributes the disturbance to a particular situation, but this turns out not to be the real problem.

The preliminary interviews, no matter how genial the rapport or clear the communications, may not begin to reveal much about the personal situation that is, nevertheless, the source of the emotional problem (Ch. 11). If the emotions are sufficiently repressed, patients cannot identify the problem, even though it emanates from a particular situation they do know about. Thus they cannot respond to your queries, even though they are trying to do so as openly as they can. Other patients have a persistent psychiatric or personality disorder that affects many aspects of life, and this cannot be identified by asking about particular situations; the focus must shift predominantly to the "intrinsic" factors, and referral for psychotherapy is usually necessary.

The patient may know very well what the problem is, but isn't ready to share, doesn't want to talk about it, and/or doesn't believe it has anything to do with the symptoms. I can recall many patients with acute anxiety, depression, and/or physical symptoms who absolutely denied any recent problems even when asked specific questions about what later turned out to be the central issue. It was only after several visits, and my insistence that the diagnosis was correct and there must be an underlying problem of some kind, that the patient disclosed, often with an outburst of emotion, the marital conflict or whatever it was. Some patients, nevertheless, will continue to "sit" on a known but concealed problem for months or years, suffering both emotionally and physically, with little or no response to symptomatic medications, even though just sharing the concerns, as with a friend, if not psychotherapy, could well have provided relief.

Thus doctor and patient must realize together that the quest for understanding, though sometimes clear and obvious, can often be an extended process in which the patient personally must become deeply involved, as in psychotherapy. We all know this, I believe, in trying to understand ourselves. With patients, a personal illness provides the incentive and direction. The initial interviews with a doctor or therapist are a beginning.

Some Common Problem Areas

Stress

There are, of course, many kinds of stressful situations, too numerous to mention. A partial list would include school problems, restricted opportunities for personal growth, a difficult job or loss of a job, interpersonal conflict, divorce, emotional isolation, inadequate personal support, loss and grief, sickness or injury, physical or sexual abuse, neglect, discrimination, and poverty, subsistence-level income, or financial reverses. Then there are the life transformations that can challenge anyone: adolescence, establishing sexuality, forming and holding relationships, leaving the parental home and starting one's own, securing a job or career, marriage, pregnancy, childbirth, raising children, retirement. Adolescence is now a particular problem because of the early introduction of sexuality, the wave of teenage pregnancy and sexually transmitted disease, the prevalent use of alcohol and access to street drugs, and the decline of the nuclear family and educational system.[9, 10]

The impact of each stage of the lifespan, whether viewed as a problem or as an opportunity for growth, has been variously described by Erikson, [11] Sheehy, [12] Ambron and Brodzinsky, [13] and Viorst.[14] One partial view of the relative impact of recent life events is defined in the social-adjustment rating scale of Holmes and Rahe.[15] It should be noted here, however, that many of the most severe stress reactions result from steady states, such as a difficult marriage or borderline socioeconomic status, not from recent changes.

The presence or absence of a stress response is determined by many factors: the magnitude of the "stressor" and its overall impact on the subject's life, the environment in which the stress occurs, and the person's appraisal of the situation, coping skills, personal resources, social support systems, and commitment to self and to life.[16, 17] We are concerned here with the direct effects of stress in causing a psychosomatic or emotional disorder, not with its long-range effects as a factor in the evolution of disease in general. Clearly, the interview will focus on the sources of stress most likely to occur in the patient's life situation.

Exhaustion

Here I will focus not on stress in general but on exhaustion in particular, because it is both common and often unrecognized. By this I mean the "breakdown" caused by excessive demands on one's time and energy, most commonly by overwork, combined with inadequate rest, recreation, and sleep. For this kind of situation, *exhaustion* is more specific than *stress*, a more general term customarily used to indicate any life situation or event that is emotionally distressing, though physical and emotional fatigue from overdoing may not be a factor.

Exploring this issue is a good way to begin the interview, for several reasons. It is common—the main cause of at least 15 percent of the 200 consecutive functional syndromes I evaluated in the medical clinic. It follows naturally an opening statement about what the patient does on a typical day. It is little threat to the patient's self-esteem to discover that this problem often afflicts the healthiest, most dependable people—mothers, workers, physicians, business executives, anyone who has taken on more responsibilities than almost anyone can handle. Symptoms often erupt even during periods of desirable intellectual concentration, emotional intensity, or physical activity, if the pursuits are sufficiently overextended.

Such patients rarely complain of fatigue. If fatigue, "no energy, too tired," is the chief complaint, with no evidence of disease, the patient can often "barely do anything." Fatigue, as a complaint, rarely results from doing too much (Chs. 6, 13). In contrast, the truly exhausted patient as described here either ignores, denies, or is simply not aware of the fatigue that most people experience under similar circumstances. Exhausted patients rarely mention their overtaxed lifestyles, which they regard as quite appropriate or inescapable, and unrelated to the symptoms.

Finally, the limits are set by muscle pains, headaches, chest pain, backaches, GI distress, or any functional syndrome, by the accentuation of the symptoms of an otherwise manageable organic disease, by depression/anxiety and related symptoms, or by any combination thereof. Fatigue may be one symptom of many, but, if so, it is rarely the dominant complaint. As with most of the personal problem areas discussed in this chapter, the particular clinical syndrome that appears is determined more by the patient's vulnerability to that form of emotional or biological expression than by the nature of the personal situation per se.

Syndromes of exhaustion will not be disclosed unless you ask specific questions: What do you actually do at work? How hard is it? Do you stand or sit? How much vigilance does it take? How much responsibility? What are the working conditions? How many hours per day, per week? When do you get home? Do you then have more work to do? Do you have another job? Can you eat with your family? What time do you go to bed? Fall asleep? Get up? How many hours do you actually sleep? How do you get to work? How long does it take? How much traffic? How much time do you have for your spouse, your children, yourself? When did you last take a vacation? What do you do for recreation? Sundays? And, of course, I have already asked about smoking, alcohol, coffee, and drugs, which tend to complicate the problem as tension mounts.

I am often appalled by what I hear. I learn that this person (actual patient who mentioned only what appeared to be a routine job on the occupational history) really holds two jobs, works 80 hours a week, drives two hours daily on a crowded freeway, averages four hours' sleep, smokes a pack or two, drinks 15 cups of coffee, has no time at all for recreation, and took his last two-week vacation five years ago to visit relatives. This is not an unusual story. Lesser grades of exhaustion, often combined with the kinds of emotional stress described previously, are, of course, more common but enough to cause symptoms. I am further appalled when the patients comment, "What's wrong with that?"

Exhaustion syndromes are well known in the military, where they are classified as combat or operational fatigue or by the medical names of the dominant symptoms.[18] In civilian life, however, they are so much a part of the American way that they usually go unrecognized. A Medline search revealed very few papers bearing on the problem. This kind of exhaustion is not even mentioned as one of the stressors listed in Selye's book,[19] in the DSM-III-R,[20] or in the life-event scales of Holmes and Rahe.[15] Type A behavior, as described by Friedman and Rosenman,[21] was thought to be a factor, but many exhausted patients do not have such a personality.

The demands may be mainly extrinsic. One must mobilize all available energy to hold a job and care for a large family with a marginal income, to cope with the challenge of a handicapped child, a sick spouse, a dying parent, or many other kinds of overwhelming situations. The basic challenge of surviving or getting ahead in a competitive society can be a problem in itself. Then too, many people are driven to extremes by intrinsic emotional forces that have never been confronted.[22] Other subjects have not learned to assert themselves or to say no, and they get over their heads trying to meet the excessive expectations of other people. Symptoms also result, not just from exhaustion, but from the emotional disharmony caused by the neglect of other personal or family needs that may be far more important.

Thus, an exhaustion syndrome may be complex at many levels. Nothing will change, however, until the exhaustion per se is recognized as the cause of the symptoms.

Health

The patient's nutrition and eating habits, weight, exercise, stress, sleep, rest and recreation, smoking, coffee/tea ingestion, use of alcohol and street or medicinal drugs are all important in terms of current health and disease prevention. A rigorous investigation is indicated, of course, in the study of any disease or functional disorder in which inimical habits are specific factors.

Here, however, let us consider that adverse health habits can accentuate the illness of *any* functional, psychiatric, or organic disorder. Thus, the patient's general pursuit of health is often a decisive element of the plan for healing. This can represent the main thrust of holistic medicine [23] or of certain alternative healing disciplines, if indeed the practitioner is dedicated to what patients must do for themselves to achieve optimal health.

The main underlying problem in a psychosomatic disorder, let us say, is a stressful job or marriage. But when the subject begins to drink or smoke more, gets fat, and stops exercising, a vicious circle of accentuated symptoms and adverse health habits ensues. Improvement in any component of this chain of events may effect relief. The physician with migraine, for example, may find it difficult to reduce a busy practice, but the headaches can be abated by limiting the use of alcohol and sleeping an additional hour. The pursuit of health can be recommended for its own sake, but if disturbed patients can be convinced to live accordingly, they may look more carefully at their lives, see that stress reduction may be as pertinent as other health habits, and, at a deeper level, consider more basic changes in their life situation. The physician with migraine, for example, might find a way to reduce his/her practice and spend more time with the family.

Interpersonal Conflict

Obviously, any important interpersonal conflict can provoke emotional tension. Most disturbing are conflicts involving marriage partners, parents and children, other family interactions, and crucial relationships at school, at work, or with friends or lovers.

Marital discord. This is but one aspect of disturbed family interrelationships. I focus here on marital discord for several reasons. In a brief interview, one can more readily ask about the marital situation than about family systems in general, and it is one of the most common stressful situations of adult life that are of sufficient emotional intensity to cause symptoms. Also, unlike many other kinds of adult conflict, the subjects may have so adjusted to the situation that they are not fully aware of the problems they deal with all the time. The patient, feeling loyal and responsive to the spouse, may well be reticent to discuss the marriage. It is private, and it is supposed "to work." The patient is disconcerted, perhaps a little ashamed, that it doesn't, particularly in regard to sexual shortcomings or dissatisfaction. And women, probably more often than men, can get into passive, trying-to-please roles in which they are simply not aware of how dissatisfied they are. Thus, if you just ask questions that invite a yes or no response—Is your marriage all right? Are there any problems?—the answer is Yes, and No, respectively. Yet there may be a problem, ranging anywhere from passive discontent to active conflict.

A better way to get into this question is to invite patients to tell their own story: Tell me about your marriage. If little is forthcoming, you might suggest: Tell me about your wife (or husband). What is she (he) like? This, of course, shifts attention from the patient to the spouse and could reveal the latter's sickness or alcoholism, a personality conflict, a difference in values or interest, the inattention of a mate who is mostly involved with other pursuits or doesn't care, hostility or violence, or many other problems, especially if you follow up on clues as they appear. Then: Tell me about yourself. What are you like, I mean in relation to your wife (or husband) and the marriage. Later, more particularly: Can you share your feelings, state your needs, be assertive if necessary, get angry, talk things over? How does she (he) respond? Can she (he) be open with you? There are many ways to proceed. I mean here only to indicate how the interview might follow its own course to get to the specific areas that are most likely to result in conflict.

Alcohol abuse and dependency are common, and the excessive or inappropriate drinking patterns of a spouse (or other family member) can have profound adverse effects on the entire family. This may be the major source of your patient's functional or psychiatric disorder, sexual distress, requests for psychoactive drugs, the developmental difficulties of the children—any of a host of emotional problems. When asked to describe the spouse, the patient may well fail to disclose the core problem, for many reasons. Thus, in addition to inquiring about the general health of the family, it is well to ask disturbed patients more specifically if they have any concerns about the spouse's drinking or any other behaviors. The spouse may be viewed as a social drinker, not a problem drinker. Nevertheless: Are there any occasions on which this can be a problem for you or anyone else?

When a problem area is disclosed, it leads naturally to a further discussion about how the couple handles or avoids it. In particular, the acquiescent patient "can't do anything about it" and gets into a variety of co-dependent behaviors that are very likely to cause symptoms.[24] (Specific questions about physical or sexual abuse are discussed later in this chapter.)

Sexuality. Sexuality is a poignant core of life experience for most people. Problems with sex can be the major cause of an emotionally induced illness (Mary S., Ch. 3) or one symptom of a more general conflict (Ruth B., Ch. 1). In both cases, it proved to be the key to understanding the whole illness.

Sexuality need not be discussed in most "medical" conditions. When it is a problem, however, as in many nervous disorders, also in chronic disease, patients often respond positively to the opportunity to talk about it with a sensitive and informed professional, or at least to ask questions. If not, you can pull back from this subject. But for many patients the very process of opening this area for discussion can be therapeutic.[25] It serves to accept the patient as a sexual person, with the understanding that concerns about sex are common and expected. The physician, with a perspective on the problems most often encountered, may be able to allay the patient's discomfort, offer helpful suggestions, or, depending on the circumstances, consider referral.

When the discussion is appropriate, it can begin in many ways. "May I ask about sexuality? Is there any problem in your marriage (or relationship)? Do you have any concerns or questions?" Or, "How has this illness (or operation) affected your sexuality?" Or, especially with women, a gentle approach could be something like this: "Some people are mainly affectionate and not so sexual; others are sexual but not so affectionate. Some are both, and some are neither. How would you describe yourself in this regard? And what about your husband or partner?" In this way the problem, if there is one, can be viewed in a wider context. I would add at any point: "It doesn't matter so much where you might fit into this spectrum of feelings; what matters is whether you feel there is a problem here in your relationship." The discussion will usually include questions of general satisfaction or dismay, the orgasmic experience, and its significance for the patient.

A particular problem, especially in women with somatoform pelvic pain, is the patient who, never having experienced a sexual response, is unaware of its absence. Sex may or may not be disagreeable, but it certainly lacks any special significance. Such patients, unlike those with other kinds of sexual problems, may be quite defensive, resisting any discussion of sexuality. When asked if they respond sexually, they may reply with an oblique answer, or say, "Always," as though that could not possibly be any part of the problem. The question here will have to be viewed in conjunction with other aspects of the marital situation.

Children/parents. The psychological and social problems of children, and the developmental disorders associated therewith, which are related in many ways to the problems of their families, are intrinsic to pediatric practice.[26] Thus, unlike doctors in adult practice who tend to be focused biomedically, those who supervise the health, growth, and development of children and adolescents are naturally concerned about the family milieu in their appraisals of health or sickness. The various aspects of parental nurture, neglect, or abuse are particularly important. And, in a complex society of alternative values, the youth must contend with many kinds of pressure and conflict.

In pediatric care, difficulties in personal growth and well-being usually emerge clinically as behavioral, social, developmental, and school problems, as sleep, feeding, and eating disorders, or as problems secondary to the sexuality and alcohol or drug use of adolescence. They also appear as psycho-physiologic or somatoform functional disorders or depression, and emotional disturbances accentuate the illnesses of organic disease. An ongoing family problem or concern may well be the hidden agenda that provokes the visit about a minor complaint.[27]

Clearly, the problems of growing up erupt clinically in many ways during childhood. Unfortunately, however, the impact of interpersonal conflicts, even major trauma, is often repressed until it surfaces as the emotional problems of adult life. Thus, parent-child interactions, and the problems of childhood development, are often the key to understanding, in both pediatrics and adult medicine. The nurture of children is a problem of overwhelming importance to the present and future life of every child and to that individual's relationship to society. This whole issue, nevertheless, is beyond the scope of this book and my own clinical experience as an internist. The reader is referred to such texts as those of Prugh [28] and Green and Haggerty,[29] and the references, for both professionals and parents, that are there recommended.[30, 31]

Sadly, society in general, as well as the care providers who want to play a more effective role in spite of the limited time and resources available to them, has much to learn about how better to understand, educate, prevent, suspect, recognize, and talk about the many difficulties of childhood, or how best to help troubled families in need, or to intervene when necessary. The schools serve a function, and parenting classes and other community resources are available, but our society as a whole needs to be far more concerned about the welfare of children.

Sexual and Physical Abuse

The abuse of children and, yes, the abuse of adult women, is a devastating situation for the victims, both during the period of maltreatment and, usually, for the rest of their lives. The problem of the physically battered child is now well recognized.[32, 33] The prevalence and impact of the sexual abuse of children and of the domestic physical violence and oppressive sexual aggression or assaults against adult women, however, has only recently been recognized. Such abuse as a significant source of many kinds of clinical distress often remains unnoticed and unattended in medical care generally. Thus the problem is introduced here as another important area to consider as we seek to understand disturbed patients.

Frank abuse, of course, is the most overt manifestation of the perpetrator's failure to nourish and respect the individuality and emotional integrity of family members. Ideally, we would become aware of the inappropriate enmeshment and more general dysfunctions in the families of disturbed patients, past or present, though this kind of understanding may emerge only in psychotherapy. Nevertheless, the abuse per se is particularly pernicious, and, if detected, provides a handle to the whole problem.

The sexual abuse of children. About three of ten women and one of six men interviewed in adult surveys had suffered sexual abuse before the age of 18, often during childhood or puberty.[34–36] The facts can be difficult to elicit during the period of abuse.[37] In the case of incest, the child is dependent on the parents, and is afraid, withdrawn, bewildered. If the father is the abuser, the mother is often defensive for many reasons, and denies the child's allegations. Still, many adults molested as children, when asked why they never said anything about it, say, "No one ever asked me." This is a delicate issue, but pediatricians are learning to be responsive to cues or allegations, and how to ask about it judiciously as one of many possible problem areas in the psychosocial survey of a disturbed child. To do this tactfully and compassionately, the health professional should, of course, be comfortable with children, create an affinitive relationship, and be familiar with the approaches of experienced clinicians.[37–41]

Adults molested as children. The dominant role of childhood sexual abuse in the etiology of "hysteria" was first noted by Freud in 1896,[42] then discounted as fantasy by Freud and the psychiatric community for most of this century, only to be documented again in the past decade or so as a major source of the functional, personality, and psychiatric disorders of adult life.[43–50] In women with the kind of chronic pelvic pain described through this book, for example, several studies have demonstrated a prominent history of childhood sexual abuse,[51–55] and of sexual trauma as adults.[51, 52] In one study, childhood physical abuse predominated.[55]

The emphasis in this chapter is on current situations, not psychodynamics. Nevertheless, at least the major traumas of childhood can be readily identified by name and asked about in a brief interview. If an adult, especially one with persistent psychosomatic or psychiatric disorders, sexual dysfunction, or difficulties in relationships, has been a victim of sexual or physical abuse, it can be important to elicit this history. Parental alcoholism or other traumatic, overriding problems, such as a major loss, separation, or neglect, can also be pervasively damaging. Until the trauma is brought to light and its effects surmounted, usually in extended psychotherapy, healing, if restricted to the "present illness," ongoing behaviors, and current situation, can only go so far.

What has happened often has profound and lasting deleterious effects on psychological, social, and physical functioning.[56] The clinical syndromes we diagnose are merely one symptom of a much deeper problem. The usual secrecy and denial in the family force the child to repress overwhelming emotions and to deny a large part of reality. The fear, pain, and confusion often result in memory blocks and permanent splits in normal personality integration. The child who needs to believe the parents to be "right" usually comes to feel that there must be "something wrong with me." As adults they suffer from impaired self-esteem and confidence, an inability to trust, and blocks in sexual responses. They are often unable to cope with anger and aggression, both in themselves and in others. They find it difficult to form and hold significant relationships, including those with professionals. In many ways they suffer from the "traumagenic" effects of premature sexualization, betrayal, disempowerment, and the stigmatization that often results.[57]

Physical and sexual violence against adult women. The abuse of women constitutes a comparable assault on personal integrity. We should by now be aware of the striking prevalence of domestic physical violence, and how to suspect, recognize, and deal more effectively with the whole problem.[58–61] And we should be concerned about domestic sexual abuse: persistent, unwanted male sexual aggression, often with threats, force, or violence, certainly without any regard for the response or feelings of the woman partner in an ongoing relationship.[62] We should also realize the far-reaching effects of adult abuse of any kind in the genesis of psychiatric and psychosomatic disorders.[43, 58, 63–65] For example, in one study of women with chronic pain (low back, abdominal/pelvic, headache, other) referred to a pain center, half or more had suffered sexual and/or physical abuse.[65] In this study, the abuse was experienced predominantly as adults, and it had usually continued for years. In another survey, one of five women patients in an emergency department had suffered domestic physical violence.[58] The visit was prompted either by the injury itself or by symptoms due in part to the stress of living in an abusive relationship.

Reshaping the interview when abuse is suspected. Because the medical world has but recently become aware of the extent of the abuse of children and women, most doctors in practice, myself included, have for the most part bypassed these problems in talking with our patients. It is now clear, however, that we should more often include this question in the interview, especially of women with persistent nervous disorders: "It is now known that many women with this kind of disturbance have suffered some kind of physical or sexual abuse. Did you by any chance experience any such abuse as a child or adolescent?" And, "Have you been subjected to any physical violence or unwanted sexual aggression in your adult life?" The patient may not wish to respond, or cannot do so in regard to childhood memories that may emerge only after a relationship is established with a sensitive clinician. But the question is a beginning. An important function of the physician is to accept and acknowledge the patient's history. The patient may then come to realize, sooner or later, the importance of dealing more effectively with an ongoing problem, or surmounting the aftermath of previous abuse.

The same issues apply to the most flagrant of all psychosomatic disorders: the battered woman in the emergency room. Unfortunately, here too, the basic problem, a serious threat to her very life, is often disregarded. It is not considered to be a relevant medical concern.[60, 66–69] In a recent analysis of the emergency department records of 52 patients who were seriously and unquestionably injured deliberately by another person, the physician in 90 percent of the interactions had asked little or nothing about the violent marital situation or previous physical or sexual abuse, and failed to address the question of the woman's safety.[67] Sometimes both the assailant and the victim, as persons, have been detached from the event as recorded in the account of the injury: "hit in mouth by fist." Failure to acknowledge the woman's abusive experience is psychologically damaging *in itself.*

At the least, someone in the emergency room, if not the physician personally, must acknowledge the violence, ask about it, and assert that such an attack is illegal and intolerable. It is simply wrong. Nothing she may have done makes her "deserve" to be beaten. And she is not alone in this experience. The staff should express concern about her safety. "Is there some place you can go—to a friend or relative—if it is too dangerous to return home? Can you get out before this happens? Are the children safe?" Often a woman will not complain until she feels the children are endangered. Most important, she should be apprised of the community-based resources available to help her. The very acknowledgment that domestic violence is going on, that it is a serious problem, and that something needs to be done about it can be a powerful and therapeutic first step.

Working with family problems, the physician is aware of the interdependence of family relationships as well as the problems, but abuse is intolerable, and, especially with problems of the intrafamilial abuse of children, both the parents and their victims can be helped in programs of individual and family therapy.[33, 39, 40, 70] To resolve a problem it must first be identified. That is the immediate goal of the interview, both at the clinical and personal levels.

Loss and Grief

Grief in response to the loss (death, sickness, separation) of a spouse, parent, child, or other significant person can impair physical as well as emotional health and social functioning in many ways.[71] Even the usual normal grief that most people experience often results in depression, anxiety, and functional disorders; "morbid" grief reactions, related to unresolved problems in the lives of the bereaved, the deceased, or the relationship, compound the problem.[72, 73] In a survey of 375 widows, 28 percent were deemed to have suffered a marked deterioration of health in the year following the death of their husbands, compared to 4.5 percent of a control series.[74] The most common physical symptoms were sleep disturbances, anorexia and weight loss, dyspnea, palpitation, chest pain, trembling, fatigue and weakness, headaches, dizziness, widespread pains, and GI disturbances.[75]

The problem in medical care is that the patient simply reports the headaches (Daphne G., Ch. 14), the dizziness (Joseph H., Ch. 1), or whatever the symptom. This person may be trying to be stoical, not to grieve, to ignore, deny, or rise above the whole problem, or, though aware of grief, regards it as a normal process unrelated to the symptoms. In any event, nothing is said about either the loss or the grief. Meanwhile, the physician, who also regards grief as a natural, self-limited response of little or no medical concern, does not think to ask about it, or, though aware of the loss from learning of the family or marital history, fails to recognize the grief reaction or its relation to the symptoms.[76]

Thus, it may be helpful to consider and ask about loss and grief as one possible cause of a personal illness. There are several important considerations here. For example, the bereaved person may not have grieved (Daphne). Although grief is a very natural expression of the love shared, many people feel somehow that it is not proper: "I never cried at the funeral or since." The family attitude is often to protect the bereaved from grief. There is a conspiracy of silence in our culture. Although psychoactive drugs can be helpful to tide the patient over a crisis, the physician may contribute to the problem with an allied medical frame of reference in which emotional distress is regarded as something that can and should be overcome or suppressed, regardless of its source or function. Nevertheless, healing usually depends on acknowledging the loss, accepting the pain, and experiencing the grief process as one works through it to a new sense of self and interactive life patterns.

The bereaved may be beset with guilt, perhaps not about what one has done but about what one could have done in a more loving way but did not. Or the bereaved may encounter the greatest loss of all, the discovery of "no self," as Joseph did (Ch. 1).

Though the loss is usually recent, within a year or so, it is sometimes distant, the grief now surfacing when precipitated by an anniversary reaction or some other current reminder. Death is the most tragic loss, but a major interpersonal loss of any kind—"exits from the social field" as described by Paykel et al., divorce, separation, family member leaving home, etc.—often precipitate depressive reactions.[77]

The general problem of loss can be construed in many other ways that are more strictly intrapersonal. Any life transformation such as retirement, for example, involves a certain loss of previous ways of being, meaning, and purpose that may, for some individuals, outweigh the new opportunities. A personal failure can be experienced as an overwhelming loss in terms of what one had hoped to achieve, as discussed under depression. In many situations, though the whole process can be difficult, it is necessary to acknowledge the loss, accept it, let it go, and move on.

Another devastating problem is the isolation, the loneliness, the lack of personal support, that so many people endure constantly. Though perhaps not due to a recent separation from family or friends, it is indeed a "loss" of what could have been. In a vulnerable person, it can be a major factor in depression and a serious mortality risk for disease in general (Ch. 7). And it can be a critical problem in the care of any disease. The physician must be aware of the patient's support system.

Clearly, loss is an inherent problem of the human condition that we must all face in many ways, sooner or later.[14] A major loss, with its attendant grief and the unexpected constellation of personal needs that falls in its place, can readily precipitate enough distress to induce a medical visit. Fortunately, loss and grief, because they are such universal predicaments, are not usually difficult to recognize or talk about, if we think to do so, and the doctor can be a distinct source of support during the process of grief and recovery. "Working through" a major loss can take a long time, and may well require professional counsel or therapy.

Contained Emotions

As we have seen in many case histories, emotional containment is virtually a universal problem underlying the functional disorders of medical practice. Whether the emotions smolder deeply suppressed or just under the surface, the patients speak only of the symptoms, nothing more. The suppression may preclude an awareness of the underlying problematic situation as well as the emotional distress it causes. Or, though aware of the situation but not the emotional reaction, patients fail to perceive how the troubling situation could cause the symptoms.

Many patients fall into the latter group, and it is not difficult to get to the source of the distress. As understanding evolves, the emotional reaction that actually causes the symptoms may or may not erupt, but the patient need not experience the emotions in order to understand the symptoms in relation to the problematic situation.

If, however, an awareness of the disturbing reality of a situation, as well as its emotional readout, are strongly dissociated from the patient's conscious view of the same situation, the interviewer will not discover the source of the illness, even though specific questions about the very situation that provokes the disturbance may have been asked. This characterized the first three interviews with Evelyn C. (Ch. 11). We have previously discussed ways to suspect and surmount such barriers to understanding, but here I return again to emotional containment as a category for consideration during the interview, so as to reemphasize its ubiquity and importance. It is especially relevant when you find nothing about the life situation of a clearly disturbed patient that could be upsetting, and there is no obvious personality problem, past or present. In such patients, two possibilities should be understood:

First, there may or may not be a significant conflict. There was no discord, for example, between Evelyn C. and her husband. Her problem was her own: a habitual suppression of what she was really feeling or needed, to such an extent that she was barely aware how she routinely subjugated her real self to the way she thought she ought to be. In contrast, Ann F. (Ch. 5) suffered a real conflict, but emotional suppression was such a dominant force in her personality that she was unable to recognize her husband's indifference or describe any problem in the marriage, when first interviewed.

Second, there may or may not be a major personality problem. It is always a problem, of course, to be out of touch with one's own feelings, but many patients are outgoing, responsive, have many interests, activities, and a sense of humor, and it is difficult to detect how they may be beset with unfilled needs and emotional containment. Others have a more pervasive passivity or dependency, but, again, this goes unrecognized because the patient is "such a good person," sincere, friendly, well-liked, one who does "what is right." At the far pole of this spectrum are those who are insecure, overly dependent on relationships for their essential meaning in life, and have a need "to look good" with a real fear of facing the negative emotions and problems of themselves and their families, along with many other related traits variously described as dependent personality disorder [78] or, more flagrantly, by Schaef [24] and others, as co-dependence. This is often a key point in the whole problem of a person with an alcohol- or drug-dependent spouse. It can be a problem in any relationship in which the subject puts up with any inappropriate behavior of another person. And it can be the main hindrance even to good relationships, such as that of Evelyn, whenever it serves to bypass problems that should be recognized and dealt with as they arise.

Because of the many difficulties encountered in getting to the emotional source of personal illnesses in interviews, it may be well here to consider some alternative approaches.

Because emotions are always expressed in the body, there is invariably a mind-body connection and, in terms of previous distress, a mind-body memory. Thus, both mind and body can act as repositories of emotional experience and as portals through which the release of emotional suppression can occur.

The mind is the conventional portal for the verbal interview when it touches on sensitive areas. Because, however, we may engage only the verbal cognitive mind of the patient, which may be quite dissociated from the real problem, the body may sometimes be a more powerful portal. This can begin with the "Tell me how you are feeling" overture to the medical history and continue with the physician's responses to the wide range of body (nonverbal) expressions of emotional distress as described in Chapter 14. It may be even more effective in some patients to focus directly on the symptomatic expression itself.

> *Marie Louise H., 42, an accounting clerk, was referred for persistent attacks of hyperventilation during the preceding year. She was aware that such a symptom could be emotional, but she couldn't say what it was, and no clear cause emerged during the interview. She was bright and responsive, and did not appear disturbed. I asked if she would be willing to hyperventilate voluntarily, not to demonstrate how this can cause secondary symptoms, but because I find that hyperventilating may reveal its emotional source more readily than verbal questioning. The hyperventilation indeed gave way to an emotional outburst. When invited to share what she was feeling, she poured out a story of previous depressions, a suicide attempt, and hospitalization, all of which had been short-circuited in the medical history. Suddenly she stopped crying and overbreathing, and with great control offered this remarkable statement:*
>
> *"I got so sick of being depressed and crying so much—I was so miserable—that I decided one day I was just not going to be depressed any more. I would not let myself cry. And I haven't. That's when I started to breathe so hard. I guess I hold it all in. But I'd rather go on the way I am, than to have to go back to all the depression."*

Breath is the one vital function we can all be aware of from moment to moment. In it are expressed a host of emotional, physical, and spiritual states. Awareness of breath is often regarded as an essential component of yoga and meditation, and it has become the central focus of several more recently developed breath-work approaches to self-awareness and personal growth. In the patient cited here, a focus on breathing, the essential physiologic function in which the distress was expressed, served to reveal its emotional basis if not the underlying personality or social disturbance. Sometimes it does both. Here the patient, apparently satisfied with the consultation, rejected my recommendation for further visits, either with me or with a psychotherapist, but she agreed to stay in touch by phone. She did, and the attacks slowly ceased over the next three months. The depression had not recurred.

The patients with somatoform coma and pseudoepilepsy described in Chapter 12 provide other examples in which the underlying emotional problem was made explicit by focusing on its symptomatic expression. This approach can also be effective in some patients with more common functional syndromes, especially when the symptoms, like chest pain, are immediate expressions of emotional tension and are also found present during the examination.

I do this by suggesting that I would like to get a better sense of the distress the patient has been suffering. If they would be willing to proceed a little differently than by talking more about it, I would like to ask them to sit quietly, close their eyes, and focus on the distress. Then, giving the patient a little time for self, I suggest, "Be aware of the intensity of this distress. Notice the tension in your chest [or whatever the symptom]." Later: "As the tension mounts, you may become aware of other feelings, thoughts, or emotions that connect with the pain. That may be important." Finally: "Feel free to share whatever you experience." At any point in this process, the patient's experience may shift from the symptom to the emotion, to the underlying problem, or both. If not, the patient simply says, "I don't feel anything but the pain." In this case, I acknowledge, "Very well, but is there anything you could add to your previous description?"

Like most physicians, I am most comfortable with verbal discourse. Though familiar with the alternative approaches described above, I use them, not often, but mainly with patients who seem open to this path to awareness.

Unfortunately, it can be difficult to reveal the essence of the problem by any approach that can be applied readily in primary practice. In terms of referral, however, psychotherapists today have many ways to help patients experience and work through suppressed emotions, as well as to achieve a more effective understanding of themselves, their life situations, and behaviors.

Closely allied to these approaches to emotional release through the body are the many disciplines in which the body as a whole is incorporated as the essential participant in personal awareness, expression, and growth,[79] or, in other words, the individual is regarded as a whole person from which the body cannot be excluded. Traditional practices include yoga, t'ai chi ch'uan, and aikido and other martial arts, to name a few. Emotions held or expressed in the body are a pivotal focus of such psychotherapeutic systems as gestalt therapy,[80] bioenergetics,[81] and the Rubenfeld synergy method.[82] Though not specifically developed as psychotherapeutic, the purpose of many other forms of "somatics" or "body work," such as the systems of Alexander, Feldenkrais, Trager, Rosen, and autogenic training, is an expansion of aware-ness of one's own body, a greater freedom of movement and release from long-standing restrictions, and a more sensitive integration of the physical with the psychosocial and emotional domains. Clearly, this can be an impor-tant goal in itself, but such work also leads to insights that call for further understanding, perhaps including psychotherapy. Or, beginning with the mental pole of the mind-body connection, some psychiatrists recommend body work as a useful adjunct to psychotherapy.

I am personally most familiar with the sensory awareness or "rediscovery of experiencing" as developed by Charlotte Selver and Charles Brooks.[83] Most of us have a diminished capacity to be fully present here and now. In this work one learns to be more open and receptive—physically, emotionally, mentally—to ongoing experience, whatever that may be: awareness of self in relation to the current situation and its setting, and/or an enhanced sensitivity to the presence, the life, the connection with another person in the relation-ship of this moment. I found this approach helpful in my practice and in my personal life.

Joy, Meaning, Purpose, and Growth

In seeking to understand the source of an enigmatic nervous disorder, there is another important area to consider, one that is often bypassed by many people in everyday life, and also in medical care and psychotherapy. Instead of something distressful happening, the problem may be something that is *not* happening, something missing in terms of personal fulfillment or the patient's feeling, or zest, for the dynamic flow of life. I know that I have often failed to understand patients by not considering their basic human needs (such as proposed in Ch. 5), which have been too sparsely experienced. Most pertinent, of course, are those that this person could do something about.

First, let us focus on the basic questions of meaning, purpose, and growth. Jean G. (Ch. 5) was a prototype of the kinds of existential voids in this area that eventually gnaw at the edges of one's being and bring patients into medical care. This is clearly a complex problem that evolves in many ways throughout the life cycle, culminating in the middle and later years in problems of the resolution of generativity vs. stagnation, and ego integrity vs. despair, as designated by Erikson,[11] and in the many other challenges of adult life delineated so well by many others.[8, 84, 85] To get into such questions at all can be difficult, but I believe it to be an issue that cannot be avoided if we hope to understand many patients.

Frankl describes "the basic striving of man to find and fulfill meaning and purpose" as a universal and primary concern.[86] Yalom defines the many forms it takes.[87] Everyone wonders at times about the meaning of life, and loss of meaning is a common complaint that confronts the psychiatrist. Jung noted: "About a third of my cases are not suffering from any clinically definable neurosis but from the senselessness and aimlessness of their lives."[88]

Many people, however, have never asked the question. They are hardly aware how they "choose" by not choosing. Like Jean, they have learned since childhood to do what is expected of them and not to act independently. They go through life, doing a job, getting married, raising kids, with few other major interests, but fail to encounter the problem of "no self" until the spouse dies, as with Joseph, or the children are gone, as with Jean, or the person simply wears down in a stalemate of sameness, nothing new. Instead of controlling their lives, they allow life events to control them. Though there may be nothing particularly "wrong" about anything, the static state, combined with a failure to evolve in other ways, steadily undermines their vitality. Any measure of dissatisfaction, whether latent or overt, about any aspect of the situation, adds to the problem. Such behavior patterns are often tied to the dependent personality and emotional containment described previously. In Erikson's perspective, there may well have been blocks to formation of the foundations for a healthy personality: basic trust, autonomy, initiative, industry, identity.[11]

Why now? This is the usual question that arises in any nervous disorder attributed to a steady state. The patient, let us say, has continued in the same mundane marriage, the same job as a telephone operator, the same hour's drive to and from work, the same evening fatigue, with few other interests, for 10, 20, 30 years (my particular patient, 27 years). You suggest that perhaps all this has something to do with the distress that has emerged, that perhaps he or she needs something more out of life. "How could that be?" the patient responds. "I have always lived this way, and I never felt sick like this before."

Probably it cannot be known just how, why, or when the fatigue, the boredom, the latent dissatisfaction, a wonder about whether it's all worthwhile, whatever it is, finally unsettles the patient's psychobiological equilibrium. But it does, and it is a common problem.

If you can get the point across—and it can be difficult—it may not take much to make a difference. Jean simply parlayed an old hobby into a small business. Another patient learned to swim. Another, who had never worked before, got a job. Another started to travel. Many people would regard other kinds of pursuits as more important: the joy of a freer participation in, and experience of, life's many possibilities; an expanded knowledge of self, the natural world, and the people in it; dedication to a cause; self-transcendence in terms of helping and caring relationships with others; some kind of creative pursuit.[87, 89] A major spiritual or philosophic transformation, however, is not necessary, but the patient does need to embrace whatever interests or activities are needed for a renewed zest for life.

Thus, some people actually have to learn that they have a right and a need for their own personal joy and growth, their own meanings and purpose, apart from their relations to others. The physician provides no answers, but, knowing the patient's life story, the achievements as well as the difficulties, and viewing the illness from this perspective, can often act as a catalyst. The psychological blocks can be formidable, however, and psychotherapy may be necessary to make any progress at all.

There is another kind of existential problem to be considered here. Jean was not dissatisfied with her situation; she needed something more, but she did not feel "stuck" in any way. Many people, however, though not constrained in terms of personal growth as was Jean, have been active, outgoing, and successful until they begin to feel stuck, mired, no longer enthusiastic about some aspect of life to which they are, nevertheless, strongly committed. This could be an educational program, a career, a job, a marriage, their way of life, where they live, many things. The patient may have been "born into" the path, or it was chosen for good reason at one time, or the involvement may have resulted from family pressures, what seemed like a good marriage, an unexpected job opportunity, many other situations. In any event, there are now compelling reasons why the commitment should continue just as it is, and why it would be a disaster to suggest or make a change, both for the individual and for the others involved. It would be difficult, if not impossible, to start all over again. Yet emotionally, if not cognitively, this person has become disenchanted, perhaps in large part unconsciously so. At some deep feeling level, he/she doesn't really want to continue, or feels that the effort required outweighs the expected returns. But, whether the problem is clear or ill-defined, the subject cannot bring him/herself to make the break, or see how the problem could be resolved in some other way. An inertia ensues.

Getting stuck in this way, I believe, is often found to be a common denominator of chronic fatigue. It can be a factor in any kind of functional syndrome.

Such individuals, however, feel OK about themselves. They are doing the right thing. In terms of personal integrity they do not feel hopeless or helpless. There is no self-reproach or guilt. In short, they are not depressed, as medically defined. And, focused on their commitment and the fatigue, or whatever symptom it is that blocks their path, they are not fully aware of their discontent, nor are they in a position to shift their attention from the symptom to their inner needs.

When this is a factor in a personal illness, it can be difficult to elicit, unless the patient is asked to elaborate on the joys and excitement of his/her life situation, whatever it is. Because of the person's commitment and the dissociation of the attendant emotions, this will be an area of controversy, and the physician proceeds tactfully. Nevertheless, if the discontent can be defined, it may be possible for the patient to do something positive about it, to adapt in a more salutary way, or to focus on other pursuits for one's essential well-being.

The Joint Interview

Interviews with significant persons in the patient's life—jointly, separately, or both—especially spouses, or parent and child, are often essential, for both the "diagnosis" and the "treatment" of the personal source of the illness.

I can suggest only some general guidelines. Discretion concerning who, how, and when to interview must be individualized. The patient should, of course, concur in the request to interview another person or set up a joint interview. In my experience such requests are rarely denied, even by patients with somatoform disorders, who may at one level be manipulating the spouse through the illness, though they are not usually fully aware of this aspect of the problem.

Such interviews are often the most effective way, perhaps the only possible way, to understand the basic problem in an inexplicable nervous disorder. Personal illnesses evolve, after all, in a family context. Whether the source of the problem lies primarily within the individual, as with alcohol dependency or exhaustion from overwork, or primarily in family interactions, as with marital discord or a parent-child conflict, the family is involved. Knowing the patient far better than you do, the family can often provide the essential information, whereas the patient may not provide a straight story even though you ask specific questions.

If the problem is interpersonal conflict (and I will focus here again on marital discord, with which I am most familiar), interviews with the spouse separately and/or jointly with the patient are often crucial. You may suspect a problem, though the patient is unable to say much about it, for many reasons. Or you set up a joint interview just to get the spouse's insight, whatever the problem may be. What happens? If there is an ongoing conflict, the participants cannot usually keep it contained in the presence of a third person, especially in the sharing ambience of the patient-doctor relationship. The conflict soon surfaces, though the discourse begins innocently: "Can you share any thoughts you may have about your spouse's illness?"

Another scenario: the patient has described the conflict and blamed the spouse. What then? To clarify the issues, I have often found a joint interview helpful, but only with the explicit proviso that my sole purpose is to hear both sides of the question. I may discover the situation to be quite the opposite of what the patient had said. In any event, it is difficult to comment at all, or even to refer for psychotherapy, until I have some notion of the balance of forces between these two people.

The problem of the somatoform disorder is unique, there being at least two individuals hooked into the illness, which, for better or for worse, may have solved a problem between them (Ch. 12). A separate interview with the spouse and/or a joint interview is often necessary to know what is really going on. Both the patient and the spouse may be aware of and upset about the underlying problem, and, therefore, they know intuitively that the illness is somehow related. Thus, as with Ruth (Ch. 1) or George (Ch. 2), it may not be difficult to talk with them or their spouses about the emotional situation. Or the spouse, if not the patient, may be quite aware of the function of the illness and only too willing to give his/her side of the story. On the other hand, both parties may be assiduously avoiding any recognition of the underlying issues, and the illness is such a fait accompli that both resent any emotional connotation whatsoever.

Thus, the problem of a somatoform disorder is to be approached judiciously, and you will want to describe the symptom more or less as suggested in Chapter 16, and then explore the various factors that could bear on the continued pain. In general, many patients and their families are sufficiently cooperative to reveal its probable source. Or it is disclosed by the abrupt resistance that is provoked when you hit on the key question, as occurred with an adolescent I interviewed: "I know you have these pains, but why don't you go to school anyway?"

Finally, just as a personal illness may evolve in a family context, that is where recovery must take place. If there is a conflict, both parties are involved in the resolution. If one spouse is alcohol-dependent or has other attributes that pose a problem for the relationship, and the other has a co-dependent personality, both must change. Even if it is the patient who must make the essential changes, as was the case with Evelyn and her inability to express herself, the spouse, understanding the problem, can obviously be of great help. In this way the spouses of Ruth, George, and Jean, for example, were enlisted as allies in the recovery process. If the spouse will be a barrier, that too needs to be known.

Clearly, a family interview may be as critical to the recovery process as it was to understanding the problem in the first place. Involving the family is often equally advantageous to the adaptation or recovery of the patient with organic disease.

Engaging the Patient

To be well, the patient with a persistent personal illness must usually bring about some effective change in stressful life situations, relationships, attitudes, behaviors, habits—whatever the underlying problem may be. Medical care, however, focused as it is on the biomedical aspects of the illness, its diagnosis and treatment, tends to block the process of change by taking over. How to collaborate—that is, coordinate the biomedical "management" of the illness with what patients must do for themselves—is the challenge of person-centered care. Every person and every problem situation is unique. Therefore, there can be no overriding systematic approach that will ensure the necessary shift in responsibility for recovery from doctor to patient, and achieving that may not be possible. Nevertheless, that is the goal of the healing plan.

ᏬᏊ In personal illness, the crowning achievement for the clinician is to make the correct diagnosis and to reach, with the patient, an understanding of the underlying problem situation. Together, clinician and patient can then begin to consider what the patient may be able to do about the situation. Following through with a collaborative approach is what I mean by engaging the patient. The physician, though in a position neither to solve the personal problems of the patient nor to make decisions for her/him, can help in many ways: accept with compassion the patient's situation as it is at the beginning of care, encourage further understanding, provide perspective, consider with the patient what might, could, must be done to be well (that is, identify her/his options for change); restore self-esteem and build upon the strengths and latent capacity of the patient to surmount the problem in some way; and if necessary, make appropriate referrals. In the last analysis, however, the patient must grapple with the problem, personally and realistically. How to help, motivate, and inspire the patient to do this is the challenge. One hopes that a committed, mutually responsive, patient/doctor relationship leads into such a path. There is no magic formula. This is often the core problem that healers must face with such patients, sooner or later. Even in extended psychotherapy, the therapist often wonders: when is this patient going to begin to do something about the problems we have been talking about?

Shifting Responsibility

Even when the problem situation has been clearly identified, all physicians know how difficult it can be for many patients to make the necessary changes. Fortunately, for both doctor and patient, the medical model provides a measure of understanding, if only for the nature of the illness and the relief of symptoms. In personal illnesses with symptoms of sufficient magnitude for a doctor to be consulted, medical care is usually unavoidable, if not essential. But the medical model is seductive. Once we get into it, it may obscure what else needs to be done. We, not the patient, have assumed responsibility for fixing what has gone wrong—that is what we are trained to do. And the patient often, though not always, is gratified that we have taken over. Ironically, doctor and patient may then join unwittingly in what constitutes a "therapeutic" block to recovery.

How then can we maintain or return to a process of collaboration while prescribing pharmacotherapy? When psychoactive or other symptomatic drugs are prescribed, preferably with the concurrence of the patient, who has been made aware of their purpose and action, it can be emphasized [1] that the drugs can be effective, but [2] that relieving symptoms is basically what they do. There are many ways to realize the placebo as well as biological effects of the drugs without allowing them to take over. In short, the physician seeks to bring about the maximal therapeutic efficacy without undermining the groundwork of what may well have to be returned to later. A canny, long-term surveillance is necessary. Otherwise, recovery is likely to disintegrate in the pursuit of symptomatic relief. The patient, though persistently symptomatic, feels dependent, nevertheless, on drugs, and the physician is embroiled in an endless chain of therapeutic trials. There are, of course, intractable physical or psychiatric disorders in which one agent may be found more effective than another, and even partial relief is imperative. But in the polypharmacy of Orvieta T. (Ch. 2) and the daily narcotics of Jean G. (Ch. 5) and innumerable other patients, the therapeutic attack is clearly futile, out of control. Whenever this problem is recognized, we need to clarify again the real source of the illness, the limitations and failure of biotherapy, and return in any way possible to a more integrated approach.

We have seen repeatedly that the main concern of many patients is simply to find out what is wrong and what can be done about it, not necessarily to get the doctor to apply a specific medical modality. But many other patients do indeed expect this, and we must either comply with their wishes or carefully explain the contrary course of action. We know that the balance of biosocial and psychosocial components in a comprehensive recovery plan varies considerably, depending on the unique situation of each patient (Ch. 2).

In the ideal scenario, understanding the underlying problem situation is sufficient. The patients are gratified to discover that symptoms that seemed so ominous are not due to disease after all, that they don't have to be treated or get further involved with the medical system. Perhaps they have been aware of the underlying problem situation, but have let it slide, as people tend to do. This has now been clarified in relation to the distress. Obviously, some changes could or should be made. Subsequent office visits are then primarily for further discussion. Meanwhile, the patients proceed to act on their own, or, if necessary, are referred for counseling, which can often be viewed less as therapy than as a means of learning better ways to handle the situation. In any event, medical therapy is optional. The symptoms are likely to subside, sometimes because of the relief that ensues from the understanding per se, or, if not that, because the patient has begun to take active steps toward resolution.

But responses are rarely so straightforward. More often, an adequate understanding has not yet been achieved and cannot be expected soon, even in psychotherapy. Or, though aware of the underlying problem situation and what *could* be done about it, the patient finds it difficult to act upon the necessary changes. For many reasons, the symptoms are likely to recur or persist. The biotherapeutic side of the collaborative interaction predominates, and it may be essential, as it so often is in the major psychiatric disorders or migraine, for example.

Clearly, for many patients, a medical superstructure—being diagnosed and treated by a doctor—is necessary. Once in care, however, patients may well appreciate the opportunity to discuss their problems. They may then respond appropriately and begin to act toward resolution. But even the most responsive patients might not return at all were it not for the necessary medical follow-up of the irritable-bowel syndrome, the back condition, the fibromyalgia, the menopause, the anxiety state, however the disorder is identified, or for the treatment of a coincidental disease such as hypertension. That, they tell themselves, their families, and their friends, is the real reason for medical care. The personal issues, which are resolved privately, are secondary considerations. In other words, the medical care, though helpful in itself, can also serve the patient as a face-saving device for not fully acknowledging what is really counseling or psychotherapeutic intervention. Patients often say, "I'm much better. The medicine has worked wonders." I try to restore the balance: "I think it's because you are feeling more secure about what you can do about the whole situation." The patient usually responds: "I know what you mean, Doctor, but it's the medicine." Nevertheless, something has been accomplished.

Referrals

Referrals have traditionally been made for frank mental disorders, or when patients request psychotherapy, but we need to expand our referral horizons. A consultation of one or two interviews, simply to assess the patient's problem situation, may be sufficient. For the more intractable problems there is a vast selection of qualified specialists to assist in treatment.

Psychological Assessment and/or Psychotherapy

In the last 50 years there has been an incredible expansion of psychological and social understanding, counseling skills, and psychotherapeutic approaches. Among many advances are the whole fields of marital and family systems therapy, behavioral modification, the humanistic, existential, cognitive, and transpersonal psychologies, the reorientation of the psychoanalytic focus from sexual and other internal drives to interpersonal relationships, and the introduction of such notions as the patient's choice, will, and responsibility in effecting change—to name just a few.

The following list of counseling skills, taken from a directory of marriage and family therapists,[1] is provided here to indicate the breadth of current concerns in psychotherapy:

Addictions	Behavior modification
Adults abused as children	Biofeedback
Adolescents	Brief therapy
Adoption issues	Child abuse
Adult children of alcoholics/	Children
dysfunctional families	Chronic illness or physical
Adults molested as children	disability
Aging and elderly	Co-dependency
Alcohol and substance abuse	Combat veterans
AIDS	Couples
Anxiety, panic attacks, and phobias	Cross-cultural issues
Behavior assessment testing	Depression

Dissociative disorders
Divorce and custody mediation
Domestic violence
Eating disorders
Family systems orientation
Families
Gay and lesbian issues
General life problems
Gestalt therapy
Grief and loss
Hypnotherapy
Intercultural/interracial relationships
Jungian therapy
Life-cycle transitions
Life-threatening illness
Men's issues
Mind, body, and energy work
Object relations
Parenting
Personality disorders

Post-traumatic stress syndrome
Pregnancy, postnatal, post-abortion
   counseling
Premarital counseling
Psychoanalytic therapy
Psychodynamic therapy
Psychosynthesis and transpersonal
   therapy
Rape survivors
Rogerian therapy
Self-esteem
Self-psychology
Sexual abuse
Sex therapy
Spiritual issues
Stress
Suicide
Vocational/career issues
Women's issues

Other skills—for example assertiveness training, cognitive therapy, and meditation—could be added to the list.

Stress Reduction

A stress-reduction program constitutes another type of integrated approach. If the patient's illness is deemed to be related to the kinds of life stresses and stress reactions that can be expected to resolve with stress reduction, as in some patients with chronic headaches,[2] or in any functional syndrome caused by exhaustion (Ch. 17), such a program may well be effective. When patients become fully aware of the particular stress that results in their symptoms, they may be able to make the necessary changes on their own. Change, however, can be blocked in many ways, whether practical or psychological. A therapeutic program is helpful. For some patients, "stress reduction" may be more pertinent, as well as more acceptable, than "psychotherapy" and it can move directly into the core of the problem in two ways.

The first effect has to do with reducing the patient's stress responses. This includes such modalities as the relaxation response in any of its many forms (progressive relaxation, autogenic training, meditation, etc.), biofeedback, healing imagery, and various other approaches to somatic or body work. Such approaches may in turn lead into the second effect, a more indirect, but more important, response: "If I can control my own body, could I not also get better control of my life?" This in turn connects the situation to the other aspects of stress reduction: an analysis of the compulsions, personality traits, behavior styles, or other dysfunctional, maladaptive mental fixes or belief systems, described so well in cognitive therapy, that either induce stress responses or hold the patient trapped in a stressful situation that could otherwise be modified. The patient's particular needs might include enhancement of self-esteem, assertiveness training, attention to co-dependency patterns, discussion of occupational issues, other forms of behavior modification, or any of many other things. All of these psychotherapeutic approaches could be introduced directly, of course, with or without an associated technique for relaxation.

A stress response involves a demanding situation (the stressor), the kinds of attitudes and behaviors the subject applies to the situation, the resulting conflict, and, finally, the stress response per se. If the therapeutic plan focuses solely on the latter, as by a relaxation or biofeedback program only, the focus is mainly symptomatic, and the illness may well persist. If, however, the plan also provides opportunities to learn better ways to revise or reclarify the stressor, the focus can be truly integrated.

In the evaluation of any functional disorder, the clinician must know the patient well, and must keep in mind that "stress" is but one of many factors. An ongoing emotional conflict as the source of headaches, for example, cannot be resolved simply by "stress reduction." And the source of Jean's (Ch. 5) and Daphne's (Ch. 14) headaches lay in different areas altogether: Jean needed a new direction in life; and Daphne needed recognition and support for her grief reaction.

Another useful approach to intractable functional syndromes—if caused by an extended period of stress on a demanding job (especially in a conscientious person whose life is way out of balance with the work demands), constant fatigue, inadequate rest, limited opportunity for other activities, and little support—is to give the patient a break. I advise such patients that I do not believe the headaches (or whatever symptom) can be brought under control with medical treatment alone. A distinct respite is necessary. Medical disability could be authorized for one or two months (more or less, whatever seems right). The purpose is not simply for the management of the illness. It is also designed to restore harmony to the patients' lives. I expect them to be active, to be with friends, do things they have been wanting to do, get into something of personal interest, mostly to consider carefully how they can return to work with a reasonable workload, and keep it in balance with their other needs as human beings.

In many other situations of extraordinary stress, whether imposed from without or the result of uncontrolled but understandable motivations on the part of the patient, the physician can either make strong recommendations or find some way to intervene in the patient's behalf. Assuming that the patients do indeed use the respite to gain a new perspective on themselves and their lives, they may well be able to return to work, to school, whatever, with the strength and insight needed for a more salutary ongoing equanimity.

Pain Syndromes and Pain Clinics

The physician must be particularly wary of the predicament of the patient with a chronic pain syndrome not due to demonstrable disease (especially if somatoform features are likely), when narcotics are prescribed for what will soon be daily use. Although narcotics (codeine, oxycodone, and stronger) are not particularly effective here, they relieve the feelings of emotional distress (which both caused the syndrome and result from it) as well as the pain, to some extent. Therefore, such patients quickly become dependent, unlike most patients with obviously organic pain syndromes. Recovery is then out of the question. This becomes a monstrous problem when the patient is ultimately referred to a pain clinic to reverse the process. When the question of narcotic use first comes up is the time to push hard for a biopsychosocial overview of the whole problem.

Pain clinics vary considerably in their approach. Some are fully prepared to work with the psychological and somatoform as well as the physical aspects of the problem. At the other extreme are those concerned predominantly with the relief of pain caused by organic pathology. In these, somatoform features may not be recognized, and in some clinics, disease diagnoses are stretched to fit the condition. If the somatic approach proves to be unworkable, the pain may be regarded as "central," and tricyclic drugs prescribed, either as analgesics or antidepressants. If the latter, the depression is regarded as secondary to the pain syndrome. A primary or separate source of emotional pain is not seriously considered.

The orientation of most pain clinics, however, falls somewhere between these two extremes. The program is interdisciplinary and thereby integrated in many ways, but the emphasis is primarily behavioral rather than psychodynamic. Although the clinical efficacy of these clinics has been demonstrated in many studies summarized in two recent reports,[2, 3] the improvement of the patient, though distinctly superior to that yielded by the medical model too strictly applied (more tests, analgesics, other drugs, or surgery), is often modest, and the outcome varies considerably. Chronic pain, often complicated by somatoform features, is inherently refractory, but the therapeutic difficulties are due in part, I believe, to the limitations of an approach based mainly on behavioral modification. The real problems of a woman with psychogenic pelvic pain, for example, may involve her background of sexual abuse, fear, distrust, or other emotional problems that manifest as marital and sexual difficulties. Or the real problems of a man with a chronic backache after an injury may have less to do with the injury than with his insecure or adverse personal situation at the time of the accident. This, combined with the disability benefits, though they may be appropriate, constitutes a barrier to recovery. Again, healing is blocked if the patient's personal needs and problems cannot be addressed definitively, and that can be a formidable problem. Psychotherapy not only is difficult, costly, and time-consuming, but it can be totally unacceptable to the patient. Physicians, in turn, need to be aware of their own bias regarding psychotherapy, and how that bias transmits to the patient. Behavioral modification combined with the other modalities of therapy may well be the most that can be done, and in spite of the barriers to recovery, this approach can be quite effective, even in the two situations described above.[2, 4] On the other hand, there are patients—several have been discussed—who will respond to a more directed approach to the emotional issues, and an even better outcome can result.

Alcohol and Drug Dependency and Substance Abuse Treatment Programs

Dependency problems belong in a special category, because they usually take precedence over other considerations. The problem must be recognized early and stated clearly, and a recovery program must be instituted as soon as possible. Though some patients can achieve abstinence under a physician's direction, most of those with an established dependency will require referral to a dependency treatment center and/or Alcoholics Anonymous. Personal support, understanding the life situation, and helping patients to make the necessary changes may well be important, but these aspects of the recovery program are not usually effective until abstinence is established.

Alternative Licensed Healing Approaches

Acupuncture and chiropractic are sometimes incorporated into medical practice, or referrals are made, although there are few controlled studies to demonstrate their objective efficacy. Nevertheless, there are innumerable anecdotal accounts that appear to demonstrate their value, and they are commonly accepted as useful by the general public. When making referrals, the doctor must decide about the potential value of each approach for the individual patient.

Helping Patients Find Their Own Path

Medical doctors have had little training in counseling skills, and they are beset by the barriers to patient-centered care described in Chapter 10. Nevertheless, at least a third of our patients need to understand the personal source of their illness. This is an enormous problem, but as we have seen, many of the problem situations in primary care are not difficult to recognize. The path the patient could take toward recovery is often fairly clear. How to engage the patient is implicit in the case histories described in this book. Here I wish only to summarize what has been said about how the physician can be helpful.

Your undivided attention, willingness to understand, and acceptance of and concern about the situation from the patient's point of view, are therapeutic in themselves. Only when patients feel accepted in this way can they begin to look at themselves more realistically, less defensively.

State as clearly as you can the patient's unrealized needs (Ch. 5), as you see them in relation to the problem situation as it unfolds. The specificity of the feedback varies, of course. Sometimes it can be straightforward, as with an exhaustion syndrome; what that patient needs is obvious, and it can be detected readily and stated clearly. What the patient can or cannot do about it, or chooses to do about it, is a separate but related issue; it is the physician's responsibility to explain the illness, not to make personal decisions for the patient.

Some kinds of problems, however, such as a patient's needs in relation to an existential problem of meaning, purpose, or growth, are not so clear. This is a value judgment that evolves only after you have spent some time with the patient. Here the feedback would be tentative, gently provocative: "I have some thoughts about your situation. Because this represents to some extent my own point of view about life, you may or may not feel that it applies in any way to you. Nevertheless, I'd like you to consider the question. Could it be, for example, that you may have a real need for some kind of personal growth or greater meaning in your life, that is, activities, interests, etc., that are mainly for yourself? You are clearly devoted to your family, your job, but perhaps. . . ." This kind of overture, of course, is in no way definitive. It is intended only to open a discussion.

The needs of a patient in relation to marital discord, and their resolution, for example, can be complex. Two people are involved. Most physicians have neither the time nor the training to get into this kind of situation very far. Referral may well be appropriate. But to get to referral, or to provide some direction, permits at least a tentative feedback about the general nature of the problem, insofar as the physician feels capable of conveying that. The first step might simply be an affirmation of what anyone should expect to experience in a satisfying, personally fulfilling relationship, focusing particularly on what appears to be missing in the patient's situation. Many individuals, beset with their own dependency needs, trying to adjust to the self-centered ways of a spouse, or embroiled in many other aspects of their own or their spouse's behavior, personality, or ways of relating, have but a vague idea of what constitutes a satisfying relationship.

A clinically symptomatic personal illness usually indicates that patients are not fully aware of the underlying problem, or, if they are, that they have not yet begun to consider how it could be resolved. The physician's role is simply to clarify the situation, provide perspective, provoke discussion, ask questions, mention options or alternatives that the patient may not have considered, and get the patient to begin thinking about what could be done. Resolution often involves consideration of the problem situation per se, as well as the behavioral style that the person brings to the situation. What could be done might involve an emphasis on one aspect or the other, or both. Any change entails pros and cons, and that should be made clear. But, if the patient is to be well, something has to change.

Even though the patient's present situation is the result of a long chain of circumstances that has not received sufficient attention, there is often some way to release the restrictive forces involved, and to provide opportunities for new learning, better ways. The process of introspection, reappraisal, and consideration of alternative pathways, as difficult and painful as that may be, can be a life-affirming, enriching experience. The growth model of personal illness, as outlined in Chapter 5, provides a general guide for a person-centered approach. Some patients will not respond, but it is better to fail than to block the healing process still further by not seeking to release the latent capacity of most patients to surmount the illness situation in some way.

It is crucial that the patient be supported throughout the period of care, regardless of what happens. Empathy and compassion for your patient's predicament are traditional functions of medical care. Support is particularly needed as the patient struggles with loss and grief, or other crises and transitions in the course of life.

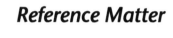

Reference Matter

Literature Cited

Preface

1. Moos RH, ed. Coping with physical illness. New York: Plenum Medical Book Co., 1977.
2. Moos RH, ed. Coping with physical illness. 2: New perspectives. New York: Plenum Medical Book Co., 1984.
3. LeMaistre J. Beyond rage. The emotional impact of chronic physical illness. Oak Park, IL: Alpine Guild, 1985.

Introduction

1. Institute of Medicine. Connor E, Mullan F, eds. Community oriented primary care. New directions for health services delivery. Washington, D.C.: National Academy Press, 1982.
2. Mawardi GH. 1956–1965 career study report. Cleveland: Case Western Reserve University School of Medicine, 1983.
3. Engel GL. The education of the physician for clinical observation. J Nerv Ment Dis 1972; 154: 159–64.
4. Takeuchi JS, Smith NM, Mortimer AM. Innovative models of medical education in the United States today: an overview with implications for curriculum and program evaluation. In: Institute of Medicine publication No. IOM-83-02, Medical education and societal needs: a planning report for the health professions. Washington, D.C.: National Academy Press, 1983.
5. Bok D. Needed: a new way to train doctors. President's report to the Harvard Board of Overseers for 1982–83. Harvard Magazine, May–June 1984: 32–71.

6. Bulger RJ, ed. Hippocrates revisited. A search for meaning. New York: Medcom Press, 1973.
7. Dubos R. Hippocrates in modern dress. Perspect Biol Med 1966; 9(Winter): 275–88.
8. Cope O. Man, mind, and medicine. The doctor's education. Philadelphia: J.B. Lippincott Co., 1968.
9. Eisenberg L. The search for care. Daedalus 1977; 106(Winter): 235–46.
10. Engel GL. The need for a new medical model: a challenge for biomedicine. Science 1977; 196: 129–35.
11. Evans LJ. The crisis in medicine education. Ann Arbor: University of Michigan Press, 1964: Ch 3. What makes human biology human? 39–57.
12. Lalonde M. A new perspective on the health of Canadians. Ottawa: Government of Canada, 1974.
13. Magraw RM. Ferment in medicine. A study of the essence of medical practice and of its new dilemmas. Philadelphia: W.B. Saunders, 1966: 1–83 (Chs 1–7).
14. McWhinney IR. Family medicine in perspective. N Engl J Med 1975; 293: 176–81.
15. Meeting the challenge of family practice. The report of the Ad Hoc Committee on Education for Family Practice of the Council on Medical Education, American Medical Association. Chicago: A.M.A., 1966.
16. Millis JS and members of the Citizens Commission on Graduate Education. The graduate education of physicians. Chicago: Council on Medical Education. American Medical Association, 1966: Ch 5, Comprehensive Health Care, 33–56.
17. White KL. Life and death and medicine. Sci Am 1973; 229: 23–33.
18. Balint M. The doctor, his patient and the illness. 2nd ed. New York: International Universities Press, Inc., 1964.
19. Blumgart HL. Caring for the patient. N Engl J Med 1964; 270: 449–55.
20. Cassell EJ. The healer's art. A new approach to the doctor-patient relationship. Philadelphia: J.B. Lippincott Co., 1976.
21. Cohen-Cole SA. The medical interview: the three-function approach. St. Louis: Mosby Year Book, 1991.
22. Leigh H, Reiser MF. The patient. Biological, psychological, and social dimensions of medical practice. 2nd ed. New York: Plenum Medical Book Co., 1985.
23. Lipkin M. The care of patients. Perspectives and practices. Revised ed. New Haven: Yale University Press, 1987.
24. Peabody FW. The care of the patient. JAMA 1927; 88: 877–82.
25. Remen N. The human patient. Garden City: Anchor Press/Doubleday, 1980.
26. Tumulty PA. The effective clinician. His methods and approach to diagnosis and care Philadelphia: W.B. Saunders Co., 1973.

Chapter 1

1. Kroenke K, Lucas CA, Rosenberg ML, et al. Causes of persistent dizziness. A prospective study of 100 patients in ambulatory care. Am Intern Med 1992; 117: 898–904.
2. Drachman DA, Hart CW. An approach to the dizzy patient. Neurology 1972; 22: 323–34.
3. Beckman HB, Frankel RM. The effect of physician behavior on the collection of data. Ann Intern Med 1984; 101: 692–6.
4. Fisher CM. Vertigo in cerebrovascular disease. Arch Otolaryngol 1967; 85: 529–34.
5. Jeffcoate TNA. Pelvic pain. Br Med J 1969; 3: 431–5.

6. Kroger WS, Freed SC. Psychosomatic gynecology. Philadelphia: W.B. Saunders Co., 1951: 338–52.

7. Liston WA, Bradford WP, Downie J, Kerr MG. Laparoscopy in a general gynecologic unit. Am J Obstet Gynecol 1972; 113: 672–7.

8. Lock FR. Functional pelvic pain. NC Med J 1959; 20: 301–2.

9. Mussey RD. Pelvic pain. Am J Obstet Gynecol 1939; 37: 729–40.

10. Benson RC. Psychologic aspects of gynecologic practice. In Benson RC, ed. Current obstetric & gynecologic diagnosis and treatment. 6th ed. Norwalk, CT: Appleton & Lange, 1978: 1044.

11. Benson RC, Hanson KH, Matarazzo JD. Atypical pelvic pain in women: gynecologic-psychiatric considerations. Am J Obstet Gynecol 1959; 77: 806–25.

12. Gidro-Frank L, Gordon T, Taylor HC. Pelvic pain and female identity. A survey of emotional factors in 40 patients. Am J Obstet Gynecol 1960; 79: 1184–1202.

13. Castelnuovo-Tedesco P, Krout BM. Psychosomatic aspects of chronic pelvic pain. Psychiatry in Medicine (now Int J Psychiatry Med) 1970–71; 1: 109–26.

14. Gross RJ, Doerr H, Caldirola D, Guzinski GM, Ripley HS. Borderline syndrome and incest in chronic pelvic pain patients. Int J Psychiatry Med 1980–81; 10: 79–96.

15. Harrop-Griffiths J, Katon W, Walker E, Holm L, Russo J, Hickok L. The association between chronic pelvic pain, psychiatric diagnoses, and childhood sexual abuse. Obstet Gynecol 1988; 71: 589–94.

16. Parsons L, Sommers SC. Gynecology. 2nd ed. Philadelphia: W.B. Saunders, 1978: 341–64.

17. Weingold AB. Pelvic pain. In: Kase NG, Weingold AB, Gershenson DM, eds. Principles and practice of clinical gynecology. 2nd ed. New York: Churchill Livingstone, 1990: 506–8.

18. Goldstein DP. Pediatric and adolescent gynecology. In: Ryan KJ, Berkowitz R, Barbieri RL, eds. Kistner's gynecology. Principles and practice. 5th ed. Chicago: Year Book Medical Publishers, Inc., 1990: 661–4.

19. Clarke-Pearson DL, Dawood MY, eds. Green's gynecology: essentials of clinical practice. 4th ed. Boston: Little, Brown and Co., 1990: 184–6.

20. Pernoll ML, ed. Current obstetric & gynecologic diagnosis & treatment. 7th ed. Norwalk, CT: Appleton & Lange, 1991: 892–3, 1130–1.

21. Walker J, MacGillivray I, Macnaughton MC, eds. Combined textbook of obstetrics and gynecology. 9th ed. Edinburgh: Churchill Livingstone, 1976.

22. Romney SL, Gray MJ, Little AB, Merrill JA, Quilligan EJ, Stander RW. Gynecology and obstetrics. The health care of women. 2nd ed. New York: McGraw-Hill Book Co., 1981.

23. Jones HW, III, Wentz AC, Burnett LS, eds. Novak's textbook of gynecology. 11th ed. Baltimore: Williams & Wilkins, 1988.

24. Wynn RM. Obstetrics and gynecology. The clinical core. 4th ed. Philadelphia: Lea & Febiger, 1988.

25. Scott JR, DiSaia PJ, Hammond CB, Spellacy WN. Danforth's obstetrics and gynecology. 6th ed. Philadelphia: J.B. Lippincott Co., 1990.

26. Willson JR, Carrington ER, et al., eds. Obstetrics and gynecology. 9th ed. St. Louis: Mosby Year Book, 1991.

27. Martin LL. Health care of women. Philadelphia: J.B. Lippincott, 1978: 281–301.

28. Gramlich EP. Pelvic pain. In: Hale RW, Krieger JA, eds. Gynecology. A concise textbook. New York: Medical Examination Pub. Co., Inc., 1983: 256–261.

29. Labrum AH. Psychosomatic aspects of gynecology. In: Swartz DP, ed. Practical points in gynecology. New York: Medical Examination Pub. Co., Inc., 1984: 348–71.

30. Engel GL. The need for a new medical model: a challenge for biomedicine. Science 1977; 196: 129–35.

Chapter 2

1. Wagner GS, Cebe B, Rozear MP. E.A. Stead, Jr. What this patient needs is a doctor. Durham: Carolina Academic Press, 1978.

2. Feinstein AR. Clinical judgment. Baltimore: Williams & Wilkins, 1967.

3. Hirschfeld AH, Behan RC. The accident process. I. Etiological considerations of industrial injuries. JAMA 1963; 186: 193–9.

4. Behan RC, Hirschfeld AH. The accident process. II. Toward more rational treatment of industrial injuries. JAMA 1963; 186: 300–6.

5. Trudel J, deWolfe VG, Young JR, LeFevre FA. Disuse phenomenon of lower extremity. JAMA 1963; 186: 1129–31.

6. Sternbach RA. Pain patients. Traits and treatment. New York: Academic Press, 1974.

7. Fordyce WE. Behavioral methods for chronic pain and illness. St. Louis: CV Mosby Co., 1976.

8. Nachemson AL. Low back pain. Its etiology and treatment. Clin Med 1971; 78: 18–24.

9. Blumgart HL. Caring for the patient. N Engl J Med 1964; 270: 449–56.

10. Welt LG. The art of medicine. Chapel Hill: The School of Medicine, University of North Carolina, 1966.

11. Engel GL. The need for a new medical model: a challenge for biomedicine. Science 1977; 196: 129–35.

12. Miller S, Remen N, Barbour A, Nakles MA, Miller S, Garell D. Dimensions of humanistic medicine. San Francisco: The Institute for the Study of Humanistic Medicine, 1975.

13. Tournier P. The meaning of persons. New York: Harper & Row, 1957: 183–202. Translated from the French, Le Personnage et la Personne, Delachaux & Niestlé, Neuchâtel and Paris.

14. Fox TF. Personal medicine. Bull NY Acad Med 1962; 38: 527–34.

15. Leigh H, Reiser MF. The patient. Biological, psychological, and social dimensions of medical practice. 2nd ed. New York: Plenum Medical Book Co., 1985: xiv.

16. Gordon JS. The paradigm of holistic medicine. In: Hastings AC, Fadiman J, Gordon JS, eds. Health for the whole person. The complete guide to holistic medicine. Boulder, Colo.: Westview Press, 1980: 3–35.

17. Basmajian JV, ed. Biofeedback. Principles and practice for clinicians. 3rd ed. Baltimore: Williams & Wilkins, 1989.

18. Rossman ML. Healing yourself. A step-by-step program for better health through imagery. New York: Pocket Books, 1987.

19. Benson H. The relaxation response. New York: Morrow, 1975.

20. Charlesworth EA, Nathan RG. Stress management. A comprehensive guide to wellness. New York: Atheneum, 1984.

21. Torrey EF. The mind game. Witchdoctors and psychiatrists. New York: Bantam Books, 1973: 106–14.

22. Pelletier KR. Mind as healer, mind as slayer. New York: Delacorte Press, 1977: 277–82.

23. Peabody FW. The care of the patient. JAMA 1927; 88: 877–82.

Chapter 3

1. Magraw RM. Ferment in medicine. A study of the essence of medical practice and of its new dilemmas. Philadelphia: W.B. Saunders Co., 1966: 12–13.
2. Angrist A. The student and the changing medical scene. JAMA 1962; 180: 952–7.
3. Feinstein AR. Clinical judgment. Baltimore: Williams & Wilkins Co., 1967: 73.
4. Menninger K. Changing concepts of disease. Ann Intern Med 1948; 29: 318–25.
5. Kety SS. From rationalization to reason. Am J Psychiatry 1974; 131: 957–63.
6. Seldin DW. The medical model: biomedical science as the basis of medicine. In: From beyond tomorrow: trends and prospects in medical science. 75th anniversary conference [of the Rockefeller Institute], March 8, 1976. New York: Rockefeller University, 1977: 34–9.
7. Rather LJ, ed. Rudolf Virchow. Collected essays on public health and epidemiology. Vol. 1. Canton, MA: Science History Publications, USA, 1985: xii–xiii.
8. American Psychiatric Association: Diagnostic and statistical manual of mental disorders. Washington, DC: APA. 1st ed., 1952: 9–13. 2nd ed., 1968: viii–ix. 3rd ed., 1980: 5–9. 3rd ed., revised, 1987: xxii–xxv.
9. Nyren O, Adami H-O, Bates S, et al. Absence of therapeutic benefit from antacids or cimetidine in non-ulcer dyspepsia. N Engl J Med 1986; 314: 339–43.
10. Peterson WL. Helicobacter pylori and peptic ulcer disease. N Engl J Med 1991; 324: 1043–8.
11. Graham DY, Lew GM, Klein PD, et al. Effect of treatment of Helicobacter pylori infection on the long-term recurrence of gastric or duodenal ulcer. A randomized, controlled study. Ann Intern Med 1992; 116: 705–8.
12. Walsh JH. Helicobacter pylori: selection of patients for treatment. Ann Intern Med 1992; 116: 770–1.
13. Spiro HM. Visceral viewpoints. Moynihan's disease? The diagnosis of duodenal ulcer. N Engl J Med 1974; 291: 567–9.
14. Vaillant GE. The natural history of alcoholism. Cambridge, MA: Harvard University Press, 1983: 1.
15. Redlich FC. Editorial reflections on the concepts of health and disease. J Med Philos 1976; 1: 269–280.
16. Brody H. The systems view of man: implications for medicine, science, and ethics. Perspect Biol Med 1973; Autumn: 71–92.

Chapter 4

1. Wagner GS, Cebe B, Rozear MP. E.A. Stead, Jr. What this patient needs is a doctor. Durham: Carolina Academic Press, 1978: 57.
2. Diamond S, Baltes BJ. Management of headache by the family physician. Am Fam Physician 1972; 5: 68–76.
3. Lance JW, Curran DA, Anthony M. Investigations into the mechanism and treatment of chronic headache. Med J Aust 1965; 2: 909–14.
4. Kroenke K, Mangelsdorff D. Common symptoms in ambulatory care: incidence, evaluation, therapy, and outcome. Am J Med 1989; 86: 262–6.
5. Sox HC Jr. The emergency department evaluation of chest pain. In Wolcott BW, Rund DA, eds. Emergency Medicine Annual. Vol. 1, 1982. Norwalk, CT: Appleton-Century-Crofts: 43–60.

6. Chaudhary NA, Truelove SC. The irritable colon syndrome. A study of the clinical features, predisposing causes, and prognosis in 130 cases. Q J Med 1962; new series 31: 307–22.

7. Switz DM. What the gastroenterologist does all day. Gastroenterology 1976; 70: 1048–50.

8. Schuster MM. Irritable bowel syndrome. In: Sleisenger MH, Fordtran JS, eds. Gastrointestinal disease. Pathophysiology, diagnosis, management. 4th ed., Vol 2. Philadelphia: W.B. Saunders Co., 1989: 1403.

9. Thompson WG, Heaton KW. Functional bowel disorders in apparently healthy people. Gastroenterology 1980; 79: 283–8.

10. Adami H-O, Agenas I, Gustavsson S, et al. The clinical diagnosis of 'gastritis.' Aspects of demographic epidemiology and health care consumption based on a nationwide sample survey. Scand J Gastroenterol 1984; 19: 755–60.

11. Nyren O, Adami H-O, Bates S, et al. Absence of therapeutic benefit from antacids or cimetidine in non-ulcer dyspepsia. N Engl J Med 1986; 314: 339–43.

12. Gomez J, Dally P. Psychologically mediated abdominal pain in surgical and medical outpatient clinics. Br Med J 1977; 1: 1451–3.

13. Mellinger GD, Balter MB, Manheimer DI, Cisin IH, Parry HJ. Psychic distress, life crisis, and use of psychotherapeutic medications. National household survey data. Arch Gen Psychiatry 1978; 35: 1045–52.

14. Bridges KW, Goldberg DP. Somatic presentation of DSM III psychiatric disorders in primary care. J Psychosom Res 1985; 29: 563–9.

15. Katon W. Panic disorder and somatization. Review of 55 cases. Am J Med 1984; 77: 101–6.

16. Katon W. The epidemiology of depression in medical care. Int J Psychiatry Med 1987; 17: 93–112.

17. Kannel WB, Dawber TR, Cohen ME. The electrocardiogram in neurocirculatory asthenia (anxiety, neurosis or neurasthenia): a study of 203 neurocirculatory asthenia patients and 757 healthy controls in the Framingham study. Ann Intern Med 1985; 49: 1351–60.

18. Dunnell K, Cartwright A. Medicine takers, prescribers, and hoarders. London: Routledge and Kegan Paul, 1972: 70.

19. Sydenham T. The works of Thomas Sydenham, M.D., translated from the Latin edition of Dr. Greenhill by Latham RG, Vol. II. London: The Sydenham Society, 1950: 85.

20. Cabot RC. Suggestions for reorganization of hospital out-patient departments with special reference to improvement of treatment. Md Med J 197; 50: 81–91.

21. Stoeckle JD, Zola IK, Davidson GE. The quantity and significance of psychological distress in medical patients. Some preliminary observations about the decision to seek medical aid. J Chronic Dis 1964; 17: 959–970.

22. Kleinman A, Eisenberg L, Good B. Culture, illness, and care. Clinical lessons from anthropologic and cross-cultural research. Ann Intern Med 1978; 88: 251–8.

23. Bauer J. Differential diagnosis of internal diseases. 3rd ed. New York: Grune and Stratton, 1967: xvi.

24. Allan FN, Kaufman M. Nervous factors in general practice. JAMA 1948; 138: 1135–8.

25. Fry J. Common diseases: their nature, incidence, and care. Philadelphia: Lippincott, 1974: 7.

26. Hodgkin K. Towards earlier diagnosis. A guide to primary care. 5th ed. Edinburgh: Churchill Livingstone, 1985: 18–19.
27. White KL. Life and death and medicine. Sci Am 1973; 229: 23–33.
28. Marsland DW, Wood M, Mayo F. A data bank for patient care, curriculum, and research in family practice: 526, 196 patient problems. J Fam Pract 1976; 3: 25–8; 37–68.
29. Schneeweiss R, Rosenblatt RA, Cherkin DC, Kirkwood CR, Hart G. Diagnostic clusters: a new tool for analyzing the content of ambulatory medical care. Med Care 1983; 21: 105–22.
30. Rosenblatt RA, Cherkin DC, Schneeweiss R, Hart LG. The content of ambulatory medical care in the United States. An interspecialty comparison. N Engl J Med 1983; 309: 892–7.
31. Ghormley RK. An etiologic study of backache and sciatic pain. Proc. of the staff meetings of the Mayo Clin (now called Mayo Clin Proc) 1951; 26: 457–63.
32. Dively RL, Kiene RN, Meyer PW. Low back pain. JAMA 1956; 160: 729–31.
33. Sarno JE. Psychogenic backache: the missing dimension. J Fam Pract 1974; 1: 8–12.
34. See Ch. 13, Backache, refs 116–17, 120, 125–31.
35. Stanford MD 1978; 17, Winter/spring: cover. The cartoon is by J M'Guinness at the suggestion of the editor, S. Andreopoulos, from an anecdote by KL White in Andreopoulos S, ed. Health care arrangements in the United States: A.D. 1972. New York: The Milbank Memorial Fund, 1972: 18.

Chapter 5

1. American Psychiatric Association: Diagnostic and statistical manual of mental disorders, third edition, revised (DSM-III-R). Washington, DC: APA, 1987: xxii–xxiii.
2. Heschel AJ. Who is man? The Raymond Fred West Memorial Lectures at Stanford University, 1963. Stanford: Stanford University Press, 1965: 3.
3. Adler A. Understanding human nature. New York: Greenberg, 1927.
4. Assagioli R. The act of will. New York: The Viking Press, 1973.
5. Brooks CVW. Sensory awareness. Rediscovery of experiencing through the workshops of Charlotte Selver. 3rd ed. Great Neck, NY: Felix Morrow, 1986.
6. Buber M. I and thou. New York: Charles Scribner's Sons, 1970.
7. Erikson EH. Identity and the life cycle. New York: International Universities Press, Inc., 1959.
8. Frankl VE. The will to meaning. Foundations and applications of logotherapy. New York: The World Pub. Co., 1969.
9. Glasser W. Reality therapy. A new approach to psychiatry. New York: Harper & Row, 1965.
10. Jung CG. The practice of psychotherapy. The collected works of C.G. Jung, Bollingen Series XX, vol. 16. New York: Pantheon Books, 1954.
11. Maslow AH. Toward a psychology of being. 2nd ed. New York: D. Van Nostrand Co., 1968.
12. Rogers CR. On becoming a person. A therapist's view of psychotherapy. Boston: Houghton Mifflin Co., 1961.
13. Satir V. The new peoplemaking. Mountain View, CA: Science and Behavior Books, Inc., 1988.
14. Viorst J. Necessary losses. The loves, illusions, dependencies, and impossible expec-

tations that all of us have to give up in order to grow. New York: Simon and Schuster, 1986.

15. Yalom ID. Existential psychotherapy. New York: Basic Books, Inc., 1980.
16. Hall CS, Lindzey G. Theories of personality. 3rd ed. New York: John Wiley & Sons, 1978.
17. Fadiman J, Frager R. Personality and personal growth. New York: Harper & Row, 1976.
18. Smith H. The religions of man. New York: Perennial Library, Harper & Row, 1965.
19. James W. The principles of psychology. (1st published in 1890.) New York: Dover Publications, Inc., 1950: vol. 1, 1–11.
20. Balint M. The doctor, his patient and the illness. Revised ed. New York: International Universities Press, Inc., 1972: 161.

Chapter 6

1. Meador CK. The art and science of nondisease. N Engl J Med 1965; 272: 92–5.
2. Bosk CL. Occupational rituals in patient management. N Engl J Med 1980; 303: 71–6.
3. Balint M. The doctor, his patient, and the illness. Revised edition. New York: International Universities Press, Inc., 1972: 69–103.
4. See Ch. 13, Backache, refs. 116–17, 120, 125–31.
5. Breck LW, Hillsman JW, Basom WC. Lumbosacral roentgenograms of 450 consecutive applicants for heavy work. Ann Surg 1944; 120: 88–93.
6. Barton PN, Biram JH. Pre-placement x-ray examination of the lower back. Industrial Medicine (now Occup Health Saf) 1964; 15: 319–22.
7. Frymoyer JW. Back pain and sciatica. N Engl J Med 1988; 318: 291–300.
8. Weiss NS. Relation of high blood pressure to headache, epistaxis, and selected other symptoms. The United States Health Examination Survey of Adults. N Engl J Med 1972; 287: 631–3.
9. Price WH. Gall-bladder dyspepsia. Br Med J 1963; 2: 138–41.
10. Hinkel CL, Moller GA. Correlation of symptoms, age, sex, and habitus with cholecystographic findings in 1000 consecutive examinations. Gastroenterology 1957; 32: 807–15.
11. Dyer NH, Pridie RB. Incidence of hiatus hernia in asymptomatic subjects. Gut 1968; 9: 696–9.
12. Pridie RB. Incidence and coincidence of hiatus hernia. Gut 1966; 7: 188–9.
13. Cohen S, Harris LD. Does hiatus hernia affect competence of the gastroesophageal sphincter? N Engl J Med 1971; 284: 1053–6.
14. Cohen S, Janowitz HD. Hiatal hernia—the great masquerader. An interview in Medical World News 1974; 15 (Nov. 22): 29–38.
15. Manousos O, Truelove SC, Lumsden K. Prevalence of colonic diverticulosis in general population of Oxford area. Br Med J 1967; 3: 762–3.
16. Horner JL. Natural history of diverticulosis of the colon. American Journal of Digestive Diseases (now Dig Dis Sci). New Series 1958; 3: 343–50.
17. Boles RS, Jordan SM. The clinical significance of diverticulosis. Gastroenterology 1958; 35: 579–82.
18. Gastineau CF. Editorial. Is reactive hypoglycemia a clinical entity? Mayo Clin Proc 1983; 58: 545–9.

19. Palardy J, Havrankova J, Lepage R, et al. Blood glucose measurements during symptomatic episodes in patients with suspected postprandial hypoglycemia. N Engl J Med 1989; 321: 1421–5.

20. Service FJ. Hypoglycemia and the postprandial syndrome. N Engl J Med 1989; 321: 1472–4.

21. Jung Y, Khurana RC, Corredor DG, et al. Reactive hypoglycemia in women. Results of a health survey. Diabetes 1971; 20: 428–34.

22. Fariss BL. Prevalence of post-glucose-load glycosuria and hypoglycemia in a group of healthy young men. Diabetes 1974; 23: 189–91.

23. Johnson DD, Dorr KE, Swenson WM, Service FJ. Reactive hypoglycemia. JAMA 1980; 243: 1151–5.

24. Malcolm AD, Boughner DR, Kostuk WJ, Ahuya SP. Clinical features and investigative findings in presence of mitral leaflet prolapse. Study of 85 consecutive patients. Br Heart J 1976; 38: 244–56.

25. Wooley DF. Where are the diseases of yesteryear? Da Costa's syndrome, soldiers heart, the effort syndrome, neurocirculatory asthenia—and the mitral valve prolapse syndrome. Circulation 1976; 53: 749–51.

26. Motulsky AG. Biased ascertainment and the natural history of diseases. N Engl J Med 1978; 298: 1196–7.

27. Markiewicz W, Stoner J, London E, Hunt SA, Popp RL. Mitral valve prolapse in one hundred presumably healthy young females. Circulation 1976; 53: 464–73.

28. Procacci PM, Savran SV, Schreiter SL, Bryson AL. Clinical frequency and implications of mitral valve prolapse in the female population. Circulation 1975; 52: Suppl 2: 78 (abstract).

29. Darsee JR, Mikolich JR, Nicoloff NB, Lesser LE. Prevalence of mitral valve prolapse in presumably healthy young men. Circulation 1979; 59: 619–22.

30. Cohen JL, Austin SM, Segel KR, Millman AE, Kim CS. Echocardiographic mitral valve prolapse in ballet dancers: a function of leanness. Am Heart J 1987; 113: 341–4.

31. Devereux RB, Kramer-Fox R, Brown WT, et al. Relation between clinical features of the mitral prolapse syndrome and echocardiographically documented mitral valve prolapse. J Am Coll Cardiol 1986; 8: 763–72.

32. Venkatesh A, Pauls DL, Crowe R, et al. Mitral valve prolapse in anxiety neurosis (panic disorder). Am Heart J 1980; 100: 302–5.

33. Wood P. Da Costa's syndrome (or effort syndrome). Br Med J 1941; 767–72.

34. Cohen ME, White PD. Life situations, emotions, and neurocirculatory asthenia (anxiety neurosis, neurasthenia, effort syndrome). Psychosom Med 1951; 13: 335–57.

35. Katon WJ. Chest pain, cardiac disease, and panic disorder. J Clin Psychiatry 1990; 51: 5 (Suppl): 27–30.

36. American Psychiatric Association: Diagnostic and statistical manual of mental disorders; third edition, revised. (DSM-III-R). Washington, DC: APA, 1987: 235–41, 251–53, 329–31.

37. Kemp HG Jr, Vokonas PS, Cohn PF, Gorlin R. The anginal syndrome associated with normal coronary arteriograms. Report of a six-year experience. Am J Med 1973; 54: 735–42.

38. Ockene IS, Shay MJ, Alpert JS, Weiner BH, Dalen JE. Unexplained chest pain in patients with normal coronary arteriograms. A follow-up study of functional status. N Engl J Med 1980; 303: 1249–52.

39. Allan FN. The differential diagnosis of weakness and fatigue. N Engl J Med 1944; 231: 414–8.
40. Morrison JD. Fatigue as a presenting complaint in family practice. J Fam Pract 1980; 10: 795–801.
41. Jerrett WA. Lethargy in general practice. Practitioner 1981; 225: 731–7.
42. Sugarman JR, Berg AO. Evaluation of fatigue in a family practice. J Fam Pract 1984; 19: 643–7.
43. Kroenke K, Wood DR, Mangelsdorff AD, Meier NJ, Powell JB. Chronic fatigue in primary care. Prevalence, patient characteristics, and outcome. JAMA 1988; 260: 929–34.
44. Detre T, Hayashi TT, Archer DF. Management of the menopause. Ann Intern Med 1978; 88: 373–8.
45. Williams TJ, Pratt JH. Endometriosis in 1,000 consecutive celiotomies: incidence and management. Am J Obstet Gynecol 1977; 129: 245–50.
46. Wentz AC. Endometriosis. In: Jones HW III, Wentz AC, Burnett LS. Novak's textbook of gynecology. 11th ed. Baltimore: Williams & Wilkins, 1988: 308.
47. Liston WA, Bradford WP, Downie J, Kerr MG. Laparoscopy in a general gynecologic unit. Am J Obstet Gynecol 1972; 113: 672–7.
48. Rapkin AJ. Adhesions and pelvic pain: a retrospective study. Obstet Gynecol 1986; 68: 13–15.
49. Harrop-Griffiths J, Katon W, Walker E, Holm L, Russo J, Hickok L. The association between chronic pelvic pain, psychiatric diagnoses, and childhood sexual abuse. Obstet Gynecol 1988; 71: 590–4.
50. Kresch AJ, Seifer DB, Sachs LB, Barrese I. Laparoscopy in 100 women with chronic pelvic pain. Obstet Gynecol 1984; 64: 672–4.
51. Merrill JA. Endometriosis. In: Danforth DN, Scott JR, eds. Obstetrics and gynecology. 5th ed. Philadelphia: J.B. Lippincott Co., 1986: 1000.
52. Barbieri R, Kistner RW. Endometriosis. In Kistner RW. Gynecology. Principles and practice. 4th ed. Chicago: Year Book Medical Publishers, Inc., 1986: 399.
53. Thompson WG. The irritable gut. Functional disorders of the alimentary canal. Baltimore: University Park Press, 1979: 191.
54. Raphael B. The crisis of hysterectomy. Aust NZ J Psychiatry 1972; 6: 106–15.
55. Barker MG. Psychiatric illness after hysterectomy. Br Med J 1968; 2: 91–5.
56. Richards DH. Depression after hysterectomy. Lancet 1973; 2: 430–2.
57. See Ch. 1, refs. 11–15.
58. Castelnuovo-Tedesco P, Krout BM. Psychosomatic aspects of chronic pelvic pain. Psychiatry in Medicine (now Int J Psychiatry Med) 1970–71; 1: 109–26.
59. Mussey RD, Wilson RB. Pelvic pain. A follow-up study. Am J Obstet Gynecol 1941; 42: 759–67.
60. Youngs DD, Wise TN. Preparing a patient for surgery. Consent, information, and emotional support. Clin Obstet Gynecol 1976; 19: 431–48.
61. Bennett RM. Fibrositis: misnomer for a common rheumatic disorder. West J Med 1981; 134: 405–13.
62. Prinzmetal M, Massumi R. The anterior wall syndrome—chest pain resembling pain of cardiac origin. JAMA 1955; 159: 177–84.
63. Kayser HL. Tietze's syndrome. A review of the literature. Am J Med 1957; 21: 982–9.
64. Munthe A. The story of San Michele. New York: E.P. Dutton & Co., Inc., paperback ed. (first published, 1929): 31–44.

65. Renfro L, Feder HM Jr., Lane TJ, Manu P, Matthews DA. Yeast connection among 100 patients with chronic fatigue. Am J Med 1989; 86: 165–8.
66. Terr AI. Position paper. Clinical ecology. American College of Physicians. Ann Intern Med 1989; 111: 168–78.
67. Kahn E, Letz G. Clinical ecology: environmental medicine or unsubstantiated theory? Ann Intern Med 1989; 111: 104–6.

Chapter 7

1. Belloc NB. Relationship of health practices and mortality. Prev Med 1973; 2: 67–81.
2. Breslow L, Enstrom JE. Persistence of health habits and their relationship to mortality. Prev Med 1980; 9: 469–83.
3. Gotto AM Jr, Farmer JA. Risk factors for coronary artery disease. In Braunwald E, ed. Heart disease. A textbook of cardiovascular medicine. 3rd. ed., vol. 2, Philadelphia: W.B. Saunders Co., 1988: 1153–90.
4. Gordon T, Kannel WB. The effects of overweight on cardiovascular diseases. Geriatrics 1973; 28: 80–8.
5. Report of the Expert Panel on Detection, Evaluation, and Treatment of High Blood Cholesterol in Adults. Bethesda, MD.: National Heart, Lung and Blood Institute, U.S. Department of Health and Human Services, Public Health Service. NIH publication No. 88-2925, 1988.
6. Fujita T, Henry WL, Bartter FC, Lake CR, Delea CS. Factors influencing blood pressure in salt-sensitive patients with hypertension. Am J Med 1980; 69: 334–44.
7. Truett J, Cornfield J, Kannel W. A multivariate analysis of the risk of coronary heart disease in Framingham. J Chronic Dis 1967; 20: 511–24.
8. Kannel WB, Castelli WP, Verter J, McNamara PM. Relative importance of factors of risk in the pathogenesis of coronary heart disease: the Framingham Study. In Russek HI, Zohman BL, eds. Coronary heart disease. Philadelphia: J.B. Lippincott Co., 1971: 97–115.
9. Farquhar JW. The American way of life need not be hazardous to your health. New York: W.W. Norton & Co., 1978: 39–43.
10. U.S. Bureau of the Census. Statistical abstract of the United States: 1986 (106th edition). Washington, DC, 1985: 73.
11. Stamler J. Primary prevention of coronary heart disease: The last 20 years. Am J Cardiol 1981; 47: 722–35.
12. Doll R, Peto R. The causes of cancer: quantitative estimates of avoidable risks of cancer in the United States today. JNCI 1986; 66: 1191–1308.
13. Fielding JE. Smoking: health effects and control (first of two parts). N Engl J Med 1985; 313: 491–8.
14. Kissin B. Alcohol abuse and alcohol-related illnesses. In Wyngaarden JB, Smith LH Jr. Cecil textbook of medicine, 18th. ed., vol. 1. Philadelphia: W.B. Saunders Co., 1988: 48–52.
15. Stat Bull, Metropolitan Life Insurance Co. (now Stat Bull, Metropolitan Life and affiliated companies) 1960; 41: Feb., 6–10, Mar., 1–4.
16. Ibid. Apr. 1–3.
17. Kahn HA. The Dorn study of smoking and mortality among U.S. Veterans: report on eight and one-half years of observation. Bethesda: National Cancer Institute Monograph No. 19, Jan. 1966: 1–27.

18. Hjermann I, Holme I, Velve Byre K, Leren P. Effect of diet and smoking intervention on the incidence of coronary heart disease. Report from the Oslo Study Group of a randomized trial in healthy men. Lancet 1981; 2: 1303–10.

19. Lipid Research Clinics' Program. The Lipid Research Clinics' coronary primary prevention trial results. I. Reduction in incidence of coronary heart disease. II. The relationships of reduction in incidence of coronary heart disease to cholesterol lowering. JAMA 1984; 251: 351–74.

20. Frick MH, Elo O, Haapa K, et al. Helsinki Heart Study: primary-prevention trial with gemfibrozil in middle-aged men with dyslipidemia. Safety of treatment, changes in risk factors, and incidence of coronary heart disease. N Engl J Med 1987; 317: 1237–45.

21. Brensike SF, Levy RI, Kelsey SF, et al. Effects of therapy with cholestyramine on progression of coronary arteriosclerosis. Results of the NHLBI [National Heart, Lung and Blood Institute] Type II Coronary Intervention Study. Circulation 1984; 69: 313–24.

22. Blankenhorn DH, Nessim SA, Johnson RL, Sanmarco ME, Azen SP, Cashin-Hemphill L. Beneficial effects of combined colestipol-niacin therapy on coronary atherosclerosis and coronary venous bypass grafts. JAMA 1987; 257: 3233–40.

23. Brown G, Albers JJ, Fisher LD, et al. Regression of coronary artery disease as a result of intensive lipid-lowering therapy in men with high levels of apolipoprotein B. N Engl J Med 1990; 323: 1289–98.

24. The Joint National Committee on Detection, Evaluation and Treatment of High Blood Pressure. The 1988 report of the Joint National Committee on Detection, Evaluation, and Treatment of High Blood Pressure. Arch Intern Med 1988; 148: 1023–38.

25. Littenberg B, Garber AM, Sox HC, Jr. Screening for hypertension. Ann Intern Med 1990; 112: 192–202.

26. Kaplan NM. Non-drug treatment of hypertension. Ann Intern Med 1985; 102: 359–73.

27. Kannel WB, Thom TJ. Declining cardiovascular mortality. Circulation 1984; 70: 331–6.

28. Goldman L, Cook EF. The decline in ischemic heart disease mortality rates. An analysis of the comparative effects of medical interventions and changes in lifestyle. Ann Intern Med 1984; 101: 825–36.

29. Sytkowski PA, Kannel WB, D'Agostino RB. Changes in risk factors and the decline in mortality from cardiovascular disease. The Framingham Heart Study. N Engl J Med 1990; 322: 1635–41.

30. Jeffery RW, Folsom AR, Luepker RV, et al. Prevalence of overweight and weight loss behavior in a metropolitan adult population: the Minnesota Heart Survey experience. Am J Public Health 1984; 74: 349–52.

31. Schoenborn C, Cohen B. Trends in smoking, alcohol consumption, and other health practices among U.S. adults, 1977 and 1983. Washington, D.C.: National Center for Health Statistics, Advanced Data No. 118. U.S. Government Printing Office, 30 June 1986.

32a. Centers for Disease Control. HIV/AIDS surveillance year-end edition, 2/93: 17.

32b. Statistical abstract of the United States 1992. The National Data Book. 112th. ed.: 124.

33. Eddy MB. Science and health. Boston: W.F. Brown, 1875.

34. Pauling L. Orthomolecular psychiatry. Science 1968; 160: 265–71.
35. Gellhorn E, Loefbourrow GN. Emotions and emotional disorders. A neurophysiological study. New York: Hoeber Medical Division, Harper & Row, 1963: 142–3.
36. Plato. Timaeus. In Jowett B. The dialogues of Plato translated into English with analysis and introductions, 3rd. ed. Oxford: Clarendon Press, 1982: vol. 3: 510–11.
37. Dunbar HF. Emotions and bodily changes. A survey of literature on psychosomatic interrelationships, 1910–1933. New York: Columbia University Press, 1935. 4th. ed. (1910–1953), 1954.
38. Alexander F. Psychosomatic medicine. Its principles and applications. New York: W.W. Norton & Co., 1950.
39. Selye H. Stress. Montreal: Acta, Inc., 1950.
40. Chen E, Cobb S. Family structure in relation to health and disease. J Chronic Dis 1960; 12: 544–67.
41. Andrews G, Tennant C, Hewson D, and Schonell M. The relation of social factors to physical and psychiatric illness. Am J Epidemiol 1978; 108: 27–35.
42. Berkman LF, Syme SC. Social networks, host resistance, and mortality: a nine-year follow-up study of Alameda County residents. Am J Epidemiol 1979; 109: 186–204.
43. House JS, Robbins C, Metzner HL. Association of social relationships and activities with mortality: prospective evidence from the Tecumseh [Michigan] Community Health Study. Am J Epidemiol 1982; 116: 123–40.
44. Cobb S. Social support as a moderator of life stress. Psychosom Med 1976; 38: 300–14.
45. House JS, Landis KR, Umberson D. Social relationships and health. Science 1988; 241: 540–5.
46. Ortmeyer CE. Variations in mortality, morbidity, and health care by marital status. In: Erhardt CL, Berlin JE, eds. Mortality and morbidity in the United States. Cambridge: Harvard University Press, 1974: 159–88.
47. Kraus AS, Lilienfeld AM. Some epidemiologic aspects of the high mortality rate in the young widowed group. J Chronic Dis 1959; 10: 207–17.
48. Dohrenwend BS, Dohrenwend BP, eds. Stressful life events: their nature and effects. New York: John Wiley & Sons, 1974: See chapters of Hinkle LE Jr, Holmes TH and Masula M, Rahe RH, and Mechanic D.
49. Klerman GL, Izen JE. The effects of bereavement and grief on physical health and general well-being. Adv Psychosom Med 1977; 9: 63–104.
50. Rosenman RH, Brand RJ, Jenkins CD, Friedman M, Straus R, and Wurm M. Coronary heart disease in the Western Collaborative Group Study. Final follow-up experience of 8 1/2 years. JAMA 1975; 233: 872–7.
51. Jenkins CD. Recent evidence supporting psychologic and social risk factors for coronary disease. N Engl J Med 1976; 294: 987–94; 1033–8.
52. The Review Panel on Coronary-prone Behavior and Coronary Heart Disease. Coronary-prone behavior and coronary heart disease: a critical review. Circulation 1981; 63: 1199–1215.
53. Marmot MG, Kogevinas M, Elston MA. Social/economic status and disease. Annu Rev Public Health 1987; 8: 111–35.
54. Zaidi SA. Poverty and disease: need for structural change. Soc Sci Med 1988; 27: 119–27.
55. Damon A. Race, ethnic group, and disease. Soc Biol 1969; 16: 69–80.

56. Vaillant GE. Natural history of male psychologic health. Effects of mental health on physical health. N Engl J Med 1979, 301: 1249–54.
57. Palmore E. Predicting longevity: A follow-up controlling for age. Gerontologist 1969; 9: 247–50.
58. Rabkin JG, Struening EL. Life events, stress, and illness. Science 1976; 194: 1013–20.
59. Pratt MW, Hutchins VL. Infant and perinatal mortality rates by age and race. United States, each state, and county, 1971–1975, 1976–1980. Vienna, VA: Maternal and Child Health Studies Project, ISRI, 1985: ii.
60. New high for expectation of life. Stat Bull Metrop Life Found 1987; 8–14.
61. Thomas CB. Precursors of premature disease and death. The predictive potential of habits and family attitudes. Ann Intern Med 1976; 85: 653–7.
62. Betz BJ, Thomas CB. Individual temperament as a predictor of health or premature disease. Johns Hopkins Med J 1979; 144: 81–9.
63. Vaillant GE, Vaillant CO. The relation of psychological adaptation to medical disability in middle aged men. In: Pfeiffer E, ed. Successful aging. Durham: Center for the Study of Aging and Human Development, Duke University, 1974: 19–32.
64. Cassel J. The contribution of the social environment to host resistance. Am J Epidemiol 1976; 104: 107–23.
65. Bovard EW. Brain mechanisms in effects of social support on viability. In Williams RB, Jr, ed. Perspectives on behavioral medicine. Vol. 2. Neuroendocrine control and behavior. Orlando: Academic Press, Inc., 1985: 103–29.
66. Solomon GF, Amkraut AA. Emotions, immunity and disease. In Temoshok L, Van Dyke CV, Zegans LS, eds. Emotions in health and illness. Theoretical and research foundations. New York: Grune & Stratton, 1983: 167–86.
67. Calabrese JR, Kling MA, Gold PW. Alterations in immunocompetence during stress, bereavement, and depression: focus on neuroendocrine regulation. Am J Psychiatry 1987; 144: 1123–34.
68. Ader R, Felten DL, Cohen N, eds. Psychoneuroimmunology. 2nd ed. San Diego: Academic Press, Inc., 1991.
69. Groopman JE, Broder S. Cancer in AIDS and other immunodeficiency states. In DeVita VT Jr, Hellman S, Rosenberg SA, eds. Cancer. Principles & practice of oncology. 3rd. ed., vol 2. Philadelphia: J.B. Lippincott Co., 1989: 1953–70.
70. Kiecolt-Glaser JK, Glaser R. Stress and immune function in humans. In ref. 68: 849–67.
71. Soll AH. Duodenal ulcer and drug therapy. In Sleisenger MH, Fordtran JS. Gastrointestinal disease. Pathophysiology, diagnosis, management. 4th. ed. Philadelphia: W.B. Saunders Co., 1989: 822–3, and 845.
72. Davies MH. Is high blood pressure a psychosomatic disorder? A critical review of the evidence. J Chronic Dis 1971; 24: 239–258.
73. Rees L. The importance of psychological, allergic and infective factors in childhood asthma. J Psychosom Res 1964; 7: 253–62.
74. Purcell K, Brady K, Chai H, et al. The effect on asthma in children of experimental separation from the family. Psychosom Med 1969; 31: 144–64.
75. Engel GL. Biologic and psychologic features of the ulcerative colitis patient. Gastroenterology 1961; 40: 313–22.
76. MacMahon SW. Alcohol and hypertension: implications for prevention and treatment. Ann Intern Med 1986; 105: 124–6.
77. Weiner H. Psychobiology and human disease. New York: Elsevier, 1977: 319–574.

78. LeShan L. Psychological states as factors in the development of malignant disease: a critical review. JNCI 1959; 22: 1–18.

79. Bahnson CB. Emotional and personality characteristics of cancer patients. In Sutnick AI, Engstrom PF, eds. Oncologic medicine. Clinical topics and practical management. Baltimore: University Park Press, 1976: 357–78.

80. Achterberg J, Simonton OC, Matthews-Simonton S. Stress, psychological factors, and cancer. An annotated collection of readings from the professional literature, with bibliography. Fort Worth: New Medicine Press, 1976.

81. Temoshok L. Personality, coping style, emotion and cancer: towards an integrative model. Cancer Surv 1987; 6: 545–67.

82. Eysenck HJ. Personality stress and cancer: Prediction and prophylaxis. Br J Med Psychol 1988; 61: 57–75.

83. Riley V. Biobehavioral factors in animal work on tumorigenesis. In Weiss SM, Herd JA, Fox BH, eds. Perspectives on behavioral medicine. New York: Academic Press, 1981: 183–214.

84. Fox BH. Premorbid psychological factors as related to cancer incidence. J Behav Med 1978; 1: 45–133.

85. Fox BH. Current theory of psychogenic effects on cancer incidence and prognosis. J Psychosoc Oncol 1983; 1: 17–31.

86. Hurst MW, Jenkins CD, Rose RM. The relation of psychological stress to onset of medical illness. Annu Rev Med 1976; 27: 301–12.

87. Surawicz FG, Brightwell DR, Weitzel WD, Othmer E. Cancer, emotions, and mental illness: the present state of understanding. Am J Psychiatry 1976; 133: 1306–9.

88. Morrison FR, Paffenbarger RA. Epidemiological aspects of biobehavior in the etiology of cancer: a critical review. In Weiss SM, Herd JA, Fox BH. Perspectives on behavioral medicine. New York: Academic Press, 1981: 135–61.

89. Wellisch DK, Yager J. Is there a cancer-prone personality? CA 1983; 33: 145–53.

90. Zonderman AB, Costa PT, Jr, McCrae RP. Depression as a risk for cancer morbidity and mortality in a nationally representative sample. JAMA 1989; 262: 1191–5.

91. Jamison RN, Burish TG, Wallston KA. Psychogenic factors in predicting survival of breast cancer patients. J Clin Oncol 1987; 5: 768–72.

92. Cassileth BR, Lusk EJ, Miller DS, Brown LL, Miller C. Psychosocial correlates of survival in advanced malignant disease? N Engl J Med 1985; 312: 1551–5.

93. Angell M. Disease as a reflection of the psyche. N Engl J Med 1985; 312: 1570–2.

94. Correspondence. N Engl J Med 1985; 313: 1354–9.

95. Council condemns journal editorial. APA Monitor 1985; 16: 6.

96. Matthews-Simonton S, Simonton OC, Creighton JL. Getting well again. A step-by-step, self-help guide to overcoming cancer for patients and their families. New York: Bantam Books, Inc., 1984 (1st published, 1978).

97. Siegel BS. Love, medicine, and miracles. Lessons learned about self-healing from a surgeon's experience with exceptional patients. New York: Perennial Library, Harper & Row, 1988 (1st published, 1986).

98. Siegel BS. Peace, love and healing. Bodymind communication and the path to self-healing: an exploration. New York: Harper & Row, 1989.

99. Simonton OC, Matthews-Simonton S, Sparks TF. Psychological intervention in the treatment of cancer. Psychosomatics 1980; 21: 226–33.

100. Simonton OC, Matthews-Simonton S. Cancer and stress. Counselling the cancer patient. Med J Aust 1981; 1: 679–83.

101. Morgenstern H, Gellert GA, Walter SD, Ostfeld AM, Siegel BS. The impact of a psychosocial support program on survival with breast cancer: the importance of selection bias in program evaluation. J Chronic Dis 1984; 37: 273–82.

102. Spiegel D, Bloom JR, Kraemer HC, Gottheil E. Effect of psychosocial treatment on survival of patients with metastatic breast cancer. Lancet 1989; 2: 888–91.

103. Panagis DM. Supportive therapy: goals and methods. In: Stoll BA, ed. Mind and cancer prognosis. Chichester: John Wiley & Sons Ltd., 1979: 139–52.

104. Silberfarb PM. Research in adaptation to illness and psychosocial intervention. An overview. Cancer 1982; 50: 1921–5.

105. Watson M. Psychosocial intervention with cancer patients: A review. Psychol Med 1983; 13: 839–46.

106. Vachon MLS. Models of group intervention for cancer patients and families. In: Day SB, ed. Cancer, stress, and death. 2nd ed. New York: Plenum Medical Book Co., 1986: 203–16.

107. Spiegel D, Bloom JR, Yalom I. Group support for patients with metastatic cancer. A randomized prospective outcome study. Arch Gen Psychiatry 1981; 38: 527–33.

108. Forester B, Kornfeld DS, Fleiss JL. Psychotherapy during radiotherapy: effects on emotional and physical distress. Am J Psychiatry 1985; 142: 22–7.

109. Gordon WA, Freidenbergs I, Diller L. Efficacy of psychosocial intervention with cancer patients. J Consult Clin Psychol 1980; 48: 743–59.

110. Heffron WA. Group therapy sessions as part of treatment of children with cancer. Pediatr Ann 1975; 4: 102–12.

111. Ferlic M, Goldman A, Kennedy BJ. Group counseling in adult patients with advanced cancer. Cancer 1979; 43: 760–6.

112. Izsac FC, Engel J, Medalie JH. Comprehensive rehabilitation of the patient with cancer. Five-year experience of a home-care unit. J Chronic Dis 1973; 26: 363–74.

113. Cain EN, Kohorn EI, Quinlan DM, Latimer K, Schwartz PE. Psychosocial benefits of a cancer support group. Cancer 1986; 57: 183–9.

114. Holland JC, Rowland JH. Psychiatric, psychosocial, and behavioral interventions in the treatment of cancer: an historical review. In Weiss SM, Herd JA, Fox BH, eds. Perspectives on behavioral medicine. New York: Academic Press, 1981: 235–60.

115. Spiegel D, Bloom JR. Group therapy and hypnosis reduce metastatic carcinoma pain. Psychosom Medicine 1983; 45: 333–9.

116. Olness K. Imagery (self-hypnosis) as adjunct therapy in childhood cancer. Clinical experience with 25 patients. Am J Pediatr Hematol Oncol 1981; 3: 313–321.

117. Ref. 96: page 75.

118. Ref. 98: page 40.

119. Constitution of the World Health Organization. In: The first ten years of the World Health Organization. Geneva: W.H.O., 1958: 459.

120. Hippocrates. On airs, waters, and places. In Adams F. The genuine works of Hippocrates. Baltimore: The Williams & Wilkins Co., 1939: 19–41.

121. Schneiderman LJ. The practice of preventive health care. Menlo Park, CA: Addison-Wesley Pub. Co., 1981.

122. U.S. Preventive Services Task Force. Guide to clinical preventive services. Baltimore: Williams & Wilkins, 1989.

123. Satir V. The new peoplemaking. Mountain View, CA: Science and Behavior Books, Inc., 1988: 20–42.

124. Branden N. Honoring the self. The psychology of confidence and respect. Toronto: Bantam Books, 1985 (1st published, 1983).
125. Toward a state of esteem. The final report of the California Task Force to Promote Self-esteem and Personal and Social Responsibility. Sacramento: Bureau of Publications, Calif. State Dept. of Education, 1990.
126. Sagan LA. The health of nations. True causes of sickness and well-being. New York: Basic Books, Inc., 1987.
127. Lalonde M. A new perspective on the health of Canadians. Ottawa: Government of Canada, 1974.
128. Smoking and health: report of the Advisory Committee to the Surgeon General of the Public Health Service. Washington, DC: US Dept. of Health, Education, and Welfare, 1964 (Public Health Service Publication 1103, Government Printing Office).
129. The Surgeon General's report on nutrition and health. Washington, DC: Department of Health and Human Services (Public Health Service) publication No. 88-50210, 1988.
130. Califano JA. The Secretary's foreword. In: Smoking and health—A report of the Surgeon General. Washington, DC: Department of Health, Education and Welfare, 1979 (Public Health Service Publication 79-50066, Government Printing Office): I–V.
131. Luce BR, Schweitzer SO. Smoking and alcohol abuse: A comparison of their economic consequences. N Engl J Med 1978; 298: 569–70.
132. Warner KE. The economics of smoking: dollars and sense. NY State J Med 1983; 83: 1273–4.
133. Knowles JH. The responsibility of the individual. Daedalus 1977 (Winter); 106: 57–80.
134. Clinical opportunities for smoking intervention. A guide for the busy physician. U.S. Department of Health and Human Services, Public Health Service, National Institutes of Health. NIH Publication No. 86-2178, 1986.
135. National Cancer Institute: The smoking digest. Progress report on a nation kicking the habit. US DHEW, Public Health Service, National Institutes of Health. National Cancer Institute, Bethesda, MD, Oct. 1977: 57–8.
136. Schachter S. Recidivism and self-cure of smoking and obesity. Am Psychol 1982; 37: 436–44.

Chapter 8

1. Srole L, Langner TS, Michael ST, Opler MK, Rennie TAC. Mental health in the metropolis: the Midtown Manhattan Study. New York: The Blakiston Division, McGraw-Hill Book Co., Inc., 1962: 138.
2. Mellinger GD, Balter MB, Manheimer DI, Cisin IH, Perry HJ. Psychic distress, life crisis, and use of psychotherapeutic medications. National household survey data. Arch Gen Psychiatry 1978; 35: 1045–52.
3. American Psychiatric Association: Diagnostic and statistical manual of mental disorders, third edition, revised (DSM-III-R). Washington, D.C.: APA, 1987.
4. Tischler GL, Heinsz JE, Myers JK, et al. Utilization of mental health services: I. Patienthood and the prevalence of symptomatology in the community. II. Mediators of service allocation. Arch Gen Psychiatry 1975; 32: 411–18.
5. Boyd JH, Burke JD, Jr, Gruenberg E, et al. Exclusion criteria of DSM-III. A study of co-occurrence of hierarchy-free syndromes. Arch Gen Psychiatry 1984; 41: 983–9.

6. Robins LN, Helzer JE, Weissman MM, et al. Lifetime prevalence of specific psychiatric disorders in three sites. Arch Gen Psychiatry 1984; 41: 949–58.

7. Blum RH & Associates. Society and drugs. Drugs I. Social and cultural observations. San Francisco: Jossey-Bass Inc., 1969: 13–16.

8. Ref. 3: 226–8.

9. Akiskal HS. Dysthymic disorder: psychopathology of proposed chronic depressive subtypes. Am J Psychiatry 1983; 140: 11–20.

10. Ref. 3: 329–31.

11. Ref. 3: 333–4.

12. Ref. 3: 255–67.

13. Brown HN, Zinberg NE. Difficulties in the integration of psychological and medical practices. Am J Psychiatry 1982; 139: 1576–80.

14. Docherty JP, Marder SR, VanKammen DP, Siris SG. Psychotherapy and pharmacotherapy; conceptual issues. Am J Psychiatry 1977; 134: 529–33.

15. Silverman D, Gartrell N, Aronson M, Steer M, Edbril S. In search of a biopsychosocial perspective: an experiment with beginning medical students. Am J Psychiatry 1983; 140: 1154–9.

16. Vasile RG, Samson JA, Bemporad J, et al. A biopsychosocial approach to treating patients with affective disorders. Am J Psychiatry 1987; 144: 341–4.

17. Parry HJ, Balter MB, Mellinger GD, Cisin IH, Manheimer DI. National patterns of psychotherapeutic drug use. Arch Gen Psychiatry 1973; 28: 769–83.

18. National Center for Health Statistics. Koch H, Campbell WH. Utilization of psychotropic drugs in office-based ambulatory care: National Ambulatory Medical Care Survey, 1980 and 1981. Advance data from vital and health statistics, No. 90. DHHS Pub. No. (PHS) 83-1250. Public Health Service, Hyattsville, Md., June 1983.

19. Regier DA, Goldberg ID, Taube CA. The de facto US mental health services system. A public health perspective. Arch Gen Psychiatry 1978; 35: 685–93.

20. Plomin R. Nature and nurture. An introduction to human behavioral genetics. Pacific Grove, CA: Brooks/Cole Pub. Co., 1990: 107–10.

21. Guze SB, Cloninger CR, Martin RL, Clayton PJ. A follow-up and family study of Briquet's syndrome. Br J Psychiatry 1986; 149: 17–23.

22. Dobzhansky T. Mankind evolving. The evolution of the human species. New Haven: Yale University Press, 1962: 98.

23. Elkins R, Rapoport JL, Lipsky A. Obsessive-compulsive disorder of childhood and adolescence. A neurobiological viewpoint. J Am Acad Child Psychiatry 1980; 19: 511–24.

24. Rapoport JL. The biology of obsessions and compulsions. Sci Am 1989; 260: 83–9.

25. Gottesman II, Shields J. Schizophrenia: the epigenetic puzzle. Cambridge: Cambridge University Press, 1982.

26. McGuffin P, Sargeant M, Hetti G, Tidmarsh S, Whatley S, Marchbanks RM. Exclusion of a schizophrenia susceptibility gene from the chromosome 5q11-q13 region: New data and a reanalysis of previous reports. Am J Hum Genet 1990; 47: 524–35.

27. Pardes H, Kaufmann CA, Pincus HA, West A. Genetics and psychiatry: past discoveries, current dilemmas, and future directions. Am J Psychiatry 1989; 146: 435–43.

28. Lander ES. Splitting schizophrenia. Nature 1988; 336: 105–6.

29. Torrey EF. Surviving schizophrenia. A family manual. Revised edition. New York: Perennial Library, Harper & Row, 1988: 129–40.

30. Mesulam M-M. Schizophrenia and the brain. N Engl J Med 1990; 322: 842–5.

31. Reveley AM, Reveley MA, Clifford CA, Murray RM. Cerebral ventricular size in twins discordant for schizophrenia. Lancet 1982; 1: 540–1.
32. Suddath RL, Christison GW, Torrey EF, Casanova MF, Weinberger DR. Anatomical abnormalities in the brains of monozygotic twins discordant for schizophrenia. N Engl J Med 1990; 322: 789–94.
33. Ref. 3: 191.
34. Ref. 3: 205–8.
35. Foulds GA, Bedford A. Hierarchy of classes of personal illness. Psychol Med 1975; 5: 181–192.
36. Weissman MM. The epidemiology of anxiety disorders: rates, risks and familial patterns. J Psychiat Res 1988; 22, suppl. 1: 99–114.
37. Humble M. Aetiology and mechanisms of anxiety disorders. Acta Psychiatr Scand 1987; 76, suppl 335: 15–30.
38. Judd FK, Burrows GD, Hay DA. Panic disorder: evidence for genetic vulnerability. Aust NZ J Psychiatry 1987; 21: 197–208.
39. McGuffin P, Katz R. The genetics of depression and manic-depressive disorder. Br J Psychiatry 1989; 155: 294–304.
40. Torgerson S. Genetic factors in anxiety disorders. Arch Gen Psychiatry 1983; 40: 1085–92.
41. Torgerson S. Genetic factors in moderately severe and mild affective disorder. Arch Gen Psychiatry 1986; 43: 222–6.
42. Blehar MC, Weissman M, Gershon ES, Hirschfeld RMA. Family and genetic studies of affective disorders. Arch Gen Psychiatry 1988; 45: 289–92.
43. Loehlin JC, Nichols RC. Heredity, environment, & personality. A study of 850 sets of twins. Austin: University of Texas Press, 1976.
44. Plomin R. Heredity and temperament: a comparison of twin data for self-report questionnaires, parental ratings, and objectively assessed behavior. Progress in clinical and biological research 1981; 69B (Twin research 3, part B, intelligence, personality, and development): 269–278.
45. Thomas A, Chess S. Temperament and development. New York: Brunner/Mazel, Publishers, 1977.
46. Eysenck HJ. The scientific study of personality. London: Routledge & Kegan Paul Ltd, 1952.
47. McClearn GE, DeFries JC. Introduction to behavioral genetics. San Francisco: W.H. Freeman and Co., 1973: 164–72.
48. Marks IM. Genetics of fear and anxiety disorders. Br J Psychiatry 1986; 149: 406–18.
49. Suomi SJ. Genetic and maternal contributions to individual differences in rhesus monkey biobehavioral development. In Krasnegor NA, Blass EM, Hofer MA, Smotherman WP, eds. Perinatal development. A psychobiological perspective. Orlando: Academic Press, Inc., 1987: 397–419.
50. Cloninger CR. A systematic method for clinical description and classification of personality variants. A proposal. Arch Gen Psychiatry 1987; 44: 573–88.
51. Kagan J, Reznick JS, Snidman N. Biological bases of childhood shyness. Science 1988; 240: 167–71.
52. Plomin R. Nature and nurture. An introduction to human behavioral genetics. Pacific Grove, CA: Brooks/Cole Pub. Co., 1990.
53. Cloninger CR. A unified biosocial theory of personality and its role in the development of anxiety states. Psychiatr Dev 1986; 4: 167–226.

54. Kagan J, Reznick JS, Snidman N, et al. Origins of panic disorder. In Ballenger JC, ed. Neurobiology of panic disorder. New York: Wiley-Liss, 1990: 71–87.
55. Cloninger CR. Neurogenetic adaptive mechanisms in alcoholism. Science 1987; 236: 410–6.
56. Cloninger CR, Sigvardsson S, Bohman M. Childhood personality predicts alcohol abuse in young adults. Alcoholism 1988; 12: 494–505.
57. Hirschfeld RMA, Klerman GL. Personality attributes and affective disorders. Am J Psychiatry 1979; 136: 67–70.
58. Akiskal HS, Hirschfeld RMA, Yerevanian, BI. The relationship of personality to affective disorders. A critical review. Arch Gen Psychiatry 1983; 40: 801–10.
59. Winokur G, Behar D, Vanvalkenburg C, Lowry M. Is a familial definition of depression both feasible and valid? J Nerv Ment Dis 1978; 166: 764–8.
60. Merikangas KR, Leckman JF, Prusoff BA, Pauls DL, Weissman MM. Familial transmission of depression and alcoholism. Arch Gen Psychiatry 1985; 42: 367–72.
61. Weissman MM, Myers JK, Harding PS. Prevalence and psychiatric heterogeneity of alcoholism in a United States urban community. J Stud Alcohol 1980; 41: 672–81.
62. Weissman MM, Boyd JH. The epidemiology of affective disorders: rates and risk factors. In Grinspoon L, ed. Psychiatry update, Vol. II. Washington, DC: American Psychiatric Press, 1983: 406–28.
63. Gilligan C. In a different voice. Psychological theory and women's development. Cambridge: Harvard University Press, 1982.
64. Miller JB. Toward a new psychology of women. 2nd ed. Boston: Beacon Press, 1986.
65. Formanek R, Gurian A, eds. Women and depression. A lifespan perspective. New York: Springer Pub. Co., 1987: See chapters of Jack D, Lewis HB, and Lerner HG, 147–99.
66. McGrath E, Keita GP, Strickland BR, Russo NF. Women and depression: risk factors and treatment issues. Washington, DC: American Psychological Asso., 1990: 22–23.
67. Schachter S, Singer JE. Cognitive, social, and physiological determinants of emotional state. Psychol Rev 1962; 69: 379–99.
68. Breggin PR. The psychophysiology of anxiety. With a review of the literature concerning adrenaline. J Nerv Ment Dis 1964; 139: 558–68.
69. Gorman JM. The biology of anxiety. In Psychiatry Update. The American Psychiatric Association Annual Review, Vol. III. Washington, DC: APA Press, 1984: 467–82.
70. Shear MK. Pathophysiology of panic: a review of pharmacologic provocative tests and naturalistic monitoring data. J Clin Psychiatry 1986; 47: 6 (Suppl): 18–25.
71. Starkman MN, Zelnik TC, Nesse RM, Cameron OG. Anxiety in patients with pheochromocytoma. Arch Int Med 1985; 145: 248–52.
72. Cannon WB. The James-Lange theory of emotions: a critical examination and an alternative theory. Am J Psychol 1927; 39: 106–24.
73. Klein DF, Gorman JM. A model of panic and agoraphobic development. Acta Psychiatr Scand 1987; 76 (suppl 335): 87–95.
74. Sheehan DV. Current concepts in psychiatry. Panic attacks and phobias. N Engl J Med 1982; 30: 156–8.
75. Ref. 3: 235–8.
76. Satir V. The new peoplemaking. Mountain View, CA: Science and Behavior Books, Inc., 1988.

77. Raskin M, Peeke HVS, Dickman W, Pinsker H. Panic and generalized anxiety disorders. Developmental antecedents and precipitants. Arch Gen Psychiatry 1982; 39: 687–9.

78. Klein DF. Delineation of two drug-responsive anxiety syndromes. Psychopharmacologia 1964; 5: 397–408.

79. Finlay-Jones R, Brown GW. Types of stressful life event and the onset of anxiety and depressive disorders. Psychol Med 1981; 11: 803–15.

80. Roy-Byrne PR, Geraci M, Uhde TW. Life events and the onset of panic disorder. Am J Psychiatry 1986; 143: 1424–7.

81. Gittelman R, Klein DF. Relationship between separation anxiety and panic and agoraphobic disorders. Psychopathology 1984; 17: Suppl. 1, 56–65.

82. Bowlby J. Separation anxiety. Int J Psychoanal 1960; 41: 89–113.

83. Ballenger JC. Toward an integrated model of panic disorder. Am J Orthopsychiatry 1989; 59: 284–93.

84. Katon W. Panic disorder in the medical setting. National Institute of Mental Health. DHHS Pub. No. (ADM) 89-1629. Washington, DC: Supt. of Docs., U.S. Govt. Print Off., 1989.

85. Ackerman SH, Sachar EJ. The lactate theory of anxiety: a review and reevaluation. Psychosom Med 1974; 36: 69–81.

86. Margraf J, Ehlers A, and Roth WT. Sodium lactate infusions and panic attacks: A review and critique. Psychosom Med 1986; 48: 23–51.

87. Katon WJ. Chest pain, cardiac disease, and panic disorder. J Clin Psychiatry 1990; 51: 5 (Suppl): 27–30.

88. Osler W. The principles and practice of medicine. 1st. ed. New York: D. Appleton and Co., 1893: 657–9.

89. Mayou R. Invited review: atypical chest pain. J Psychosom Res 1989: 33: 393–406.

90. Zigler E, Phillips L. Psychiatric diagnosis: a critique. J of Abnormal and Social Psychology (now J Abnorm Psychology) 1961; 63: 607–18.

91. Freudenberg RK, Robertson SPS. Symptoms in relation to psychiatric diagnosis and treatment. Archives of Neurology and Psychiatry (now Arch Neurol) 1956; 76: 14–22.

92. Schulterbrandt JG, Raskin A, Reatig N. Further replication of factors of psychopathology in the interview, ward behavior and self reported ratings of hospitalized depressed patients. Psychol Rep 1974; 34: 23–32.

93. Surtees PG, Kendall RE. The hierarchy model of psychiatric symptomatology: an investigation based on Present State Examination ratings. Br J Psychiatry 1979; 135: 438–43.

94. Sturt E. Hierarchical patterns in the distribution of psychiatric symptoms. Psychol Med 1981; 11: 783–94.

95. Robins LN, Helzer JE, Croughan J, Ratcliff KS. National Institute of Mental Health Diagnostic Interview Schedule. Its history, characteristics, and validity. Arch Gen Psychiatry 1981; 38: 381–9.

96. Tsuang MT, Woolson RF, Winokur G, Crowe RR. Stability of psychiatric diagnosis. Schizophrenia and affective disorders followed up over a 30- to 40-year period. Arch Gen Psychiatry 1981; 38: 535–9.

97. Tsuang MT, Winokur G, Crowe RR: Morbidity risks of schizophrenia and affective disorders among first degree relatives of patients with schizophrenia, mania, depression and surgical conditions. Br J Psychiatry 1980; 137: 497–504.

98. Test MA, Wallisch LS, Allness DJ, Ripp K. Substance use in young adults with schizophrenic disorders. Schizophr Bull 1989; 15: 465–76.

99. Prusoff B, Klerman G. Differentiating depressed from anxious neurotic outpatients. Arch Gen Psychiatry 1974; 30: 302–8.

100. American Psychiatric Association: Diagnostic and statistical manual of mental disorders, third edition (DSM-III). Washington, DC: APA, 1980: 5–9.

101. Ref. 3: xxiii–xxiv.

102. Ref. 3: 192.

103. Milne AA. Now we are six. New York: E.P. Dutton, 1927: from Sneezles, 12–14.

104. Ref. 3: 208.

105. Rogers CR. Client-centered therapy. Its current practice, implications, and theory. Boston: Houghton Mifflin Co., 1951.

106. Satir V. Conjoint family therapy. A guide to theory and technique. Revised edition. Palo Alto: Science and Behavior Books, Inc., 1967 (original edition, 1964).

107. James W. The varieties of religious experience. A study in human nature. New York: Random House (The Modern Library), 1902: 10.

Chapter 9

1. Weissman MM, Boyd JH. The epidemiology of affective disorders: rates and risk factors. In Grinspoon L, ed. Psychiatry update, Vol. II. Washington, DC: American Psychiatric Press, 1983: 406–28.

2. American Psychiatric Association: Diagnostic and statistical manual of mental disorders, third edition, revised (DSM-III-R). Washington, DC: APA, 1987: 359–62.

3. Ref. 2: 329–31.

4. Ref. 2: 230–3.

5. Chodoff P. The depressive personality. A critical review. Arch Gen Psychiatry 1972; 27: 666–73.

6. Akiskal HS, Rosenthal TL, Haykal RF, Lemmi H, Rosenthal RH, Scott-Strauss A. Characterological depressions. Clinical and sleep EEG findings separating subaffective dysthymias from character spectrum disorders. Arch Gen Psychiatry 1980; 37: 777–83.

7. Spitzer RL, Endicott J, Robins E. Research diagnostic criteria. Rationale and reliability. Arch Gen Psychiatry 1978; 35: 773–82.

8. Ref. 2: 222–4, 228–30.

9. Spitz RA, Wolf KM. Anaclitic depression: an inquiry into the genesis of psychiatric conditions in early childhood, II. In Emde RN, ed. Rene A. Spitz: dialogues from infancy. Selected papers. New York: International Universities Press, Inc., 1983: 28–52.

10. Malmquist CP. Depressions in childhood and adolescence. N Engl J Med 1971; 284: 887–93, 955–61.

11. Blazer D. Depression in the elderly. N Engl J Med 1989; 320: 164–6.

12. Karasu TB. Toward a clinical model of psychotherapy for depression, II: an integrative and selective treatment approach. Am J Psychiatry 1990; 147: 269–78.

13. Perris C. Towards an integrating theory of depression focusing on the concept of vulnerability. Integr Psychiatry 1987; 5: 27–39.

14. Kline NS. Uses of reserpine, the newer phenothiazines, and iproniazid. Res Publ Assoc Res Nerv Ment Dis 1959; 37: 218–44.

15. Muller JC, Pryor WW, Gibbons JE, Orgain ES. Depression and anxiety occurring during Rauwolfia therapy. JAMA 1955; 159: 836–9.
16. Andreasen NC, Grove WM, Maurer R. Cluster analysis and the classification of depression. Br J Psychiatry 1980; 137: 256–65.
17. Carroll BJ, Feinberg M, Greden JF, et al. A specific laboratory test for the diagnosis of melancholia: standardization, validation and clinical utility. Arch Gen Psychiatry 1981; 38: 15–22.
18. Berger M, Doerr P, Lund R, Bronisch T, von Zerssen D. Neuroendocrinological and neurophysiological studies in major depressive disorders: are there biological markers for the endogenous subtype? Biol Psychiatry 1982; 17: 1217–42.
19. Stokes PE, Stoll PM, Koslow SH, et al. Pretreatment DST and hypothalamic-pituitary-adrenocortical function in depressed patients and comparison groups. A multicenter study. Arch Gen Psychiatry 1984; 41: 257–67.
20. Schweizer EE, Swenson CM, Winokur A, Rickels K, Maislin G. The dexamethasone suppression test in generalized anxiety disorder. Br J Psychiatry 1986; 149: 320–2.
21. Gerner RH, Gwirtsman HE. Abnormalities of dexamethasone suppression test and urinary MHPG in anorexia nervosa. Am J Psychiatry 1981; 138: 650–3.
22. Mitchell JE, Seim HC, Colon E, Pomeroy C. Medical complications and medical management of bulimia. Ann Intern Med 1987; 107: 71–7.
23. Edelstein CK, Roy-Byrne P, Fawzy FI, Dornfield L. Effects of weight loss on the dexamethasone suppression test. Am J Psychiatry 1983; 140: 338–41.
24. Morgan MY. Alcohol and the endocrine system. Br Med Bull 1982; 38: 35–42.
25. Raskind M, Peskind E, Rivard MF, Veith R, Barnes R. Dexamethasone suppression test and cortisol circadian rhythm in primary degenerative dementia. Am J Psychiatry 1982; 139: 1468–71.
26. Connolly CK, Gore MBR, Stanley N, Wills MR. Single-dose dexamethasone suppression in normal subjects and hospital patients. Br Med J 1968; 2: 665–7.
27. Mason JW. A review of psychoendocrine research on the pituitary-adrenal cortical system. Psychosom Med 1968; 30: 576–607.
28. Rose RM. Overview of endocrinology of stress. In Brown GM, Koslow SH, Reichlin S, eds. Neuroendocrinology and psychiatric disorder. New York: Raven Press, 1984: 95–122.
29. Sachar EJ. Twenty-four hour cortisol secretory patterns in depressed and manic patients. Prog Brain Res 1975; 42: 81–91.
30. Kupfer DJ. REM latency: a psychobiologic marker of primary depressive disease. Biol Psychiatry 1976; 11: 159–74.
31. Zarcone VP, Jr, Benson KL, Berger PA. Abnormal rapid eye movement latencies in schizophrenia. Arch Gen Psychiatry 1987; 44: 45–8.
32. Keshavan MS, Reynolds CF, Kupfer DJ. Electroencephalographic sleep in schizophrenia: a critical review. Compr Psychiatry 1990; 31: 34–47.
33. Hudson JI, Lipinski JF, Frankenburg FR, Grochocinski VJ, Kupfer DJ. Electroencephalographic sleep in mania. Arch Gen Psychiatry 1988; 45: 267–73.
34. Insel TR, Gillin JC, Moore A, Mendelson WB, Loewenstein RJ, Murphy DL. The sleep of patients with obsessive-compulsive disorder. Arch Gen Psychiatry 1982; 39: 1372–7.
35. McNamara E, Reynolds CF, III, Soloff PH. EEG sleep evaluation of depression in borderline patients. Am J Psychiatry 1984; 141: 182–6.
36. Montplaisir J, Billiard M, Takahashi S, Bell IR, Guilleminault C, Dement WC.

Twenty-four-hour recording in REM-narcoleptics with special reference to nocturnal sleep disruption. Biol Psychiatry 1978; 13: 73–89.

37. Sasaki M, Endo S. Disturbances of the circadian sleep-wake rhythm after time zone changes. Sangyo Ika Daigaku Zasshi 1985; 7 Suppl: 141–50.

38. Gillin JC, Sitaram N, Wehr T, et al. Sleep and affective illness. In Post RM, Ballenger JC, eds. Neurobiology of mood disorders. Baltimore: Williams & Wilkins, 1984: 157–89.

39. Campbell SS, Zulley J. Induction of depressive-like sleep patterns in normal subjects. In Halaris A, ed. Chronobiology and psychiatric disorders. New York: Elsevier, 1987: 117–32.

40. Janowsky DS, Davis JM, El-Yousef MK, Sekerke HJ. A cholinergic-adrenergic hypothesis of mania and depression. Lancet 1972; 2: 632–5.

41. McCarley RW. REM sleep and depression: common neurobiological control mechanisms. Am J Psychiatry 1982; 139: 565–70.

42. Hess WR. The functional organization of the diencephalon. New York: Grune & Stratton, 1957: 23–53.

43. Schildkraut JJ. The catecholamine hypothesis of affective disorders: a review of supporting evidence. Am J Psychiatry 1965; 122: 509–22.

44. Leong SS, Brown WA. Acetylcholine and affective disorder. J Neural Transm 1987; 70: 295–312.

45. Gold PW, Goodwin FK, Chrousos GP. Clinical and biochemical manifestations of depression. Relation to the neurobiology of stress. N Engl J Med 1988; 319: 348–53, 413–20.

46. Siever LJ, Davis KL. Overview: toward a dysregulation hypothesis of depression. Am J Psychiatry 1985; 142: 1017–31.

47. James W. The principles of psychology. Vol. 2. New York: Dover Pubs., Inc., 1950 (1st published, 1890): The emotions, 442–85.

48. Cannon WB. The James-Lange theory of emotions: a critical examination and an alternative theory. Am J Psychol 1927; 39: 106–24.

49. Viorst J. Necessary losses. The loves, illusions, dependencies, and impossible expectations that all of us have to give up in order to grow. New York: Simon and Schuster, 1986.

50. Arieti S, Bemporad J. Severe and mild depression. The psychotherapeutic approach. New York: Basic Books, 1978.

51. Klerman GL, Weissman MM, Rounsaville BJ, Chevron ES. Interpersonal psychotherapy of depression. New York: Basic Books, 1984.

52. Beck AT, Rush AJ, Shaw BF, Emery G. Cognitive therapy of depression. New York: The Guilford Press, 1979.

53. Burns DD. Feeling good. New York: William Morrow and Co., Inc., 1980.

54. Burns, DD. The feeling good handbook. Using the new mood therapy in everyday life. New York: William Morrow and Co., Inc., 1989.

55. Ref. 50: 5.

56. Gershon ES, Dunner DL, Goodwin FK. Toward a biology of affective disorders. Genetic contributions. Arch Gen Psychiat 1971; 25: 1–15.

57. Ref. 2: 18.

58. Robinson LA, Berman JS, Neimeyer RA. Psychotherapy for the treatment of depression: a comprehensive review of controlled outcome research. Psychol Bull 1990; 108: 30–49.

59. Elkin I, Shea T, Watkins JT, et al. National Institute of Mental Health Treatment of Depression Collaborative Research Program. General effectiveness of treatments. Arch Gen Psychiatry 1989; 46: 971–83.

60. Klerman GL. Psychotherapies and somatic therapies in affective disorders. Psychiatr Clin North Am 1983; 6: 85–103.

61. Conte HR, Platchik R, Wild KV, Karasu TB. Combined psychotherapy and pharmacotherapy for depression. A systematic analysis of the evidence. Arch Gen Psychiatry 1986; 43: 471–9.

62. Paykel ES, Prusoff B, Klerman GL. The endogenous-neurotic continuum in depression. J Psychiatr Res 1971; 8: 73–90.

63. Prusoff BA, Weissman MM, Klerman GL, Rounsaville BJ. Research Diagnostic Criteria subtypes of depression. Their role as predictors of differential response to psychotherapy and drug treatment. Arch Gen Psychiatry 1980; 37: 796–801.

64. Klein DF. Endogenomorphic depression. A conceptual and terminological revision. Arch Gen Psychiatry 1974; 31: 447–54.

65. American Psychiatric Association: Diagnostic and statistical manual of mental disorders, third edition (DSM-III). Washington, DC: APA, 1980: 205.

66. Ref. 2: 213–53.

67. Ref. 2: 481–3.

68. Barlow DH. Anxiety and its disorders. The nature and treatment of anxiety and panic. New York: The Guilford Press, 1988: 67–9; 276–8.

69. Ibid.: 66–7; 278–82.

70. Mendels J, Weinstein N, Cochrane C. The relationship between depression and anxiety. Arch Gen Psychiatry 1972; 27: 649–53.

71. Lipman RS. Differentiating anxiety and depression in anxiety disorders: use of rating scales. Psychopharmacol Bull 1982; 18: 69–77.

72. Kraepelin E. Lectures on clinical psychiatry. New York, William Wood, 1904: 1–10.

73. Roth M, Gurney C, Garside RF, Kerr TA. Studies in the classification of affective disorders. The relationship between anxiety states and depressive illness. I. Br J Psychiatry 1972; 121: 147–61.

74. Prusoff B, Klerman G. Differentiating depressed from anxious neurotic outpatients. Arch Gen Psychiatry 1974; 30: 302–8.

75. Derogatis LR, Lipman RS, Covi L, Rickels K. Factorial invariance of symptom dimensions in anxious and depressive neuroses. Arch Gen Psychiatry 1972; 27: 659–65.

76. Darwin C. The expression of the emotions in man and animals. New York: D. Appleton and Co., 1890 (1st published, 1872): 178.

77. Mellinger GD, Balter MB, Manheimer DI, Cisin IH, Perry HJ. Psychic distress, life crisis, and use of psychotherapeutic medications. National household survey data. Arch Gen Psychiatry 1978; 35: 1045–52.

78. Overall JE, Hollister LE, Johnson M, Pennington V. Nosology of depression and differential response to drugs. JAMA 1966; 195: 946–8.

79. Lipman RS, Covi L, Rickels K, et al. Imipramine and chlordiazepoxide in depressive and anxiety disorders. I. Efficacy in depressed out-patients. Arch Gen Psychiatry 1986; 43: 68–77.

80. Breier A, Charney DS, Heninger GR. The diagnostic validity of anxiety disorders and their relationship to depressive illness. Am J Psychiatry 1985; 142: 787–97.

81. Stein MB, Uhde TW. Panic disorder and major depression. A tale of two syndromes. Psychiatr Clin North Am 1988; 11: 441–61.

82. Boyd JH, Burke JD, Jr, Gruenberg E, et al. Exclusion criteria of DSM-III. A study of co-occurrence of hierarchy-free syndromes. Arch Gen Psychiatry 1984; 41: 983–89.
83. Lesse S. The relationship of anxiety to depression. Am J Psychother 1982; 36: 332–49.
84. Schatzberg AF, Cole JO. Benzodiazepines in depressive disorders. Arch Gen Psychiatry 1978; 35: 1359–65.
85. Kahn RJ, McNair DM, Lipman RS, et al. Imipramine and chlordiazepoxide in depressive and anxiety disorders. II. Efficacy in anxious outpatients. Arch Gen Psychiatry 1986; 43: 79–85.
86. Tyrer P, Murphy S, Kingdon D, et al. The Nottingham study of neurotic disorder: comparison of drug and psychological treatments. Lancet 1988; 2: 235–40.
87. Modigh K. Antidepressant drugs in anxiety disorders. Acta Psychiatr Scand 1987; 76 (suppl 335): 57–71.
88. Krishnan KRR, France RD. Antidepressants in chronic pain syndromes. Am Fam Physician 1989; 39: 233–7.
89. France RD, Krishnan KRR: Psychotropic drugs in chronic pain. In: France RD, Krishnan KRR, eds. Chronic pain. Washington, DC: American Psychiatric Press, Inc., 1988: 322–46.
90. Murphy DL, Zohar J, Benkelfat C, Pato MT, Pigott TA, Insel TR. Obsessive-compulsive disorder as a 5-HT subsystem-related behavioral disorder. Br J Psychiatry 1989; 155(suppl. 8): 15–24.
91. Baldessarini RJ. Current status of antidepressants: clinical pharmacology and therapy. J Clin Psychiatry 1989; 50: 117–26.
92. Akiskal HS. Dysthymic disorder: psychopathology of proposed chronic depressive subtypes. Am J Psychiatry 1983; 140: 11–20.
93. Paykel ES, Rowan PR, Parker RR, Bhat AV. Response to phenelzine and amitriptyline in subtypes of outpatient depression. Arch Gen Psychiatry 1982; 39: 1041–9.
94. Raskin A, Schulterbrandt JG, Reatig N, McKeon JJ. Differential response to chlorpromazine, imipramine, and placebo. Arch Gen Psychiatry 1970; 23: 164–73.
95. Morris JB, Beck AT. The efficacy of antidepressant drugs. Arch Gen Psychiatry 1974; 30: 667–74.
96. Georgotas A. Affective disorders: pharmacotherapy. In Kaplan HI, Sadock BJ, eds. Comprehensive textbook of psychiatry/IV, vol. I, 4th ed. Baltimore: Williams & Wilkins, 1985: 823.
97. Ref. 50: 37–38.
98. Papolos DF, Papolos J. Overcoming depression. New York: Harper & Row, Perennial Library, 1988 (first published, 1987): 139–52.
99. Quitkin F, Rifkin A, Klein DF. Prophylaxis of affective disorders. Current status of knowledge. Arch Gen Psychiatry 1976; 33: 337–41.

Chapter 10

1. Magraw RM. Ferment in medicine. A study of the essence of medical practice and of its new dilemmas. Philadelphia: W.B. Saunders Co., 1966: 17–18.
2. Castelnuovo-Tedesco P. The twenty-minute hour. A guide to brief psychotherapy for the physician. Boston: Little, Brown and Co., 1965.
3. Blanchard LB, Kurtz B. The social worker in a family practice setting. Primary care 1978; 5: 173–80.

Chapter 11

1. Arnold MB. Emotion and personality. Vol. 1. Psychological aspects. New York: Columbia University Press, 1960: 170–177.
2. Cannon WB. The James-Lange theory of emotions: A critical examination and an alternative theory. Am J Psychol 1927; 39: 106–24. See also ref. 43.
3. Darwin C. The expression of the emotions in man and animals. New York: D. Appleton & Co., 1913 (1st published, 1872).
4. Ekman P, ed. Darwin and facial expression. A century of research in review. New York: Academic Press, 1973.
5. MacLean PD. Psychosomatic disease and the "visceral brain." Recent developments bearing on the Papez theory of emotion. Psychosom Med 1949; 11: 338–53.
6. MacLean PD. Studies on limbic system ("visceral brain") and their bearing on psychosomatic problems. In Wittkower ED, Cleghorn RA, eds. Recent developments in psychosomatic medicine. Philadelphia, Lippincott, 1954: 101–25.
7. MacLean PD. The limbic system with respect to self-preservation and the preservation of the species. J Nerv Ment Dis 1958; 127: 1–11.
8. MacLean PD. Sensory and perceptive factors in emotional functions of the triune brain. In: Levi L, ed. Emotions. Their parameters and measurement. New York: Raven Press, 1975: 71–92.
9. Papez JW. A proposed mechanism of emotion. Arch Neurol and Psychiat (now Arch Neurol) 1937; 38: 725–43.
10. Livingston RB. Some brain stem mechanisms relating to psychosomatic functions. Psychosom Med 1955; 17: 347–54.
11. Hess WR. The functional organization of the diencephalon. New York: Grune & Stratton, 1957.
12. Arnold MB. Emotion and personality. Vol. 2. Neurological and physiological aspects. New York: Columbia University Press, 1960: 3–132.
13. Lindsley DB. The role of nonspecific reticulo-thalamo-cortical systems in emotion. In: Black P, ed. Physiological correlates of emotion. New York: Academic Press, 1970: 147–88.
14. Redmond DE, Jr. New and old evidence for the involvement of a brain norepinephrine system in anxiety. In: Fann WE, Karacan I, Porkorny AD, Williams RL, eds. Phenomenology and treatment of anxiety. New York: Spectrum Publications, 1979: 153–203.
15. Ballenger JC. Toward an integrated model of panic disorder. Am J Orthopsychiatry 1989; 59: 284–93.
16. Hsiao JK, Potter WZ. Mechanisms of action of antipanic drugs. In: Ballenger JC, ed. Clinical aspects of panic disorder. New York: Wiley-Liss, 1990: 297–317.
17. Kelly GA. The psychology of personal constructs. Vol. 1, A theory of personality. Vol. 2, Clinical diagnosis and psychotherapy. New York: Norton, 1955.
18. Frank JD. Persuasion and healing. A comparative study of psychotherapy. New York: Schocken Books, 1963 (1st published, 1961).
19. Ellis A. Humanistic psychotherapy. The rational-emotive approach. New York: McGraw-Hill Book Co., 1974 (1st published, 1973).
20. Beck AT. Cognitive therapy and emotional disorders. New York: New American Library, 1979.

21. Burns DD. Feeling good. The new mood therapy. New York: William Morrow and Co., Inc., 1980.

22. Brooks, CVW. Sensory awareness. Rediscovery of experiencing through the workshops of Charlotte Selver. 3rd ed. New York: Felix Morrow, 1986 (first published 1974).

23. Lazarus RS, Averill VR, Opton EM, Jr. Towards a cognitive theory of emotion. In: Arnold MB, ed. Feelings and emotions. New York: Academic Press, 1970: 190–205.

24. Leeper RW. A motivational theory of emotion to replace "emotion as a disorganized response." Psychol Rev 1948; 55: 5–21. See also ref. 43.

25. Hilgard ER. Divided consciousness: Multiple controls in human thought and action. New York: John Wiley & Sons, 1977: 185–256.

26. Aristotle. De Anima. Translated by Smith JA. In: Ross WD, ed. The works of Aristotle. Vol. III. London: Oxford University Press, 1931: 402b.

27. Breuer J, Freud S. Studies in hysteria. New York: Nervous and Mental Disease Pub. Co., 1936 (1st published, 1895).

28. Levy J, Trevarthen C, Sperry RW. Perception of bilateral chimeric figures following hemispheric deconnexion. Brain 1972; 95: 61–78.

29. Sperry RW. Hemisphere deconnection and unity in conscious awareness. Am Psychol 1968; 23: 723–33.

30. Bogen JE. The other side of the brain I: dysgraphia and dyscopia following cerebral commissurotomy. Bull Los Angeles Neurol Soc 1969; 34: 73–105.

31. Bogen JE. The other side of the brain II: an oppositional mind. Bull Los Angeles Neurol Soc 1969; 34: 135–62.

32. Bogen JE, Bogen GM. The other side of the brain III: the corpus callosum and creativity. Bull Los Angeles Neurol Soc 1969; 34: 191–220.

33. Bogen JE, DeZure R, Tenhouten WD, Marsh JF. The other side of the brain IV. The A/P ratio. Bull Los Angeles Neurol Soc 1972; 37: 49–61.

34. Galin D. Implications for psychiatry of left and right cerebral specialization. A neurophysiological context for unconscious processes. Arch Gen Psychiatry 1974; 31: 572–83.

35. Davidson RJ. Affect, repression, and cerebral asymmetry. In Temoshok L, Van Dyke C, Zegans LS, eds. Emotions in health and illness. Theoretical and research foundations. New York: Grune & Stratton, 1983: 123–35.

36. Beahrs JO. Unity and multiplicity. Multilevel consciousness of self in hypnosis, psychiatric disorder and mental health. New York: Brunner/Mazel, Publishers, 1982.

37. Miller A. The drama of the gifted child. How narcissistic parents form and deform the emotional lives of their talented children. New York: Basic Books, Inc., Publishers, 1981 (1st published, 1979).

38. Haronian F. The repression of the sublime. In Fadiman J. The proper study of man. Perspectives on the social sciences. New York: The Macmillan Co., 1971: 239–46.

39. Peters RS. Emotion, passivity and the place of Freud's theory in psychology. In: Wolman BB, Nagel E, eds. Scientific psychology: principles and approaches. New York: Basic Books, 1965: 365–83. See also ref. 43.

40. Frankl VE. Man's search for meaning: an introduction to logotherapy. New York: Washington Square Press, 1963.

41. Perls F, Hefferline RF, Goodman P. Gestalt therapy. Excitement and growth in the human personality. New York: Dell Pub. Co., Inc., 1951: 25–9.

42. Assagioli R. Psychosynthesis. A manual of principles and techniques. New York: The Viking Press, 1971 (1st published, 1965): 116–25.
43. Note: References 2, 24, and 39 are reprinted in Pribram KH, ed. Brain and behavior 4. Adaptation. Selected readings. Baltimore: Penguin Books, Inc., 1969.

Chapter 12

1. American Psychiatric Association: Diagnostic and statistical manual of mental disorders, third edition (DSM-III). Washington, DC: APA, 1980: 241–52.
2. Ibid., 8, 303–4.
3. American Psychiatric Association: Diagnostic and statistical manual of mental disorders, third edition, revised (DSM-III-R). Washington, DC: APA, 1987: 264–6.
4. Engel GL. "Psychogenic" pain and the pain-prone patient. Am J Med 1959; 26: 899–918.
5. Fordyce WE. Behavioral methods for chronic pain and illness. St. Louis: C.V. Mosby Co., 1976.
6. Ref. 3: 257–9.
7. Ref. 3: 261–4.
8. Ziegler FJ, Imboden JB, Meyer E. Contemporary conversion reactions: A clinical study. Am J Psychiatry 1960; 116: 901–10.
9. Selye H. Stress. Montreal: Acta, Inc., 1950: 688–707.
10. Alexander F. Psychosomatic medicine. Its principles and applications. New York: W.W. Norton, 1950: 39–44.
11. Walters A. Psychogenic regional pain alias hysterical pain. Brain 1961; 84: 1–18.
12. Szasz TS. The myth of mental illness. Foundations of a theory of personal conduct. New York: Dell Publishing Co., Inc., 1961.
13. Ziegler FS, Imboden JB. Contemporary conversion reactions. II. A conceptional model. Arch Gen Psychiatry 1962; 6: 279–87.
14. Chodoff P. The diagnosis of hysteria: An overview. Am J Psychiatry 1974; 131: 1073–8.
15. Sternbach RA. Pain patient traits and treatment. New York: Academic Press, 1974.
16. Hilgard ER. Divided consciousness: Multiple controls in human thought and action. New York: John Wiley & Sons, 1977.
17. Balint M. The doctor, his patient and the illness. Revised ed. New York: International Universities Press, Inc., 1972: 161.
18. Ref. 5: 32.
19. Purtell JJ, Robins E, Cohen ME. Observations on clinical aspects of hysteria. A quantitative study of 50 hysteria patients and 156 control subjects. JAMA 1951; 146: 902–9.
20. Perley MJ, Guze SB. Hysteria—the stability and usefulness of clinical criteria. A quantitative study based on a follow-up period of six to eight years in 39 patients. N Engl J Med 1962; 266: 421–6.
21. Woodruff RA, Clayton PJ, Guze SB. Hysteria. Studies of diagnosis, outcome, and prevalence. JAMA 1971; 215: 425–8.
22. Breuer J, Freud S. Studies in hysteria. New York: Nervous and Mental Disease Pub. Co., 1936 (1st. published, 1895): 97.
23. Munro A. Two cases of delusions of worm infestation. Am J Psychiatry 1978; 135: 234–5.

Chapter 13

1. Billings RF. Psychological aspects of chest pain. Chest pain related to emotional disorders. In Levene DL, Billings RF, Davies GM, Edmeads J, Saibil FG, eds. Chest pain: An integrated diagnostic approach. Philadelphia: Lea & Febiger, 1977: 16–21, 133–49.

2. Kroenke K, Mangelsdorff D. Common symptoms in ambulatory care: incidence, evaluation, therapy, and outcome. Am J Med 1989; 86: 262–6.

3. Sox HC, Jr. The emergency department evaluation of chest pain. In Wolcott BW, Rund DA, eds. Emergency Medicine Annual. Vol. 1, 1982. Norwalk, CT: Appleton-Century-Crofts: 43–60.

4. Christie LG, Conti CR. Systematic approach to evaluation of angina-like chest pain: pathophysiology and clinical testing with emphasis on objective documentation of myocardial ischemia. Am Heart J 1981; 102: 897–912.

5. Walters A. Psychogenic regional pain alias hysterical pain. Brain 1961; 84: 1–18.

6. Wood P. Da Costa's syndrome (or effort syndrome). Br Med J 1941; 1: 767–72.

7. Cohen ME, White PD. Life situations, emotions, and neurocirculatory asthenia (anxiety neurosis, neurasthenia, effort syndrome). Psychosom Med 1951; 13: 335–57.

8. Singer EP. The hyperventilation syndrome in clinical medicine. NY State J Med 1958; 58: 1494–1500.

9. Evans DW, Lum LC. Hyperventilation: an important cause of pseudoangina. Lancet 1977; 1: 155–7.

10. Channer KS, James MA, Papouchado M, Rees JR. Anxiety and depression in patients with chest pain referred for exercise testing. Lancet 1985; 2: 820–3.

11. Bass C, Wade C. Chest pain with normal coronary arteries: a comparative study of psychiatric and social morbidity. Psychol Med 1984; 14: 51–61.

12. Katon W, Hall ML, Russo J. Chest pain: relationship of psychiatric illness to coronary arteriographic results. Am J Med 1988; 84: 1–9.

13. Cormier LE, Katon W, Russo J, Hollifield M, Hall ML, Vitaliano PP. Chest pain with negative cardiac diagnostic studies. Relationship to psychiatric illness. J Nerv Ment Dis 1988; 176: 351–8.

14. Dunnell K, Cartwright A. Medicine takers, prescribers, and hoarders. London: Routledge and Kegan Paul, 1972: 11.

15. Levene DL, Billings RF, Davies GM, Edmeads J, Saibil FG, eds. Chest pain: An integrated diagnostic approach. Philadelphia: Lea & Febiger, 1977.

16. Likoff W, Segal BL, Kasparian H. Paradox of normal selective coronary arteriograms in patients considered to have unmistakable coronary heart disease. N Engl J Med 1967; 276: 1063–6.

17. Waxler EB, Kimbiris D, Dreifus LS. The fate of women with normal coronary arteriograms and chest pain resembling angina pectoris. Am J Cardiol 1971; 28: 25–32.

18. Kemp HG, Vokonas PS, et al. The anginal syndrome associated with normal coronary arteriograms. Report of a six year experience. Am J Med 1973; 54: 735–42.

19. Ockene IS, Shay MJ, Alpert JS, Weiner BH, Dalen JE. Unexplained chest pain in patients with normal coronary arteriograms. A follow-up study of functional status. N Engl J Med 1980; 303: 1249–52.

20. Weiner DA, Ryan TJ, McCabe CH. Exercise stress testing. Correlations among history of angina, ST-segment response and prevalence of coronary-artery disease in the coronary artery surgery study (CASS). N Engl J Med 1979; 301: 230–5.

21. Rutherford JD, Braunwald E, Cohn PF. Chronic ischemic heart disease. In Braunwald

E., ed. Heart disease. A textbook of cardiovascular medicine. 3rd ed. Philadelphia: W.B. Saunders Co., 1988: Vol. 2: 1323. See also Beleslin BD, Ostojic M, et al. Stress echocardiography in the detection of myocardial ischemia. Head-to-head comparison of exercise, dobutamine, and dipyridamole tests. Circulation 1994; 90:1168–76.

22. Diamond GA, Forrester JS. Analysis of probability as an aid in the clinical diagnosis of coronary-artery disease. N Engl J Med 1979; 300: 1350–8.

23. Kemp HG, Elliott WC, Gorlin R. The anginal syndrome with normal coronary arteriography. Trans Assoc Am Physicians 1967; 80: 59–70.

24. Proudfit WL, Shirey EK, Sones FM, Jr. Selective cine coronary arteriography. Correlation with clinical findings in 1000 patients. Circulation 1966; 33: 901–10.

25. Wielgosz AT, Fletcher RH, McCants CB, McKinnis RA, Haney TL, Williams RB. Unimproved chest pain in patients with minimal or no coronary disease: a behavioral phenomenon. Am Heart J 1984; 108: 67–72.

26. McLaurin LP, Raft D, Tate S, Harrell L. Chest pain with normal coronaries—a psychosomatic illness? Circulation 1977; 55–56 Abstracts: Supp III-174.

27. Bass C, Wade C, et al. Unexplained breathlessness and psychiatric morbidity in patients with normal and abnormal coronary arteries. Lancet 1983; 1: 605–9.

28. Beitman BD, Basha I, Flaker G, et al. Atypical or nonanginal chest pain. Panic disorder or coronary artery disease? Arch Intern Med 1987; 147: 1548–52.

29. Wulsin LR, Hillard JR, Geier P, Hissa D, Rouan GW. Screening emergency room patients with atypical chest pain for depression and panic disorder. Int J Psychiatry Med 1988; 18: 315–23.

30. Katz PO, Dalton CB, Richter JE, Wallace CW, Castell DO. Esophageal testing of patients with noncardiac chest pain or dysphagia. Results of three years' experience with 1161 patients. Ann Intern Med 1987; 106: 593–7.

31. DeMeester TR, O'Sullivan GC, Bermudez G, Midell AI, Cimochowski GE, O'Drobinak J. Esophageal function in patients with angina-type chest pain and normal coronary angiograms. Ann Surg 1982; 196: 488–98.

32. de Caestecker JS, Brown J, Blackwell JN, Heading RC. The oesophagus as a cause of recurrent chest pain: which patients should be investigated and which tests should be used? Lancet 1985; 2: 1143–6.

33. Rapaport E. Angina and oesophageal pain. Eur Heart J 1986; 7: 824–7.

34. Vantrappen G, Janssens J. Angina and oesophageal pain—a gastroenterologist's point of view. Eur Heart J 1986; 7: 828–34.

35. Richter JE, Bradley LA, Castell DO. Esophageal chest pain: current controversies in pathogenesis, diagnosis, and therapy. Ann Intern Med 1989; 110: 66–78.

36. Clouse RE, Lustman PJ. Psychiatric illness and contraction abnormalities of the esophagus. N Engl J Med 1983; 309: 1337–83.

37. Schuster MM. Esophageal spasm and psychiatric disorder. N Engl J Med 1983; 309: 1382–3.

38. Greenberg MA, Grose RM, Neuburger N, Silverman R, Strain JE, Cohen MV. Impaired coronary vasodilator responsiveness as a cause of lactate production during pacing-induced ischemia in patients with angina pectoris and normal coronary arteries. J Am Coll Cardiol 1987; 9: 743–51.

39. Opherk D, Zebe H, Weihe E, et al. Reduced coronary dilatory capacity and ultrastructural changes of the myocardium in patients with angina pectoris but normal coronary arteriograms. Circulation 1981; 63: 817–25.

40. Cannon RO, III, Leon MB, Watson RM, Rosing DR, Epstein SE. Chest pain and "nor-

mal" coronary arteries—role of small coronary arteries. Am J Cardiol 1985; 55: 50B–60B.

41. Bemiller CR, Pepine CJ, Rogers AK. Long-term observations in patients with angina and normal coronary arteriograms. Circulation 1973; 47: 36–43.

42. Cannon RO, III, Watson RM, Rosing DR, Epstein SE. Angina caused by reduced vasodilator reserve of the small coronary arteries. J Am Coll Cardiol 1983; 1: 1359–73.

43. James TN. Editorial. Angina without coronary disease (sic). Circulation 1970; 42: 189–91.

44. Richardson PJ, Livesley B, Oram S. Angina pectoris with normal coronary arteries. Transvenous myocardial biopsy in diagnosis. Lancet 1974; 2: 677–80.

45. Cannon RO, III, Bonow RO, Bacharach SL, et al. Left ventricular dysfunction in patients with angina pectoris, normal epicardial coronary arteries, and abnormal vasodilator reserve. Circulation 1985; 71: 218–26.

46. Cannon RO, III. Angina pectoris with normal coronary arteriograms. Cardiology Clinics 1991; 9: 157–66.

47. Ducrotte P, Berland J, Denis P, et al. Coronary sinus lactate estimation and esophageal motor anomalies in angina with normal coronary angiogram. Dig Dis Sc 1984; 29: 305–10.

48. Cannon RO, III, Cattau EL, Jr, Yakshe PN, et al. Coronary flow reserve, esophageal motility, and chest pain in patients with angiographically normal coronary arteries. Am J Med 1990; 88: 217–22.

49. Roy-Byrne PP, Schmidt P, Cannon RO, Diem H, Rubinow DR. Microvascular angina and panic disorder. Int J Psychiatry Med 1989; 19: 315–25.

50. Sax FL, Cannon RO, III, Hanson C, Epstein SE. Impaired forearm vasodilator reserve in patients with microvascular angina. Evidence of a generalized disorder of vascular function? N Engl J Med 1987; 317: 1366–70.

51. Cannon RO, III, Peden DP, Berkebile C, Schenke WH, Kaliner MA, Epstein SE. Airway hyperresponsiveness in patients with microvascular angina. Evidence for a diffuse disorder of smooth muscle responsiveness. Circulation 1990; 82: 2011–7.

52. Demeter SL, Cordasco EM. Hyperventilation syndrome and asthma. Am J Med 1986; 81: 989–94.

53. Epstein SE, Gerber LH, Borer JS. Chest wall syndrome. A common cause of unexplained cardiac pain. JAMA 1979; 241: 2793–7.

54. Peyton FW. Unexpected frequency of idiopathic costochondral pain. Obstet Gynecol 1983; 62: 605–8.

55. Tietze A. Ueber eine eigen artige haufung von follen mit dystrophie der rippenknorpel. Berliner Klinische Wochenschrift 1921; 58: 829–31.

56. Kayser HL. Tietze's syndrome. A review of the literature. Am J Med 1956; 21: 982–9.

57. Prinzmetal M, Massumi RA. The anterior chest wall syndrome—chest pain resembling pain of cardiac origin. JAMA 1955; 159: 177–84.

58. Katon WJ. Chest pain, cardiac disease, and panic disorder. J Clin Psychiatry 1990; 51: 5(Suppl): 27–30.

59. Ballenger JC. Pharmacotherapy of the panic disorders. J Clin Psychiatry 1986; 47: 6(Suppl): 27–32.

60. Beitman BD, Basha IM, Trombka LH, et al. Pharmacotherapeutic treatment of panic disorder in patients presenting with chest pain. J Fam Pract 1989; 28: 177–80.

61. Blacklock SM. The symptom of chest pain in family practice. J Fam Pract 1977; 4: 429–33.

62. Asnes RS, Santulli R, Bemporad JR. Psychogenic chest pain in children. Clin Pediatr 1981; 20: 788–91.
63. Bass C, Wade C, Hand D, Jackson G. Patients with angina with normal or near normal coronary arteries; clinical and psychosocial state 12 months after angiography. Br Med J 1983; 287: 1505–8.
64. Pasternak RC, Thibault GE, Savoia M, DeSanctis RW, Hutter AM, Jr. Chest pain with angiographically insignificant coronary arterial obstruction. Clinical presentation and long term follow-up. Am J Med 1980; 68: 813–17.
65. Proudfit WL, Bruschke AGV, Sones FM, Jr. Clinical course of patients with normal or slightly or moderately abnormal coronary arteriograms: 10-year follow-up of 521 patients. Circulation 1980; 62: 712–7.
66. Isner JM, Salem DN, Banas JS, Jr, Levine, HJ. Long term clinical course of patients with normal coronary arteriography: follow-up study of 121 patients with normal or nearly normal coronary arteriograms. Am Heart J 1981; 102: 645–53.
67. Lantinga LJ, Sprafkin RP, McCroskery JH, Baker MT, Warner RA, Hill NE. One-year psychosocial follow-up of patients with chest pain and angiographically normal coronary arteries. Am J Cardiol 1988; 62: 209–13.
68. Katon W. Panic disorder and somatization. Review of 55 cases. Am J Med 1984; 77: 101–6.
69. Apley J, Naish N. Recurrent abdominal pains: a field survey of 1,000 school children. Arch Dis Child 1958; 33: 165–70.
70. Thompson WG, Heaton KW. Functional bowel disorders in apparently healthy people. Gastroenterology 1980; 79: 283–8.
71. Stone RT, Barbero GJ. Recurrent abdominal pain in childhood. Pediatrics 1970; 45: 732–8.
72. Gomez J, Dally P. Psychologically mediated abdominal pain in surgical and medical outpatient clinics. Br Med J 1977; 1: 1451–3.
73. Dodge JA. Recurrent abdominal pain in children. Br Med J 1976; 1: 385–7.
74. Drossman DA. Patients with psychogenic abdominal pain: six years' observation in the medical setting. Am J Psychiatry 1982; 139: 1549–57.
75. Chaudhary NA, Truelove SC. The irritable colon syndrome. A study of the clinical features, predisposing causes, and prognosis in 130 cases. QJ Med 1962; new series 31: 307–22.
76. Kirsner JB. Clinical challenge of functional gastrointestinal disorders. Postgrad Med 1966; 39: 565–75.
77. Thompson WG. The irritable gut. Functional disorders of the alimentary canal. Baltimore: University Park Press, 1979.
78. Lennard-Jones JE. Current concepts. Functional gastrointestinal disorders. N Engl J Med 1983; 308: 431–6.
79. Drossman DA. The physician and the patient. Review of the psychosocial gastrointestinal literature with an integrated approach to the patient. In Sleisenger MH, Fordtran JS, eds. Gastrointestinal disease. Pathophysiology, diagnosis, management. 4th. ed., Vol. 1. Philadelphia: W.B. Saunders Co., 1989: 3–20.
80. Schuster MM. Irritable bowel syndrome. In Sleisenger MH, Fordtran JS, eds. Gastrointestinal disease. 4th. ed., Vol. 2. Philadelphia: W.B. Saunders Co., 1989: 1402–18.
81. Drossman DA, McKee DC, Sandler RS, et al. Psychosocial factors in the irritable bowel syndrome. A multivariate study of patients and nonpatients with irritable bowel syndrome. Gastroenterology 1988; 95: 701–8.

82. Whitehead WE, Bosmajian L, Zonderman AB, Costa PT, Jr, Schuster MM. Symptoms of psychologic distress associated with irritable bowel syndrome. Comparison of community and medical clinic samples. Gastroenterology 1988; 95: 709–14.

83. Stoeckle JD, Zola IK, Davidson GE. The quantity and significance of psychological distress in medical patients. Some preliminary observations about the decision to seek medical aid. J Chronic Dis 1964; 17: 959–70.

84. Dunnell K, Cartwright A. Medicine takers, prescribers, and hoarders. London: Routledge and Kegan Paul, 1972: 6.

85. Ref. 77: 27–39.

86. Jones VA, Shorthouse M, McLaughlan P, Workman E, Hunter JO. Food intolerance: a major factor in the pathogenesis of irritable bowel syndrome. Lancet 1982; 2: 1115–7.

87. Heyman MB. Food sensitivity and eosinophilic gastroenteropathies. In Sleisenger MH, Fordtran JS, eds. Gastrointestinal disease. 4th. ed., Vol. 2. Philadelphia: W.B. Saunders Co., 1989: 1119–1122.

88. Methods for diagnosis of adverse reactions to foods. In: Adverse reactions to foods. American Academy of Allergy and Immunology Committee on Adverse Reactions to Foods. National Institute of Allergy and Infectious Diseases. U.S. Department of Health and Human Services. Public Health Service. National Institutes of Health. NIH Publication No. 84-2442, 1984: 123–60.

89. Ref. 77: 153–63.

90. Adami H-O, Agenas I, Gustavsson S, et al. The clinical diagnosis of gastritis: Aspects of demographic epidemiology and health care consumption based on a nationwide sample survey. Scand J Gastroenterol 1984; 19: 755–60.

91. Nyren O, Adami H-O, Bates S, et al. Absence of therapeutic benefit from antacids or cimetidine in non-ulcer dyspepsia. N Engl J Med 1986; 314: 339–43.

92. Peterson WL. Helicobacter pylori and peptic ulcer disease. N Engl J Med 1991; 324: 1043–8.

93. Van Dyke JA, Stanley RJ, Berland LL. Pancreatic imaging. Ann Intern Med 1985; 102: 212–217.

94. Grendell JH, Cello JP. Chronic pancreatitis. In Sleisenger MH, Fordtran JS., eds. Gastrointestinal disease. 4th. ed., Vol. 2. Philadelphia: W.B. Saunders Co., 1989: 1842–72.

95. Kruis W, Thieme CH, Weinzierl M, Schussler P, Holl J, Paulus W. A diagnostic score for the irritable bowel syndrome. Its value in the exclusion of organic disease. Gastroenterology 1984; 87: 1–7.

96. Manning AP, Thompson WG, Heaton KW, Morris AF. Towards positive diagnosis of the irritable bowel. Br Med J 1978; 2: 653–4.

97. Talley NJ, Phillips SF, Melton J, Wiltgen C, Zinsmeister AR. A patient questionnaire to identify bowel disease. Ann Intern Med 1989; 111: 671–4.

98. Drossman DA. A questionnaire for functional bowel disorders. Ann Intern Med 1989; 111: 627–9.

99. Thompson WG, Patel DG, Tao H, Nair RC. Does uncomplicated diverticular disease produce symptoms? Dig Dis Sci 1982; 27: 605–8.

100. Mussey RD, Wilson RB. Pelvic pain. A follow-up study. Am J Obstet Gynecol 1941; 42: 759–67.

101. Lock FR, Donnelly J. The incidence of psychosomatic disease from a private referred gynecologic practice. Am J Obstet Gynecol 1947; 54: 783–90.

102. Cohen ME, Robins E, Purtell JJ, Altmann MW. Excessive surgery in hysteria. Study

of surgical procedures in 50 women with hysteria and 190 controls. JAMA 1953; 151: 977–86.

103. Taylor HC, Jr. Vascular congestion and hyperemia. Their effect on structure and function in the female reproductive system. Am J Obstet Gynecol 1949; 57: 211–230, 637–53, 654–68.

104. Gidro-Frank L, Gordon T, Taylor HC, Jr. Pelvic pain and female identity. A survey of emotional factors in 40 patients. Am J Obstet Gynecol 1960; 79: 1184–1202.

105. Lundberg WI, Wall JE, Mathers JE. Laparoscopy in evaluation of pelvic pain. Obstet Gynecol 1973; 42: 872–6.

106. Castelnuovo-Tedesco P, Krout BM. Psychosomatic aspects of chronic pelvic pain. Psychiatry In Medicine (now Int J Psychiatry Med) 1970; 1: 109–26.

107. Levitan Z, Eibschitz I, de Vries K, Hakim M, Sharf M. The value of laparoscopy in women with chronic pelvic pain and a "normal pelvis." Int J Gynecol Obstet 1985; 23: 71–74.

108. Liston WA, Bradford WP, Downie J, Kerr MG. Laparoscopy in a general gynecologic unit. Am J Obstet Gynecol 1972; 113: 672–77.

109. Benson RC, Hanson KH, Matarazzo JD. Atypical pelvic pain in women: gynecologic-psychiatric considerations. Am J Obstet Gynecol 1959; 77: 806–25.

110. Beard RW, Belsey EM, Lieberman BA, Wilkinson JCM. Pelvic pain in women. Am J Obstet Gynecol 1977; 128: 566–70.

111. Gross RJ, Doerr H, Caldirola D, Guzinski G, Ripley HS. Borderline syndrome and incest in chronic pain patients. Int J Psychiatry Med 1980/81; 10: 79–86.

112. Renaer M. Chronic pelvic pain without obvious pathology in women. Personal observations and a review of the problems. Eur J Obstet Gynecol Reprod Biol 1980; 10: 415–63.

113. Pearce S, Knight C, Beard RW. Pelvic pain—a common gynecological problem. J Psychosom Obstet Gynaecol 1982; 1: 12–7.

114. Peters AAW, van Dorst E, Jellis B, van Zuuren E, Hermans J, Trimbos JB. A randomized clinical trial to compare two different approaches to women with chronic pelvic pain. Obstet Gynecol 1991; 77: 740–4.

115. Hirsch C, Jonsson B, Lewin T. Low-back symptoms in a Swedish female population. Clin Orthop 1969; 63: 171–176.

116. Hult L. The Munkfors investigation. Acta Orthop Scand, Suppl 16, 1954: 39.

117. Hult L. Cervical, dorsal and lumbar spinal syndromes. Acta Orthop Scand, Suppl 17, 1955: 38.

118. Coxhead CE, Meade TW, Inskip H, North WRS, Troup JDG. Multicentre trial of physiotherapy in the management of sciatic symptoms. Lancet 1981; 1: 1065–8.

119. Dillane JB, Fry J, Kalton G. Acute back syndrome—a study from general practice. Br Med J 1966; 2: 82–84.

120. Horal J. The clinical appearance of low back disorders in the city of Gothenberg, Sweden. Comparisons of incapacitated probands with matched controls. Acta Orthop Scand, Suppl 118, 1969: 61–2.

121. Wood KM. New approaches to treatment of back pain. West J Med 1979; 130: 394–8.

122. Williams ME, Hadler NM. The illness as the focus of geriatric medicine. N Engl J Med 1983; 308: 1357–60.

123. Weinreb JC, Wolbarsht LB, Cohen JM, Brown CEL, Maravilla KR. Prevalence of lumbosacral intervertebral disk abnormalities on MR images in pregnant and asymptomatic nonpregnant women. Radiology 1989; 170: 125–8.

124. Wiesel SW, Tsourmas N, Feffer HL, Citrin CM, Patronas N. A study of computer-assisted tomography. I. The incidence of positive CAT scans in an asymptomatic group of patients. Spine 1984; 9: 549–51.

125. Splithoff CA. Lumbosacral junction. Roentgenographic comparison of patients with and without backaches. JAMA 1953; 152: 1610–3.

126. Hussar AE, Guller EJ. Correlations of pain and the roentgenographic findings of spondylosis of the cervical and lumbar spine. Am J Med Sci 1956; 232: 518–27.

127. Fullenlove TM, Williams AJ. Comparative roentgen findings in symptomatic and asymptomatic backs. Radiology 1957; 68: 572–4.

128. Torgerson WR, Dotter WE. Comparative roentgenographic study of the asymptomatic and symptomatic lumbar spine. J Bone Joint Surg 1976; 58-A: 850–3.

129. Magora A, Schwartz A. Relation between the low back pain syndrome and x-ray findings. I. Degenerative osteoarthritis. Scand J Rehabil Med 1976; 8: 115–125.

130. Magora A, Schwartz A. Relation between low back pain and x-ray changes. 4. Lysis and olisthesis. Scand J Rehabil Med 1980; 12: 47–52.

131. Nachemson AL. The lumbar spine. An orthopaedic challenge. Spine 1976; 1: 59–71.

132. Deyo RA, Bigos SJ, Maravilla KR. Diagnostic imaging procedures for the lumbar spine. Ann Intern Med 1989; 111: 865–7.

133. Finneson BE. Low back pain, 2nd ed. Philadelphia: J.B. Lippincott Co., 1980: 320–7.

134. Ref. 116: 40.

135. Fernbach JC, Langer F, Gross AE. The significance of low back pain in older adults. Can Med Assoc J 1976; 115: 898–900.

136. Schutte HE, Park WM. The diagnostic value of bone scintigraphy in patients with low .back pain. Skeletal Radiol 1983; 10: 1–4.

137. Deyo RA, Diehl AK. Cancer as a cause of back pain: frequency, clinical presentation, and diagnostic strategies. J Gen Intern Med 1988; 3: 230–8.

138. Calin A, Kaye B, Sternberg M, Antell B, Chan M. The prevalence and nature of back pain in an industrial complex. A questionnaire and radiographic and HLA analysis. Spine 1980; 5: 201–5.

139. Blackburn WD, Alarcon GS, Bull GV. Evaluation of patients with back pain of suspected inflammatory nature. Am J Med 1988; 85: 766–70.

140. McKenzie R. Treat your own back. 4th ed. Waikanae, New Zealand: Spinal Publications Ltd., 1988: 1.

141. Ref. 133: the whole book.

142. Cailliet R. Low back pain syndrome. Edition 4. Philadelphia: F.A. Davis Co., 1988.

143. Ref. 140: the whole book.

144. Cailliet R. Understand your backache. A guide to prevention, treatment, and relief. Philadelphia: F.A. Davis Co., 1984.

145. Lagerwerff EB, Perlroth KA. Mensendieck your posture and your pains. Garden City: Anchor Press/Doubleday, 1973.

146. Ref. 133: 179.

147. Sarno J. Mind over back pain. A radically new approach to the diagnosis and treatment of back pain. New York: William Morrow and Co., Inc., 1984.

148. Norrelund N, Hollnagel H. Fatigue among 40-year-olds. Ugeskr Laeger 1979; 141: 1425–9.

149. Buchwald D, Sullivan JL, Komaroff AL. Frequency of chronic active Epstein-Barr virus infection in a general medical practice. JAMA 1987; 257: 2303–7.

150. Kroenke K, Wood DR, Mangelsdorff AD, Meier NJ, Powell JB. Chronic fatigue in

primary care. Prevalence, patient characteristics, and outcome. JAMA 1988; 260: 929–34.

151. Allan FK. The differential diagnosis of weakness and fatigue. N Engl J Med 1944; 231: 414–8.

152. Allan FK. The clinical management of weakness and fatigue. JAMA 1945; 127: 957–60.

153. American Psychiatric Association: Diagnostic and statistical manual of mental disorders, third edition, revised (DSM-III-R). Washington, DC: APA, 1987: 219.

154. Katon W, Kleinman A, Rosen G. Depression and somatization: A review. Am J Med 1982; 72: Part I, 127–35; Part II, 241–7.

155. Lane TJ, Manu P, Matthews DA. Depression and somatization in the chronic fatigue syndrome. Am J Med 1991; 91: 335–44.

156. Rockwell DA, Burr BD. The tired patient. J Fam Pract 1977; 5: 853–7.

157. Morrison JD. Fatigue as a presenting complaint in family practice. J Fam Pract 1980; 10; 795–801.

158. Jerrett WA. Lethargy in general practice. Practitioner 1981; 225: 731–7.

159. Sugarman JR, Berg AO. Evaluation of fatigue in a family practice. J Fam Pract 1984; 19: 643–7.

160. Solberg LI. Lassitude. A primary care evaluation. JAMA 1984; 251: 3272–6.

161. Lane TJ, Matthews DA, Manu P. The low yield of physical examinations and laboratory investigations of patients with chronic fatigue. Am J Med Sci 1990; 299: 313–8.

162. Robinson JO. Symptoms and the discovery of high blood pressure. J Psychosom Res 1969; 13: 157–61.

163. Schooley RT. Chronic fatigue syndrome: a manifestation of Epstein-Barr virus infection? In: Remington JS, Swartz MN, eds. Current clinical topics in infectious diseases. Vol. 9. New York: McGraw-Hill Book Co., 1988: 126–46.

164. Holmes GP, Kaplan JE, Stewart JA, Hunt B, Pinsky PF, Schonberger LB. A cluster of patients with a chronic mononucleosis-like syndrome. Is Epstein-Barr virus the cause? JAMA 1987; 257: 2297–2302.

165. Holmes GP, Kaplan JE, Gantz NM, et al. Chronic fatigue syndrome: a working case definition. Ann Intern Med 1988; 108: 387–9.

166. Kruesi MJP, Dale J, Straus SE. Psychiatric diagnoses in patients who have chronic fatigue syndrome. J Clin Psychiatry 1989; 50: 53–6.

167. Buchwald D, Goldenberg DL, Sullivan JL, Komaroff AL. The "chronic, active Epstein-Barr virus infection" syndrome and primary fibromyalgia. Arthritis Rheum 1987; 30: 1132–6.

168. Wessely S, Powell R. Fatigue syndromes: a comparison of chronic "postviral" fatigue with neuromuscular and affective disorders. J Neurol Neurosurg Psychiatry 1989; 52: 940–8.

169. Imboden JB, Canter A, Leighton EC. Convalescence from influenza. A study of the psychological and clinical determinants. Arch Intern Med 1961; 108: 393–9.

170. Imboden JB. Psychosocial determinants of recovery. Adv Psychosom Med 1972; 8: 142–55.

171. Straus SE, Dale JK, Tobi M, et al. Acyclovir treatment of the chronic fatigue syndrome. Lack of efficacy in a placebo-controlled trial. N Engl J Med 1988; 319: 1692–8.

172. Steere AC, Schoen RT, Taylor E. The clinical evolution of Lyme arthritis. Ann Intern Med 1987; 107: 725–31.

173. Herzer P. Joint manifestations of Lyme borreliosis in Europe. Scand J Infec Dis 1991; Supplementum 77: 55–63.

174. Gamstorp I. Lyme borreliosis from a patient's view-point. Scand J Infect Dis 1991; Supplementum 77: 15–16.

175. Kristoferitsch W. Neurological manifestations of Lyme borreliosis: clinical definition and differential diagnosis. Scand J Infect Dis 1991; Supplementum 77: 64–73.

176. Halperin JJ. North American Lyme neuroborreliosis. Scand J Infec Dis 1991; Supplementum 77: 74–80.

177. Craft JE, Grodzicki RL, Steere AC. Antibody response in Lyme disease: evaluation of diagnostic tests. J Infect Dis 1984; 149: 789–95.

178. Rose CD, Fawcett PT, Singsen BH, Dubbs SB, Doughty RA. Use of Western blot and enzyme-linked immunosorbent assays to assist in the diagnosis of Lyme disease. Pediatrics 1991; 88: 465–70.

179. Hanrahan JP, Benach JL, Coleman JL, et al. Incidence and cumulative frequency of endemic Lyme disease in a community. J Infect Dis 1984; 150: 489–96.

180. Steere AC, Taylor E, Wilson ML, Levine JF, Spielman A. Longitudinal assessment of the clinical and epidemiological features of Lyme disease in a defined population. J Infect Dis 1986; 154: 295–300.

181. Fahrer H, Linden Svd, Sauvain M-J, et al. "Lyme Borreliosis": an epidemiologic study in a Swiss risk population. Arthritis Rheum 1987; 30: S50, abstract A73.

182. Sigal LH. Summary of the first 100 patients seen at a Lyme disease referral center. Am J Med 1990; 88: 577–81.

183. Steere AC. Lyme disease. N Engl J Med 1989; 321: 586–96.

184. Rahn DW, Malawista SE. Lyme disease: recommendations for diagnosis and treatment. Ann Intern Med 1991; 114: 472–81.

185. Graham W. The fibrositis syndrome. Bull Rheum Dis 1953; 3: 51–2.

186. Smythe HA. Non-articular rheumatism and the fibrositis syndrome. In Hollander JL, McCarty DJ, Jr, eds. Arthritis and allied conditions. 8th ed., Philadelphia: Lea & Febiger, 1972: 874–84.

187. Moldofsky H, Scarisbrick P, England R, Smythe H. Musculoskeletal symptoms and non-REM sleep disturbance in patients with "fibrositis syndrome" and healthy subjects. Psychosom Med 1975; 37: 341–51.

188. Yunus M, Masi AT, Calabro JJ, Miller KA, Feigenbaum SL. Primary fibromyalgia (fibrositis): clinical study of 50 patients with matched normal controls. Semin Arthritis Rheum 1981; 11: 151–71.

189. Campbell SM, Clark S, Tindall EA, Forehand ME, Bennett RM. Clinical characteristics of fibrositis. I. A "blinded," controlled study of symptoms and tender points. Arthritis Rheum 1983; 26: 817–24.

190. Wolfe F, Hawley DJ, Cathey MA, Caro X, Russell IJ. Fibrositis: symptom frequency and criteria for diagnosis. An evaluation of 291 rheumatic disease patients and 58 normal individuals. J Rheumatol 1985; 12: 1159–63.

191. Bennett RM. Fibrositis: misnomer for a common rheumatic disorder. West J Med 1981; 134: 405–13.

192. Wolfe F, Smythe HA, Yunus MB. The American College of Rheumatology 1990 criteria for the classification of fibromyalgia. Report of the Multicenter Criteria Committee. Arthritis Rheum 1990; 33: 160–72.

193. Hadler NM. A critical reappraisal of the fibrositis concept. Am J Med 1986; 81(3A): 26–30.

194. Buchwald D, Goldenberg DL, Sullivan JL, Komaroff AL. The "chronic, active Ep-

stein-Barr virus infection" syndrome and primary fibromyalgia. Arthritis Rheum 1987; 30: 1132−6.

195. Holmes GP, Kaplan JE, Gantz NM, et al. Chronic fatigue syndrome: A working case definition. Ann Intern Med 1988; 108: 387−9.

196. Smythe H. "Fibrositis" and other diffuse musculoskeletal syndromes. In Kelley WN, Harris ED, Jr, Ruddy S, Sledge CB. Textbook of rheumatology, vol. 1, 2nd ed. Philadelphia: W.B. Saunders Co., 1985: 484.

197. Vitali C, Tavoni A, Rossi B, et al. Evidence of neuromuscular hyperexcitability features in patients with primary fibromyalgia. Clinical Exp Rheumatol 1989; 7: 385−90.

198. Kraft GH, Johnson EW, LaBan MM. The fibrositis syndrome. Arch Phys Med Rehabil 1968; 49: 155−62.

199. Bengtsson A, Henriksson KG, Jorfeldt L, Kagedal B, Lennmarken C, Lindstrom F. Primary fibromyalgia. A clinical and laboratory study of 55 patients. Scand J Rheumatol 1986; 15: 340−7.

200. Arroyo P, Jr. Electromyography in the evaluation of reflex muscle spasm. Simplified method for direct evaluation of muscle-relaxant drugs. J Fla Med Assoc 1966; 53: 29−31.

201. Fricton JR, Auvinen MD, Dykstra D, Schiffman E. Myofascial pain syndrome: electromyographic changes associated with local twitch response. Arch Phys Med Rehabil 1985; 66: 314−7.

202. Elert JE, Dahlqvist SBR, Henriksson-Larsen K, Gerdle B. Increased EMG activity during short pauses in patients with primary fibromyalgia. Scand J Rheumatol 1989; 18: 321−3.

203. Ferraccioli G, Ghirelli L, Scita F, et al. EMG-biofeedback training in fibromyalgia syndrome. J Rheumatol 1987; 14: 820−5.

204. Holmes TH, Wolff HG. Life situations, emotions and backache. Psychosom Med 1952; 14: 18−33.

205. Campbell SM. Is the tender point concept valid? Am J Med 1986; 81(3A): 33−7.

206. Masi AT, Yunus MB. Concepts of illness in populations as applied to fibromyalgia syndromes. Am J Med 1986; 81(3A): 19−25.

207. Hauri P, Hawkins DR. Alpha-delta sleep. Electroencephalogr Clin Neurophysiol 1973; 34: 233−7.

208. Watson R, Liebmann K-O, Jenson J. Alpha-delta sleep: EEG characteristics, incidence, treatment, psychophysiological correlates and personality. Sleep Research 1985; 14: 226.

209. Moldofsky H. Sleep and musculoskeletal pain. Am J Med 1986; 81(3A): 85−9.

210. Halliday JL. The concept of psychosomatic rheumatism. Ann Intern Med 1941; 15: 666−77.

211. Ellman P, Savage OA, Wittkower E, Rodger TF. Fibrositis. A biographical study of fifty civilian and military cases, from the rheumatic unit, St. Stephen's Hospital (London County Council), and a military hospital. Ann Rheum Dis 1943; 3: 56−76.

212. Reynolds MD. Clinical diagnosis of psychogenic rheumatism. West J Med 1978; 128: 285−90.

213. Payne TC, Leavitt F, Gerron DC, et al. Fibrositis and psychological disturbance. Arthritis Rheum 1982; 25: 213−7.

214. Ahles TA, Yunus MB, Riley SD, Bradley JM, Masi AT. Psychological factors associated with primary fibromyalgia syndrome. Arthritis Rheum 1984; 27: 1101−6.

215. Wolfe F, Cathey MA, Kleinheksel SM, et al. Psychological status in primary fibrositis and fibrositis associated with rheumatoid arthritis. J Rheumatol 1984; 11: 500−6.

216. Hudson JI, Hudson MS, Pliner LF, Goldenberg DL, Pope HG, Jr. Fibromyalgia and major affective disorder: A controlled phenomenology and family history study. Am J Psychiatry 1985; 142: 441–5.

217. Clark S, Campbell SM, Forehand ME, Tindall EA, Bennett RM. Clinical characteristics of fibrositis II. A "blinded," controlled study using standard psychological tests. Arthritis Rheum 1985; 28: 132–7.

218. Bille B. Migraine in childhood and its prognosis. Cephalalgia 1981; 1: 71–5.

219. Sillanpaa M. Prevalence of headache in prepuberty. Headache 1983; 23: 10–14.

220. Diamond S, Medina J, Diamond-Falk J, DeVeno T. The value of biofeedback in the treatment of chronic headache: A five-year retrospective study. Headache 1979; 19: 90–96.

221. Ford MR, Stroebel CF, Strong P, Szarek BL. Quieting response training: long-term evaluation of a clinical biofeedback practice. Biofeedback Self Regul 1983; 8: 265–78.

222. Cutler RWP. Headache. In Rubenstein E, Federman DD, eds. New York: Scientific American, Inc. Scientific American medicine: 11, Neurology: XI Headache, 1–5, (1985).

223. Martin MJ. Muscle-contraction (tension) headache. Psychosomatics 1983; 24: 319–24.

224. Ziegler DK. Headache syndromes: problems of definition. Psychosomatics 1979; 20: 443–7.

225. Bakal DA. The psychobiology of chronic headache. New York: Springer Pub. Co., Inc., 1982.

226. Adler CS, Adler SM, Packard RC. Psychiatric aspects of headache. Baltimore: Williams & Wilkins, 1987.

227. Masland WS, Friedman AP, Buchsbaum HW. Computerized axial tomography of migraine. Res Clin Stud Headache 1978; 6: 136–40.

228. Larson EB, Omenn GS, Lewis H. Diagnostic evaluation of headache. Impact of computerized tomography and cost-effectiveness. JAMA 1980; 243: 359–62.

229. Deck M. Radiologic imaging procedures. In Wyngaarden JB, Smith LH Jr, Bennett JC, eds. Cecil textbook of medicine. 19th ed. Philadelphia: W.B. Saunders Co., 1992: 2038–40.

230. Solomon S, Cappa KG. The headache of temporal arteritis. J Am Geriatr Soc 1987; 35: 163–5.

231. Jaffee JH. Drug dependence: opioids, nonnarcotics, nicotine (tobacco), and caffeine. In: Kaplan HI, Sadock BJ, eds. Comprehensive textbook of psychiatry. 5th ed., vol. 1. Baltimore: Williams & Wilkins, 1989: 683–4.

232. The Boston Collaborative Drug Surveillance Program, Boston University Medical Center. Psychiatric side effects of nonpsychiatric drugs. Seminars in Psychiatry 1971; 3: 406–20.

233. The Boston Collaborative Drug Surveillance Program. Acute adverse reactions to prednisone in relation to dosage. Clin Pharmacol Ther 1972; 13: 694–8.

234. Ling MHM, Perry PJ, Tsuang MT. Side effects of corticosteroid therapy. Psychiatric aspects. Arch Gen Psychiatry 1981; 38: 471–7.

235. Bridges KW, Goldberg DP. Somatic presentation of DSM III psychiatric disorders in primary care. J Psychosom Res 1985; 29: 563–9.

236. Tunbridge WMG, Evered DG, Hall R, et al. The spectrum of thyroid disease in a community: The Whickham Survey. Clin Endocrinol 1977; 7: 481–93.

237. Starkman MN, Zelnik TC, Nesse RM, Cameron OG. Anxiety in patients with pheochromocytoma. Arch Intern Med 1985; 145: 248–52.

238. Hall RCW. Symptoms of anxiety. In: Hall RCW, ed. Psychiatric presentations of medical illness. Somatopsychic disorders. New York: Spectrum Publications, Inc., 1980: 26–9.
239. Doniach D, Hudson RV, Roitt IM. Human auto-immune thyroiditis: clinical studies. Br Med J 1960; 1: 365–73.
240. Reilly EL, Wilson WP. Mental symptoms in hyperparathyroidism (a report of three cases). Diseases of the Nervous System 1965; 26: 361–3.
241. Tunbridge WMG, Brewis M, French JM, et al. Natural history of autoimmune thyroiditis. Br Med J 1981; 282: 258–62.
242. Goudie RB, Anderson JR, Gray KG. Complement-fixing antithyroid antibodies in hospital patients with asymptomatic thyroid lesions. J Pathol and Bacteriol (now J Pathol) 1959; 77: 389–400.
243. Williams ED, Doniach I. The post mortem incidence of focal thyroiditis. J Pathol and Bacteriol (now J Pathol) 1962; 83: 255–64.
244. Boonstra CE, Jackson CE. Serum calcium survey for hyperparathyroidism: results in 50,000 clinic patients. Am J Clin Pathol 1971; 55: 523–6.
245. Boonstra CE, Jackson CE. Hyperparathyroidism detected by routine serum calcium analysis. Prevalence in a clinic population. Ann Int Med 1965; 63: 468–74.
246. Benson DF, Blumer D, eds. Psychiatric aspects of neurological disease. New York: Grune & Stratton, Inc., 1975: 137–217; Vol. 2, 1982: 25–91.
247. Frohlich ED, Tarazi RC, Dustan HP. Hyperdynamic beta-adrenergic circulatory state. Increased beta-receptor responsiveness. Arch Int Med 1969; 123: 1–7.
248. Kroenke K, Mangelsdorff D. Common symptoms in ambulatory care: incidence, evaluation, therapy, and outcome. Am J Med 1989; 86: 262–6.
249. Regier DA, Boyd JH, Burke JD Jr, et al. One-month prevalence of mental disorders in the United States based on five epidemiologic catchment area sites. Arch Gen Psychiatry 1988; 45: 977–86.
250. Coulehan JL, Zettler-Segal M, Block M, McClelland M, Schulberg HC. Recognition of alcoholism and substance abuse in primary care patients. Arch Int Med 1987; 147: 349–52.
251. Cleary PD, Miller M, Bush BT, Warburg MM, Delbanco TL, Aronson MD. Prevalence and recognition of alcohol abuse in a primary care population. Am J Med 1988; 85: 466–71.
252. Buchsbaum DG, Buchanan RG, Lawton MJ, Schnoll SH. Alcohol consumption patterns in a primary care population. Alcohol 1991; 26: 215–20.
253. Buchsbaum DG, Buchanan RG, Centor RM, Schnoll SH, Lawton MJ. Screening for alcohol abuse using CAGE scores and likelihood ratios. Ann Intern Med 1991; 115: 774–7.
254. Clark WD, McIntyre JR. The generalist and alcoholism: dilemmas and progress. In: Noble J, ed. Textbook of general medicine and primary care. Boston: Little, Brown and Co., 1987: 1619–44.
255. Beresford TP, Blow FC, Brower KJ, Singer K. Screening for alcoholism. Prev Med 1988; 17: 653–63.
256. Ewing JA. Detecting alcoholism. The CAGE questionnaire. JAMA 1984; 252: 1905–7.
257. Mattson RH. Value of intensive monitoring. In: Wade JA, Penry JK, eds. Advances in epileptology: The Tenth Epilepsy International Symposium. New York: Raven Press, 1980: 43–51.
258. Jeavons PM. Choice of drug therapy in epilepsy. Practitioner 1977; 219: 542–56.

259. Kapoor WN. Hypotension and syncope. In: Braunwald E, ed. Heart disease. A text-book of cardiovascular medicine. 4th ed., vol. 1. Philadelphia: W.B. Saunders Co., 1992: 875–86.

260. Riley TL, Roy A, eds. Pseudoseizures. Baltimore: Williams & Wilkins, 1982.

261. Gross M, ed. Pseudoepilepsy. The clinical aspects of false seizures. Lexington, MA: Lexington Books, D.C. Heath and Co., 1983.

262. Scott DF. The use of EEG in pseudoseizures. In ref. 260: 113–121.

263. Feldman RG, Paul NL, Cummins-Ducharme J. Videotape recording in epilepsy and pseudoseizures. In ref. 260: 122–31.

264. Desai BT. Video-telemetry in the diagnosis of psychogenic seizures. In ref. 261: 49–58.

265. Ramani SV, Quesney LF, Olson D, Gumnit RJ. Diagnosis of hysterical seizures in epileptic patients. Am J Psychiatry 1980; 137: 705–9.

Chapter 14

1. Hesse H. Siddhartha. New York: New Directions Publishing Corp., 1957: 113.

2. Bird B. Talking with patients. 2nd ed. Philadelphia: J.B. Lippincott Co., 1973.

3. Blacklow RS. The study of symptoms. In Blacklow RS. MacBryde's signs and symptoms. Applied pathologic physiology and clinical interpretation. 6th ed. Philadelphia: J.B. Lippincott Co., 1983: 1–16.

4. Cassell EJ. Talking with patients. Vol. 1: The theory of doctor-patient communication. Vol. 2: Clinical technique. Cambridge, MA: The MIT Press, 1985.

5. Cohen-Cole SA. The medical interview. The three-function approach. St. Louis: Mosby Year Book, 1991.

6. Coulehan JL, Block MR. The medical interview: a primer for students of the art. 2nd ed. Philadelphia: F.A. Davis Co., 1992.

7. Enelow AJ, Swisher SN. Interviewing and patient care. 3rd ed. New York: Oxford University Press, 1986.

8. Engel GL, Morgan WL Jr. Interviewing the patient. London: W.B. Saunders Co. Ltd., 1973.

9. Morgan WL Jr, Engel GL. The clinical approach to the patient. Philadelphia: W.B. Saunders Co., 1969: 1–79.

10. Green M. The pediatric interview and history. In Green M, Haggerty RJ. Ambulatory pediatrics IV. (4th ed.) Philadelphia: W.B. Saunders Co., 1984: 578–92.

11. Ivey AE, Authier J. Microcounseling. Innovations in interviewing, counseling, psychotherapy, and psychoeducation. 2nd ed. Springfield: Charles C. Thomas.

12. Lipkin M Jr. The medical interview and related skills. In: Branch WT Jr, ed. Office practice of medicine. 2nd ed. Philadelphia: W.B. Saunders Co., 1987: 1287–1306.

13. Reiser DE, Schroder AK. Patient interviewing. The human dimension. Baltimore: Williams & Wilkins, 1980.

14. Reik T. Listening with the third ear. New York: Farrar, Straus and Co., 1948: 131–156.

15. Creative listening. This descriptive phrase was suggested by a friend and patient, Phyllis Hogan.

16. Wakefield JS, Yarnall SR. The history database. Computer-processed and other medical questionnaires. Seattle: Medical Computer Services Association, 1975.

17. Inui TS, Jared RA, Carter WB, et al. Effects of a self-administered health history on new-patient visits in a general medical clinic. Med Care 1979; 27: 1221–8.

18. McDowell I, Newell C. Measuring health: a guide to rating scales and questionnaires. New York: Oxford University Press, 1987.

19. You and Your Health.© Health History Questionnaire.© Patient Data Base System.© Miller Communications Inc., Libertyville, IL.

20. Goldberg DP. The detection of psychiatric illness by questionnaire. A technique for the identification and assessment of non-psychotic psychiatric illness. London: Oxford University Press, 1972.

21. Goldberg DP, Blackwell B. Psychiatric illness in general practice. A detailed study using a new method of case identification. Br Med J 1970; 2: 439–43.

22. Goldberg DP, Hillier VF. A scaled version of the General Health Questionnaire. Psychol Med 1979; 9: 139–45.

23. Tennant C. The General Health Questionnaire: a valid index of psychological impairment in Australian populations. Med J Aust 1977; 2: 392–4.

24. Beck AT, Ward CH, Mendelson M, Mock J, Erbaugh J. An inventory for measuring depression. Arch Gen Psychiatry 1961; 4: 561–71.

25. Zung WWK. A self-rating depression scale. Arch Gen Psychiatry 1965; 12: 63–70.

26. Burns DD. The feeling good handbook. Using the new mood therapy in everyday life. New York: William Morrow and Co., Inc., 1989: 36–42.

27. Salkind MR. Beck Depression Inventory in general practice. J R Coll Gen Pract 1969; 18: 267–71.

28. Beck AT, Beck RW. Screening depressed patients in family practice. A rapid technic. Postgrad Med 1972; 52: 81–85.

29. Nielsen AC III, Williams TA. Depression in ambulatory medical patients. Prevalence by self-report questionnaire and recognition by nonpsychiatric physicians. Arch Gen Psychiatry 1980; 37: 999–1004.

30. Zung WWK. A rating instrument for anxiety disorders. Psychosomatics 1971; 12: 371–9.

31. Ref. 26: 32–35.

Chapter 15

1. McWhinney IR. Beyond diagnosis. An approach to the integration of behavioral science and clinical medicine. N Engl J Med 1972; 287: 384–7.

2. Magraw RM. The patient's presenting complaint—signpost or goal? I. Philosophical considerations. Minnesota University Hospital Bulletin 1958; 29: 329–36.

3. Stimson GV. Doctor-patient interaction and some problems for prescribing. J R Coll Gen Pract 1976; 26 (Supplement 1): 88–96.

4. Cartwright A. Patients and their doctors. London: Routledge and Kegan Paul, 1967: 28, 119, 126–7.

5. Packard RC. What does the headache patient want? Headache 1979; 19: 370–4.

6. Wartman SA, Morlock LL, Malitz FE, Palm E. Do prescriptions adversely affect doctor-patient interactions? Am J Public Health 1981; 71: 1358–61.

7. Mellinger GD, Balter MB, Manheimer DI, Cisin IH, Parry HJ. Psychic distress, life crisis, and use of psychotherapeutic medications. National household survey data. Arch Gen Psychiatry 1978; 35: 1045–52.

8. Parish PA. Sociology of prescribing. Br Med Bull 1974; 30: 214–7.

9. Stoeckle JD, Zola IK, Davidson GE. The quantity and significance of psychological

distress in medical patients. Some preliminary observations about the decision to seek medical aid. J Chronic Dis 1964; 17: 959–970.

10. Parsons T. The social system. Glencoe: The Free Press, 1951: 433–47.
11. Mechanic D, Volkart E. Stress, illness behavior and the sick role. Am Sociol Rev 1961; 26: 51–8.
12. Stoeckle JD, Zola IK, Davidson GE. On going to see the doctor, the contributions of the patient to the decision to seek medical aid. J Chronic Dis 1963; 16: 975–89.
13. Mechanic D. Discussion of research programs on relations between stressful life events and episodes of physical illness. In: Dohrenwend BS, Dohrenwend BP, eds. Stressful life events. Their nature and effects. New York: John Wiley & Sons, 1974: 87–97.
14. Calkins DR, Rubenstein LV, Cleary PD, et al. Failure of physicians to recognize functional disability in ambulatory patients. Ann Intern Med 1991; 114: 451–4.
15. Berlin EA, Fowkes WC Jr. A teaching framework for cross-cultural health care. Application in family practice. West J Med 1983; 139: 934–8.

Chapter 16

1. Balint M. The doctor, his patient and the illness. 2nd ed. New York: International Universities Press, Inc., 1964: 21–68.
2. Torrey EF. The mind game. Witch doctors and psychiatrists. New York: Bantam Books, 1973: 15–33.

Chapter 17

1. Reiser DE, Schroder AK. Patient interviewing. The human dimension. Baltimore: Williams & Wilkins, 1980.
2. Green M. The pediatric interview and history. In: Green M, Haggerty RJ. Ambulatory pediatrics IV. (4th. ed.) Philadelphia: W.B. Saunders Co., 1984: 578–92.
3. McWhinney IR. Beyond diagnosis. An approach to the integration of behavioral science and clinical medicine. N Engl J Med 1972; 287: 384–7.
4. Ireton HR, Cassata D. A psychological systems review. J Fam Pract 1976; 3: 155–9.
5. Osler W. Aequanimitas. 3rd. ed. Philadelphia: The Blakiston Co., 1932: 368–9.
6. Kirsner JB. Clinical challenge of functional gastrointestinal disorders. Postgrad Med 1966; 39: 565–75.
7. Allan FN, Kaufman M. Nervous factors in general practice. JAMA 1948; 138: 1135–8.
8. Vaillant GE. Adaptation to life. Boston: Little, Brown and Co., 1977.
9. Neinstein LS, Stewart DC. Adolescent health care. A practical guide. Baltimore-Munich: Urban & Schwarzenberg, 1984.
10. Litt IF. Evaluation of the adolescent patient. Philadelphia: Hanley & Belfus, Inc., Mosby Year Books, 1990.
11. Erikson EH. Identity and the life cycle. New York: International Universities Press, Inc., 1959.
12. Sheehy G. Passages. Predictable crises of adult life. New York: E. P. Dutton & Co., Inc., 1976.
13. Ambron SR, Brodzinsky D. Lifespan human development. 2nd. ed. New York: Holt Rinehart and Winston, 1982.
14. Viorst J. Necessary losses. The loves, illusions, dependencies and impossible expecta-

tions that all of us have to give up in order to grow. New York: Simon and Schuster, 1986.

15. Holmes TH, Rahe RH. The social readjustment rating scale. J Psychosom Res 1967; 11: 213–8.

16. Cohen F. Stress and bodily illness. Psychiatr Clin North Am 1981; 4: 269–86.

17. Walker EA, Katon WJ. Psychological factors affecting physical conditions and responses to stress. In: Stoudemire A, ed. Clinical psychiatry for medical students. Philadelphia: J.B. Lippincott Co., 1990: 295–314.

18. Grinker RR, Spiegel JP. Men under stress. Philadelphia: Blakiston, 1945.

19. Selye H. Stress. Montreal: Acta, Inc., 1950: 27–51.

20. American Psychiatric Association. Diagnostic and statistical manual of mental disorders, third edition, revised (DSM-III-R). Washington, DC: APA, 1987: 11, 18–20, 359–62.

21. Friedman M, Rosenman RH. Type A behavior and your heart. New York: Knopf, 1974.

22. Rhoads JM. Overwork. JAMA 1977; 237: 2615–8.

23. Pelletier KR. Holistic medicine. From stress to optimum health. New York: Delacorte Press/Seymour Lawrence, 1979.

24. Schaef AW. Co-dependence. Misunderstood—mistreated. San Francisco: Harper & Row, 1986.

25. Wiens A, Brazman R. A rationale and method for the sexual history in family practice. J Fam Pract 1977; 5: 213–5.

26. Committee On Psychosocial Aspects Of Child And Family Health, American Academy Of Pediatrics. Guidelines for health supervision: II. (2nd ed.) Elk Grove Village, IL: American Academy of Pediatrics, 1988.

27. Yudkin S. Six children with coughs. The second diagnosis. Lancet 1961; 2: 561–3.

28. Prugh DG. The psychosocial aspects of pediatrics. Philadelphia: Lea & Febiger, 1983.

29. Green M, Haggerty RJ. Ambulatory pediatrics IV. (4th ed.) Philadelphia: W.B. Saunders Co., 1990.

30. Ref. 28: 87–91.

31. Green M, Haggerty RJ. Ambulatory pediatrics III. (3rd. ed.) Philadelphia: W.B. Saunders Co., 1984: 227–8.

32. Kempe CH, Silverman FN, Steele BF, Droegemueller W, Silver HK. The battered-child syndrome. JAMA 1962; 181: 17–24.

33. Helfer RE, Kempe RS, eds. The battered child. 4th. ed., revised and expanded. Chicago: The University of Chicago Press, 1987.

34. Russell DEH. The incidence and prevalence of intrafamilial and extrafamilial sexual abuse of female children. Child Abuse Negl 1983; 7: 133–146.

35. Russell DEH. The secret trauma: incest in the lives of girls and women. New York: Basic Books, 1986.

36. Finkelhor D, Hotaling G, Lewis IA, Smith C. Sexual abuse in a national survey of adult men and women: prevalence, characteristics, and risk factors. Child Abuse Negl 1990; 14: 19–28.

37. Kempe CH. Sexual abuse, another hidden pediatric problem. Pediatrics 1978; 62: 382–9.

38. National Center for the Prevention and Treatment of Child Abuse and Neglect, Denver, CO. Guidelines for the hospital and clinic management of child abuse and neglect. Washington, DC: DHEW Publication no. (OHDS) 79-30167, 1978.

39. Bentovim A, Elton A, Hildebrand J, Tranter M, Vizard E, eds. Child sexual abuse within the family: assessment and treatment. London: Wright, 1988.

40. Walker CE, Bonner BL, Kaufman KL. The physically and sexually abused child. Evaluation and treatment. New York: Pergamon Press, 1988.

41. Pediatr Clin North Am 1990; 37: 943–1011. This entire issue is about child abuse. See papers of Newberger EH, Alexander RC, Dubowitz H, and Krugman RD.

42. Freud S. The aetiology of hysteria (1896). In Jones E, ed. Collected papers. Vol. 1, 2nd. ed. London: Hogarth Press, 1940: 183–219.

43. Carmen E(H), Rieker PP, Mills T. Victims of violence and psychiatric illness. Am J Psychiatry 1984; 141: 378–83.

44. Browne A, Finkelhor D. Initial and long-term effects: a review of the research. In: Finkelhor D, Araji S, Baron L, Browne A, Peters SD, Wyatt GE. A source book on child sexual abuse. Beverly Hills, CA: Sage Pubs., 1986: 143–79.

45. Bryer JB, Nelson BA, Miller JB, Krol PA. Childhood sexual and physical abuse as factors in adult psychiatric illness. Am J Psychiatry 1987; 144: 1426–30.

46. Domino JV, Haber JD. Prior physical and sexual abuse in women with chronic headache: clinical correlates. Headaches 1987; 27: 310–4.

47. Bachmann GA, Moeller TP, Benett J. Childhood sexual abuse and the consequences in adult women. Obstet Gynecol 1988; 71: 631–42.

48. Morrison J. Childhood sexual histories of women with somatization disorder. Am J Psychiatry 1989; 146: 239–41.

49. Drossman DA, Leserman J, Nachman G, et al. Sexual and physical abuse in women with functional or organic gastrointestinal disorders. Ann Intern Med 1990; 113: 829–33.

50. Hurley DL. Women, alcohol and incest: an analytical review. J Stud Alcohol 1991; 52: 253–68.

51. Harrop-Griffiths J, Katon W, Walker E, Holm L, Russo J, Hickok L. The association between chronic pelvic pain, psychiatric diagnoses, and childhood sexual abuse. Obstet Gynecol 1988; 71: 589–94.

52. Reiter RC, Gambone JC. Demographic and historic variables in women with idiopathic chronic pelvic pain. Obstet Gynecol 1990; 75: 428–32.

53. Gross RJ, Doerr H, Caldirola D, Guzinski GM, Ripley HS. Borderline syndrome and incest in chronic pelvic pain patients. Int J Psychiatry Med 1980/81; 10: 79–86.

54. Wood DP, Wiesner MG, Reiter RC. Psychogenic chronic pelvic pain: diagnosis and management. Clin Obstet Gynecol 1990; 33: 179–95.

55. Rapkin AJ, Kames LD, Darke LL, Stampler FM, Naliboff BD. History of physical and sexual abuse in women with chronic pelvic pain. Obstet Gynecol 1990; 76: 92–6.

56. Ref. 40: 111–4.

57. Finkelhor D, Browne A. Initial and long-term effects: a conceptual framework. In: same source as ref. 44: 180–98.

58. Goldberg WG, Tomlanovich MC. Domestic violence victims in the emergency department. New findings. JAMA 1984; 251: 3259–64.

59. Burge SK. Violence against women as a health care issue. Fam Med 1989; 21: 368–73.

60. Randall T. Domestic violence intervention calls for more than treating injuries. JAMA 1990; 264: 939–40; Domestic violence begets other problems of which physicians must be aware to be effective. Ibid: 940–4.

61. Stark E, Flitcraft A, Zuckerman D, Grey A, Robison J, Frazier W. Wife abuse in the

medical setting. An introduction for health personnel. Rockville, MD: National Clearinghouse on Domestic Violence Monograph Series #7, 1981.

62. Russell DEH. Rape in marriage. Expanded and revised edition with a new introduction. Bloomington, IN: Indiana University Press, 1990.

63. Jaffe P, Wolfe DA, Wilson S, Zak L. Emotional and physical health problems of battered women. Can J Psychiatry 1986; 31: 625–9.

64. Kerouac S, Taggart ME, Lescop J, Fortin MF. Dimensions of health in violent families. Health Care Women Int 1986; 7: 413–26.

65. Haber JD, Roos C. Effects of spouse abuse and/or sexual abuse in the development and maintenance of chronic pain in women. Advances in pain research and therapy 1985; 9: 889–95.

66. McLeer SV, Anwar RAH, Herman S, Maquiling K. Education is not enough: a systems failure in protecting battered women. Ann Emerg Med 1987; 18: 651–3.

67. Warshaw C. Limitations of the medical model in the care of battered women. Gender and Society 1989; 3: 506–17.

68. Mehta P, Dandrea LA. The battered woman. Am Fam Physician 1988; 37: 193–9.

69. Candib LM. Violence against women: no more excuses. Fam Med 1989; 21: 339–42.

70. Giarretto H. Integrated treatment of child sexual abuse. A treatment and training manual. Palo Alto: Science and Behavior Books, Inc., 1982.

71. Klerman GL, Izen JE. The effects of bereavement and grief on physical health and general well-being. Adv. Psychosom Med 1977; 9: 63–104.

72. Lindemann E. Symptomatology and management of acute grief. Am J Psychiatry 1944; 101: 141–8.

73. Parkes CM. The first year of bereavement. A longitudinal study of the reaction of London widows to the death of their husbands. Psychiatry 1970; 33: 444–67.

74. Maddison D, Viola A. The health of widows in the year following bereavement. J Psychosom Res 1968; 12: 297–306.

75. Clayton P, Desmarais L, Winokur G. A study of normal bereavement. Am J Psychiatry 1968; 125: 168–78.

76. Engel GL. Is grief a disease? A challenge for medical research. Psychosom Med 1961; 23: 18–22.

77. Paykel ES, Meyers JK, Dienelt MN, Klerman GL, Lindenthal JS, Pepper MP. Life events and depression. A controlled study. Arch Gen Psychiatry 1969; 21: 753–60.

78. Ref. 20: 353–4.

79. Frager R, Fadiman J. Personality and personal growth. 2nd. ed. New York: Harper & Row, 1984: Body-oriented systems of growth, 193–214.

80. Perls F, Hefferline RF, Goodman P. Gestalt therapy. Excitement and growth in the human personality. New York: Dell Pub. Co., Inc., 1951: 82–105.

81. Lowen A. Bioenergetics. New York: Penguin Books, 1975.

82. Rubenfeld I. Beginner's hands: twenty-five years of simple. Rubenfeld synergy—the birth of a therapy. Somatics 1988; 6, Spring/Summer: 4–12.

83. Brooks CVW. Sensory awareness. Rediscovery of experiencing through the workshops of Charlotte Selver. 3rd ed. Great Neck, NY: Felix Morrow, 1986.

84. Neugarten BL, ed. Middle age and aging. A reader in social psychology. Chicago: University of Chicago Press, 1968.

85. Kimmel DC. Adulthood and aging. An interdisciplinary developmental view. 2nd. ed. New York: John Wiley & Sons, 1980.

86. Frankl VE. The will to meaning. Foundations and applications of logotherapy. New York: The World Pub. Co., 1969.
87. Yalom ID. Existential psychotherapy. New York: Basic Books, 1980: 419–83.
88. Jung CG. The practice of psychotherapy. The collected works of C. G. Jung, Bollingen Series XX, Vol. 16. New York: Pantheon Books, 1954: 41.
89. James M, James J. Passion for life. Psychology and the human spirit. New York: Dutton, 1991: 79.

Chapter 18

1. Membership Directory. Cupertino: Santa Clara Valley Chapter, California Association of Marriage and Family Therapists, 1993.
2. Maruta T, Swanson DW, McHardy MJ. Three year follow-up of patients with chronic pain who were treated in a multidisciplinary pain management center. Pain 1990; 41: 47–53.
3. Peters JL, Large RG. A randomized control trial evaluating in- and outpatient pain management programmes. Pain 1990; 41: 283–93.
4. Kames LD, Rapkin AJ, Naliboff BD, Afifi S, Ferrer-Brechner T. Effectiveness of an interdisciplinary pain management program for the treatment of chronic pelvic pain. Pain 1990; 41: 41–6.

Index

Abdominal pain, chronic, 60, 87, 215–20
Abuse, as factor in personal illness, 312–16.
  See also Sexual abuse; Substance abuse
Accident process, 35–36
Acupuncture, 334
Addison's disease, 245
Adhesions, diagnosis of, 91–92
Adjustment disorder: terminology and, 115;
  with depressed mood, 136, 148
Adler, Alfred, 77
Adrenergic discharge, 247–48
Age, identification of symptoms with, 90
Agoraphobia, 127
AIDS, 100
Alameda County study, 96–97
Alcoholics Anonymous, 111, 157, 334
Alcoholism, 249; concept of disease and,
  52–54; genetics and, 121–22; CAGE
  screening test and, 250–51. See also
  Drinking, excessive
Alternative healing practices, 42, 334
American Psychiatric Association (APA),
  48
Andrew T. (case study), 191–92
Anesthesias, 184–85, 251

Anginal syndrome associated with normal
  coronary arteriograms, diagnosis of,
  88–89
Angina pectoris, and psychogenic chest
  pain, 207–8
Animals, emotional behavior in, 164–66
Ann F. (case study), 70, 73, 174, 305, 318
Anorexia nervosa, 61, 104, 216
Antidepressants, 116, 138, 143; specificity of,
  147, 148–50. See also Psychopharmacology
Anxiety: as common functional disorder,
  60–61; spurious correlation between
  symptoms and diagnosis for, 87–89;
  as psychiatric diagnosis, 115–16;
  psychotropic drugs and, 116; biologic
  pathways and, 119–20; family clustering
  and, 119–20; as disease vs. emotional
  distress, 122–28; continuum of
  depression and, 145–48
Anxiolytics, 147
Aristotle, 169
Arteriosclerosis, diagnosis of, 90
Asthma, 103
Autoimmune thyroiditis, 246

Backache, chronic: comprehensive approach to, 33–37; as personal illness, 59, 61–62, 226–28; disease model diagnosis of, 63–64; spurious correlation between symptoms and diagnosis for, 86; differential diagnosis of, 223–28; treatment of, 224; common spinal abnormalities and, 224–25; neurologic deficit and, 225; disease of the spine and, 226; systemic disease and, 226; collaborative approach and, 290–91

Balint, Michael, 84, 292

Barriers to person-centered care: physician's perspective and, 151–53; patient's perspective and, 153–55; organization of medical practice and, 155–59; patient/doctor relationship and, 301–3

BDI, *see* Beck Depression Inventory

Beck, Aaron T., 142, 148

Beck Depression Inventory (BDI), 276

Behavioral model approach, 36

Belief systems, and healing, 286

Benzodiazepines, 116, 147. *See also* Psychopharmacology

Biliary colic, 218

Biological fault, and psychiatric diagnosis, 115, 118

Biopsychosocial medicine, 41

Bipolar (manic-depressive) disorder, 114–15, 119

Body work, 320–21

Bowel syndromes, *see* Gastrointestinal syndromes, functional

Brain disease, and emotional disorders, 122–28

Briquet's syndrome, *see* Somatization disorder

British Royal College of General Practitioners, Coded Classification of Disease, USA Modifications of, 65

Brooks, Charles, 321

Bulimia, 61, 104

Burns Anxiety Inventory, 276

Burns Depression Checklist, 276

Caffeine, 244–45

CAGE screening test, 250–51

California Task Force to Promote Self-Esteem and Personal and Social Responsibility, 110

Canada, Minister of National Health and Welfare for, 110

Cancer: risk factors for, 97–98; as psychosomatic disease, 104, 105–8; antecedents of, 105–6; course of, 106–8; abdominal pain and, 218

"Cancer-prone personality" hypothesis, 105–6

Care: meaning of, 43–44; concept of, and personal illness, 67–80. *See also* Barriers to person-centered care; Person-centered care

Case studies: Marjorie L., 9f; Joseph H., 10–15, 90, 133, 249, 264, 289, 304f, 317, 322; Ruth B., 15–18, 23, 43, 90, 179, 189, 194, 196, 200, 304f, 325; Janet F., 18–21, 23, 28, 91, 189, 202, 294, 304f; Robert B., 24–25, 28; George B., 35–37, 43, 179, 185–96 *passim*, 284, 325; Orvieta T., 38–40, 76, 128, 130, 159, 273, 289, 304, 328; Mary S., 48–49, 59, 102, 164, 174, 181, 248, 289, 295, 304f; Sarah T., 56; Walter G., 56–57; Ann F., 70, 73, 174, 305, 318; Jean G., 73–76, 305, 321–28 *passim*, 332; Evelyn C., 168–77 *passim*, 194, 206, 214f, 304f, 318f, 325; Seymour, 169; Irene F., 174, 206, 214f, 221; Martha O., 187; Richard D., 188, 227; Andrew T., 191–92; Mario L., 201–2, 215, 299; Rosetta C., 221, 271–72, 273; Cynthia S., 263, 273; Diane B., 266–67, 304; Daphne G., 269–70, 332; John T., 273; Roger H., 281–82; Marie Louise H., 319

Case Western Reserve University School of Medicine (Ohio), 3

Centers for Disease Control (CDC), 231–33

Cerebral hemispheres, and cognitive/emotional dissociation, 170–72

CFS, *see* Chronic fatigue syndrome

Change model, 41–42

Characterologic depression, 137, 148

Chest pain, chronic: as common functional disorder, 59; disease and, 59, 88–89; nonischemic, 88, 127–28, 208f; spurious correlation between symptoms and diagnosis for, 88–89; panic disorder and, 127–28; differential diagnosis of, 205–15; angina pectoris and, 207–8; noncoronary causes of, 209–12; with negative arteriograms, 210; chest wall syndrome and, 212–13; diagnostic process for, 213–15

Chest tension syndrome, 214–15

Chest wall syndrome, 212–13

Chief complaint, in medical history, 263, 268

Children: problems of, 311–12; abuse of, 312–14

Chiropractic, 334

Cholesterol level, and coronary disease, 97, 99

Chronic fatigue syndrome (CFS), 228; problems with concept of, 231–35; functional nature of, 232–33; psychogenic fatigue and, 293

Chronic pain syndromes, 60, 190, 333–34. *See also* Abdominal pain, chronic; Backache, chronic; Chest pain, chronic; Chronic fatigue syndrome; Diffuse pain, chronic; Fatigue, chronic; Pelvic pain in women, chronic

Cirrhosis of the liver, 104

"Clinical ecology," 93

Clinical judgment, 32–33; chronic backache and, 33–37; medical history in perspective and, 271–74, 276–77; positive explanation of personal illness and, 291. *See also* Diagnosis

Co-dependency, 318, 325

Cognitive/emotional dissociation: as cause of clinical symptoms, 168–70; major vs. minor hemisphere and, 170–72; effects of, 172–73; dilemmas posed by functional disorders and, 173–76; personality integration and, 176–78; patient/doctor interaction and, 193–95; split personality of patient and, 193–95

Collaboration: vs. treatment, 31–33, 34; understanding and, 40–41; personal growth and, 74–77; cancer survival and, 108; treatment of backache and, 224, 226–28; medical history and, 260–61; communication in personal illness and,

287–300; naming the illness and, 291–95; workup and, 295–96; patient resistance and, 296–300; pharmacotherapy and, 328–30. *See also* Patient/doctor relationship; Personal interview; Personal responsibility

Communication, 167, 287–300. *See also* Collaboration; Patient/doctor relationship; Personal interview

Comprehensive approach: diagnosis and, 12–15, 28–30; doctor's diagram and, 31–38; caring and, 43–44; psychiatric diagnosis and, 116. *See also* Clinical judgment; Collaboration; Patient visits, concerns in; Person-centered care

Consciousness, substance abuse and, 53–54

Conventional disease model, 36

Conversion, process of, 182, 187–88; as communication, 191–92; as unwitting drama, 192–93; doctor's responses and, 195; effectiveness of, 196–97; as monosymptomatic, 197. *See also* Somatoform disorder

Conversion disorder, 182. *See also* Somatoform disorder

Coronary artery disease: risk factors for, 97–98; psychogenic chest pain and, 208–9

Cost of medical care, 94, 155–59

Covert issues: symptoms and, 278–79; common, 279–83; secondary gain and, 283–86; alternate belief systems and, 286

Cure vs. healing, 31–33, 34

Cushing's syndrome, 245

Cyclothymia, 115

Cynthia S. (case study), 263, 273

Daphne G. (case study), 269–70, 332

Darwin, Charles, 165

Death, 49–50. *See also* Mortality rate

Denial, and concept of conversion, 188

Depression: disease concept and, 54–55, 135–50; as common functional disorder, 60–61; biomedical model and, 114–15, 120; as psychiatric diagnosis, 115–16; biology of, 119–20, 138–41; temperament and, 121f; genetic factors and, 135–36, 137–38; spectrum of symptoms in, 136–

38, 148; anxiety and, 137, 145–48; HPA response and, 139; psychobiological unit and, 140; psychological basis of, 141–43; psychotherapy and, 143–44; endogenous, 144–45; pharmacotherapy and, 148–50
Depressive neurosis (dysthymia), 115, 136–37
Diagnosis: analytic process in, 10, 273–74; problems in, 10–12, 81–97; obscure diseases and, 13, 18, 82; role of workup in, 14; for pelvic pain in women, 18–23; naming vs. understanding and, 20–21; doctor's diagram and, 31–38; vs. clinical judgment, 32–34; clinician's point of view and, 63–65; categories in, and common functional disorders, 65–66; in psychiatry, 113–14, 128–34; of somatoform pain disorder, 188–90; overview of chronic chest pain and, 213–15; in medical history, 272–73. *See also* Clinical judgment; Comprehensive approach; Diagnostic practice; Differential diagnosis
Diagnostic and Statistical Manual of Mental Disorders, 48; terminology in, 68, 145, 181–82; classification in, 114, 117, 129f, 145; symptoms and, 114, 131; depression and, 228–29
Diagnostic practice: strategies with unrecognized personal illness and, 81–95; problem of nondiagnosis and, 82–84; spurious correlation between symptoms and diagnosis and, 85–92; disease terminology used for functional disorders and, 92–93
Diane B. (case study), 266–67, 304
Differential diagnosis, 58; diseases with symptoms similar to functional disorders and, 61–66; of chest pain, 205–15; of chronic abdominal pain, 215–20; of chronic pelvic pain, 220–23; of backache, 223–28; of chronic fatigue, 228–35; of chronic diffuse pain, 235–41
Diffuse pain, chronic: as common functional disorder, 60; disease terminology and, 93; differential

diagnosis of, 235–41. *See also* Fibromyalgia
Disability, and secondary gains, 285–86
Disease, concept of: as pathological reality vs. conceptual model, 46; as specific etiology, 46–47; as structural disturbance, 47–52; as question of control over pathogenic forces, 52–54; treatability and, 54–55; systems view of the ill person and, 55–57; depression and, 135–50; medical history and, 258–59
Disease, organic: distinguished from illness, 9–10; distinguished from disorder, 10; diagnosis of, and bypass of human situation, 24–28; multiple causal factors and, 27–28; personal effects of, 28; doctor's diagram and, 31–38; human situations in development of, 49–50, 100–108; source vs. consequences of, 50; stress and, 101–4; demands of, as barrier to person-centered care, 151–52; response to, and psychosocial state, 233–34. *See also* Differential diagnosis; *specific diseases*
Disorder: distinguished from disease, 10; functional, defined, 10; psychological, defined, 10. *See also* Functional disorder
Diverticulosis, 87, 220
Dizziness: case studies involving, 9, 10–12, 24; organic bases for, 9, 13; emotional aspects of, 11–12, 13
Doctor's diagram, 31–38
Domestic violence, 314f
Drinking, excessive: mortality rates and, 99; psychosomatic disease and, 104; differential diagnosis and, 249–51; personal interview and, 310. *See also* Alcoholism
Drug dependency: concept of disease and, 53; nervous tension and, 244–45; CAGE screening test and, 251; covert issues in patient visit and, 283; treatment of pain syndromes and, 333; referral and, 334
Drugs, *see* Drug dependency; Prescriptions; Psychopharmacology
Duodenal ulcer, 103

Dyspepsia, 51, 60, 86, 217–18
Dysthymia (depressive neurosis), 115, 136–37

Eating disturbances, 61, 104, 216
EBV, *see* Epstein-Barr virus
Eddy, Mary Baker, 100
Education model, 41–42
Emotional distress: as common functional
    disorder, 60–61, 112–13; diagnostic
    terminology and, 115–16; biochemical
    fault and, 118; physiological variation in
    reactivity and, 118; life situation and,
    119f, 121–22; as psychogenic disorder,
    120, 127–28; temperament and, 121–22;
    depression as type of, 138. *See also*
    specific psychiatric disorders
Emotionally induced symptoms, 179–203;
    patients' descriptions of, 197–201;
    spectrum of patients with, 201–3.
    See also Psychogenic pain; Psycho-
    physiologic reaction; Somatoform
    disorder
Emotions: blocking of expression of, 48–
    49; concept of disease and, 54; human
    needs and, 70, 73; physical definition of,
    141; vagaries of, and person-centered
    care, 152; evolutionary function of, 163f;
    animal behavior and, 164–66; human
    behavior and, 166–68; cognitive mind
    and, 171–72; medical history taking and,
    269–71; contained, as factor in personal
    illness, 317–21. *See also* Cognitive/
    emotional dissociation; Psychogenic
    pain
Endocrine disorder, 245–47
Endogenous, as term, 83–84, 144–45
Endometriosis, diagnosis of, 90–92
Engel, George L., 29, 41, 261
Epigastric distress, 25–26, 86, 217–18
Epilepsy, and pseudoseizures, 93, 251–53
Epstein-Barr virus (EBV), 231
Erikson, Erik H., 306, 322
Esophageal pain, 210–11
Etiology of illness vs. disease, 49–50.
    See also Unknown etiology
Evelyn C. (case study), 168–77 *passim*, 194,
    206, 214f, 304f, 318f, 325

"Evolutional melancholia," 136
Exercise, 97
Exhaustion syndrome, 307–9

Family clustering: psychosocial distress
    and, 119–20; problem drinking and, 249,
    251
Family life: health and, 71, 109–10;
    interpersonal conflict and, 309–12;
    abuse and, 312–16; joint interview and,
    324–26
Fatigue, chronic: psychogenic, 61, 230–31;
    spurious correlation between symptoms
    and diagnosis for, 89; differential
    diagnosis of, 228–35; naming of illness
    and, 293; exhaustion syndrome and,
    307–9; personal fulfillment and, 323–24.
    See also Chronic fatigue syndrome
Feelings, and medical history taking, 263–
    64. *See also* Emotions
Fibromyalgia: Lyme disease and, 235–37;
    nature of, 237–38; physical basis of, 238–
    40; secondary, 239; psychosocial basis of,
    240–41
Figure/ground concept, 177, 188
Frankl, Victor, 176, 322
Freud, Sigmund, 142, 167, 169, 171, 176–77,
    194, 313
Frontal lobe lesions, 247
Functional disorder: defined, 10; diagnostic
    problems and, 14, 23–24, 50–52;
    understanding and, 15; structural
    disturbance and, 47–52, 55–57;
    physiological disorder as form of, 58;
    examples of, with physical symptoms,
    59–60; examples of, with emotional
    symptoms, 60–61; incidence of, 61–63;
    diseases causing similar symptoms and,
    61–66; dilemma of, and cognitive/
    emotional dissociation, 173–76;
    symptoms of, 179–80, 202–3. *See also*
    Differential diagnosis; Human situation;
    Personal illness; Somatoform disorder
Functional overlay, as term, 83–84

Galen, 105
Gallstones, 86

Gastrointestinal syndromes, functional, 60
Gender: identification of symptoms with, 90; emotional distress and, 121–22; types of functional disorders and, 185; diagnosis of coronary disease and, 209
General Health Questionnaire, 275–76
Genetic factors, 117–22, 135–36, 137–38
George B. (case study), 35–37, 43, 179, 185–96 *passim*, 284, 325
Graves' disease, 104
Grief, 316–17
Growth model, 41–42, 77–80. *See also* Personal growth
Gynecology, 21–23. *See also* Pelvic pain in women, chronic; Surgery

Harmful practices, *see* Alcoholism; Drinking, excessive; Drug dependency; Life expectancy; Smoking
Headache, 59, 61–62, 73–77, 241–44. *See also* Migraine; Tension headache
Healing: vs. cure, 31–33, 34; clinical judgment and, 37; person-centered care and, 42–43; learning and, 75–76, 77; change in life situation and, 104; health practices and, 109; alternate belief systems and, 286
Health: vs. sickness, emphasis on, 31–33, 35, 37; systems analysis and, 56; definition of, 108–9; preventable disease and, 109; family life and, 109–10
Health Care of Women (Martin), 22
Health-care system, costs in, 155–59
Health-history questionnaires, 274–77
Health practices, 109, 309; life expectancy and, 96–100
Heartburn, 86, 210–11
Heschel, Abraham J., 70
Hesse, Hermann, *Siddhartha*, 257f
Hiatal hernia, 25–26, 86–87, 218
Hidden agenda, *see* Covert issues
Hilgard, Ernest R., 167, 171, 193, 195
Holistic medicine, 42–43
HPA response, *see* Hypothalamic-pituitary-adrenocortical response
Humanistic medicine, 41
Human needs, and concept of personal illness, 70–73

Human situation: symptoms resulting from, 10–12; illness as expression of, 12–15; medical model and, 23–28; bypass of, with diagnosis of disease, 24–28; doctor's understanding of, 38–40, 50; development of organic disease and, 49–50, 100–108; mortality rate and, 101–3; change in, and healing, 104; psychiatric diagnosis and, 113–14, 119f, 121–22, 133–34; continuum of depression and anxiety and, 145–48; identification of, 257, 303–4; common problem areas and, 306–24. *See also* Functional disorder; Personal illness
Humor, 176
Hypercortisolism, 139
Hyperdynamic beta-adrenergic circulatory state, 247–48
Hyperparathyroidism, 246–47
Hypertension, 24; multiple causal factors and, 27–28; spurious correlation between symptoms and diagnosis of, 86; coronary disease and, 97; health habits and, 99; as psychosomatic disease, 103f; chronic fatigue and, 231
Hypnotics, 116
Hypoparathyroidism, 245
Hypothalamic-pituitary-adrenocortical (HPA) response, 139
Hypothyroidism, 89, 93, 231, 245
Hysterectomy, 92
Hysteria, *see* Somatoform disorder

Iatrogenicity, 93–95
IBS, *see* Irritable-bowel syndrome
Idiopathic, as term, 83
Illness: distinguished from disease, 9–12, 31–33; as expression of human predicament, 12–15; doctor's diagram and, 31–38; medical history and, 259–60
Injury: somatoform disorder and, 186–87; secondary gains and, 284–86
Insomnia, *see* Sleep disturbance
Intermittent depressive disorder, 137
International Classification of Diseases (ICD-9-CM), 145
Interpersonal conflict: as factor in personal illness, 309–12; joint interview and, 324–25

Intracranial disease, 243–44
Irene F. (case study), 174, 206, 214f, 221
Irritable-bowel syndrome (IBS), 215, 216–17, 218–20

James, William, 77, 133, 141
Janet F. (case study), 18–21, 23, 28, 91, 189, 202, 294, 304f
Jean G. (case study), 73–76, 305, 321–28 *passim,* 332
John T. (case study), 273
Joseph H. (case study), 10–15, 90, 133, 249, 264, 289, 304f, 317, 322
Jung, Carl, 77, 322

Learning, and healing, 75–76, 77. *See also* Personal growth
LEARN model, 286
Life expectancy, 96–100
Life situation, *see* Human situation
Listening: person-centered care and, 4–5; diagnosis of illness and, 16–18; medical history and, 258–61, 265–68; creative, 265–68; nonverbal clues and, 269–71. *See also* Understanding
Loss, 316–17
Lumbosacral spine, abnormalities of, 86
Lyme disease, 235–37

Manic-depressive disorder, *see* Bipolar disorder
MAO inhibitors, *see* Monoamine oxidase inhibitors
Marie Louise H. (case study), 319
Mario L. (case study), 201–2, 215, 299
Marital discord, 309–10, 324–25. *See also* Family life
Marjorie L. (case study), 9f
Martha O. (case study), 187
Martin, Leonide, 22
Mary S. (case study), 48–49, 59, 102, 164, 174, 181, 248, 289, 295, 304f
Massachusetts General Hospital Clinic, 62
Medical care, cost of, 94, 155–59
Medical history, 257–77; listening and, 258–61, 265–68; opening questions in, 262–64; terms used by physician and, 262–64; terms used by patient and, 264–

65; emotions and, 269–71; nonverbal clues and, 269–71; clinical judgment and, 271–74, 276–77; in perspective, 271–74. *See also* Health-history questionnaires; Personal interview
Medical model: ideal, 1–2; biomedical focus in, 2–3, 15–23, 47; person-centered care and, 3–4, 152–53; limitations of, 9–30; steps in medical analysis and, 10, 28–29; mind-body split in, 15–23; naming and, 20–21; human situation as bypassed by, 23–28; biopsychosocial model and, 29–30; doctor's diagram and, 31–38; growth model and, 77–80; iatrogenicity of, 93–95; psychiatry and, 113–16, 129; covert advantages of, 152–53
Medical theory, and psychosomatic disease, 100–101
Medication, *see* Antidepressants; Prescriptions; Psychopharmacology
Menopause, 25, 90
Mental disorder, *see* Personal illness; Psychological disorder
Metabolic disorder, 245–47
Microvascular angina (MVA), 211–12
Migraine, 26, 59, 62, 241f, 244
Mind, concept of, 68
Mind/body distinction: biomedical model and, 15–23; human emotions and, 167, 169–70, 319–21
Mitral-valve prolapse, 88, 93
Monoamine oxidase (MAO) inhibitors, 141, 148f. *See also* Antidepressants
Mortality rate: health practices and, 96–100; personal situation and, 101–3
MVA, *see* Microvascular angina (MVA)

Naming, 92–93, 153, 237; understanding and, 20–21, 26; collaboration and, 291–95. *See also* Nomenclature; Terminology
Narcotics, 333
National Ambulatory Medical Care Survey, 63
Nervous tension, differential diagnosis of, 244–49
Neuroendocrine function, 122–24
Neurotransmitter systems, and depression, 140–41, 148–50

NIMH Diagnostic Interview Schedule, 129
Nomenclature, 46, 295. *See also* Naming; Terminology
Nondiagnosis, problem of, 82–84
Nonverbal clues, and medical history, 269–71

Orvieta T. (case study), 38–40, 76, 128, 130, 159, 273, 289, 304, 328
Ovarian cyst, 90
Overt myxedema, 245
Overweight, 97f

Pain: as common functional disorder, 62; nondiagnosis of, 83; emotional, relief of, 176; somatoform disorders and, 195. *See also* Diffuse pain, chronic; Psychogenic pain; *specific anatomical locations*
Pain behavior, 36, 182. *See also* Somatoform pain disorder
Pain clinics, 333–34
Pain syndromes, *see* Chronic pain syndromes
Panic disorder: biomedical model and, 114–15; biologic pathways and, 119–20; as disease vs. emotional distress, 122–28; chest pain and, 127–28; psycho-pharmacology and, 147
Parent-child interactions, 312
Patient/doctor relationship: person-centered care and, 3–5; psychiatry and, 114, 126–27; antidepressants and, 150; directed interview and, 301–3. *See also* Collaboration; Communication; Medical history; Personal interview
Patient visits, concerns in: medical history and, 263–64, 268; covert issues and, 278–86; treatment vs. understanding and, 279–80; relief vs. reassurance and, 280–81; secondary gains and, 283–86. *See also* Medical history; Personal interview
Pelvic pain in women, chronic, 18–23, 60, 90–92, 220–23, 311
Personal growth, 70–73, 74–77, 138, 321–24. *See also* Growth model
Personal illness: common examples of, 58–

66; concept of care and, 67–80; concept of, 68–69; human needs of patient and, 70–73; learning and growth in, 73–77; medical vs. growth model and, 77–80; diagnostic strategies for, 81–95; unrecognized, and diagnostic strategies, 81–95; chronic backache as, 226–28; medical history taking and, 260–61; interactions between doctor and patient about, 287–300; overtures to collaboration and, 289–91; naming and, 291–95. *See also* Functional disorder; Human situation
Personal interview: patient/doctor relationship and, 301–3; patient's personal situation and, 303–4; flow of, 304–6; common problem areas and, 306–24; joint interview and, 324–26. *See also* CAGE screening test; Medical history
Personality: cancer-prone, 105–6; psychosocial distress and, 121–22; depressive, 136–37, 148; integration of, 176–78; split, and somatoform disorders, 193–95; "fibrositic," 239; headache and, 242; dependent, 318, 322
Personal medicine, 41
Personal responsibility: treatment of alcoholism and, 52, 53–54; personal growth and, 72; health as problem of, 110–11; attraction of medical model to patient and, 153–55; back pain and, 227; interviews and, 261; pharmacotherapy and, 328–30. *See also* Collaboration
Personal situation, *see* Human situation
Person-centered care: medical model and, 3–4; distinction between disease and functional disorder and, 50; health-history questionnaire and, 274–77; role of physician in, 334–36. *See also* Barriers to person-centered care; Comprehensive approach
Pharmacotherapy, *see* Psycho-pharmacology; *specific psychoactive drugs*
Pheochromocytoma, 246
Plato, 100
PPR, *see* Psychophysiologic reaction

Premenstrual tension syndrome, 246
Prescriptions, 279–80. *See also*
Antidepressants; Psychopharmacology
Present illness, and medical history taking, 263f, 273
Pseudoseizure, 182, 184, 195, 251–53
Psychiatric disorders: genetic background of, 117–22; biologic pathways and, 118–22; temperament and, 121–22; psychobiological unit and, 128–34; sleep disturbance and, 139–40; cognitive/emotional dissociation and, 168–70; chest pain and, 214–15; chronic fatigue syndrome and, 231–32; communication and, 295
Psychiatry: cleavage between medicine and, 17, 69; medical model of, 113–16
Psychobiological unit, 128–34, 140
Psychodynamic model, 36
Psychogenic fatigue, 293. *See also* Chronic fatigue syndrome
Psychogenic pain, types of, 19–21; chronic pelvic pain in women and, 18–23; chronic backache and, 35–37. *See also* Functional disorder; Personal illness; Somatoform disorder
Psychological assessment, referral and, 330–31
Psychological disorder: defined, 10. *See also* Functional disorder; Personal illness; Psychophysiologic reaction
"Psychological factors affecting physical condition," 115
Psychopathology, as term, 176
Psychopharmacology: treatment of psychosocial distress and, 114, 116; psychiatric treatment and, 114f; emphasis on, 117; depression and, 138, 140f, 143, 147–48; anxiety and, 147–48; communication between doctor and patient and, 295; personal responsibility and, 328–30. *See also* Antidepressants; *specific psychoactive drugs*
Psychophysiologic reaction (PPR): differences between somatoform disorder and, 180–81; function of, 181; as term, 181–82; prevalence of, 183–85;

physiological pathways and, 185–88; patient's description of symptoms in, 197–201. *See also* Psychological disorder
Psychosocial distress, *see* Emotional distress
Psychosocial evaluation, 157–58. *See also* Personal interview; Referral
Psychosomatic disease, 100–101, 103–4, 105–8
Psychotherapy: concept of personal illness and, 69, 74, 76–77; depression and, 143–44, 149; referral and, 330
Pulmonary disease, 98

Rare conditions, 13, 18, 66, 236, 247, 251
Reactive hypoglycemia, 87–88
Referral: emphasis on disease vs. illness and, 37–38; nondiagnosis and, 84; barriers to person-centered care and, 157–58; directed interview and, 301–3; psychotherapy and, 330; psychological assessment and, 330–31; stress reduction and, 331–33; pain clinics and, 333–34; alternative healing practices and, 334. *See also* Support groups
Repression, 171
Reproductive tract, lesions of, 90, 91–92
Research Diagnostic Criteria, 137
Review of systems, 265, 268, 272f
Rheumatoid arthritis, 104
Richard D. (case study), 188, 227
Robert B. (case study), 24–25, 28, 85
Roger H. (case study), 281–82
Rogers, Carl, 132
Rosetta C. (case study), 221, 271–72, 273
Ruth B. (case study), 15–18, 23, 43, 90, 179, 189, 194, 196, 200, 304f, 325

Sagan, Leonard, 110
Sarah T. (case study), 56
Satir, Virginia, 132
Schizophrenia, 114–15, 119, 129f, 131–32
SD, *see* Somatoform disorder
Secondary gain, 283–86
Sedatives, 116, 138
Self-esteem, 138, 141–43. *See also* Personal growth

Selver, Charlotte, 321

Senility, diagnosis of, 90

Sex, *see* Gender; Sexual behavior; Sexual response, disturbances of

Sexual abuse: anxiety disorders and, 122, 126; of women, 313f; of children, 313–14

Sexual behavior, 100

Sexual response, disturbances of, 61, 311

Seymour (case study), 169

Shortened rapid eye movement latency (SRL), 139–40

Sickness, eradication of, vs. achievement of health, 31–33

Sleep disturbance, 61, 139–40, 239

Smoking, 98, 104, 110, 244–45

Somatization disorder, 183

Somatoform disorder (SD): as form of psychogenic pain, 19; psychosocial distress diagnosed as, 115; differences between psychophysiologic reaction and, 180–81; function of, 180–81, 191–97; as term, 182–83; types of, 182–83; prevalence of, 183–85; physiologic pathways and, 186; as communication, 191–92; conversion process in, 191–97; reality of symptoms in, 196; monosymptomatic, 197; patient's description of symptoms in, 197–201; joint interview and, 325

Somatoform pain disorder: as type of somatoform disorder, 182; frequency of, 184, 251; diagnosis of, 188–90, 272; patients' descriptions of symptoms in, 198–99; abdominal pain and, 215; fibromyalgia and, 240; communication between doctor and patient and, 294–95

SRL, *see* Shortened rapid eye movement latency

Stanford MD (journal), 64

Stead, E. A., Jr., 31

Stead's maxim, 31, 41

Stress: coronary disease and, 97; organic disease and, 101–4; biological response to, 120; depression and, 140–41; abdominal pain and, 216; headache and, 242; as factor in personal illness, 306–7; exhaustion syndrome and, 307–9; referral and, 331–33

Stress reduction program, 331–33

Stroke, 97–98, 99

Substance abuse, 52–54. *See also* Alcoholism; Drinking, excessive; Drug dependency

Support groups, 107f, 125, 156–57. *See also* Referral

Surgeon General's report on smoking, 110

Surgery, 20, 91–92, 221–23, 225

Symptoms: diagnostic problems and, 10–12, 21–23; spurious correlations with special tests and, 20; multiple, 60–61, 273–74; common, and diagnostic categories, 65–66; medical model in psychiatry and, 113–14; family clustering and, 119–20; clustering of, and psychiatric diagnosis, 128–34; classification of, in psychiatric diagnosis, 129–30; spectrum of, in depression, 136–38; cognitive/emotional dissociation as cause of, 168–70; atypical, 179–80; of conversion disorder, 182; in somatoform disorder, 196f; chronic fatigue syndrome and, 232; isolated, 248–49; medical history and, 257, 258–59, 263, 264–65, 269–74 *passim;* diagnostic terms for, 264–65, 273; nonverbal clues and, 269; covert issues and, 278–79; vs. normality standard as problem, 281–82; suppressed emotions and, 317–18. *See also* Emotionally induced symptoms

Systemic disease: chronic backache and, 226; chronic headache and, 243–44

Systems analysis, 55–57

Szasz, Thomas S., 191, 193

Teenage pregnancy, 100

Temperament, 121–22. *See also* Personality

Temporal lobe epilepsy, 247

Temporal lobe lesions, 247

Tension headache, 59, 180, 241

Terminology: concept of disease and, 46; in *Diagnostic and Statistical Manual of Mental Disorders*, 68, 145, 181–82; concept of personal illness and, 68–69; problem of nondiagnosis and, 83; in diagnostic practice, 92–93; colloquial, 93; emotional distress and, 115–16;

medical history taking and, 263–65.
See also Naming; Nomenclature
Therapeutic imperative, 154
Therapy, and nondiagnosis, 84
Thyrotoxicosis, 245
Time, as barrier to person-centered care,
155–56, 159. *See also* Cost of medical care
Training, medical, 2f, 13, 18, 22–23
Treatability, and concept of disease, 54–55
Treatment: of disease resulting from life
situation, 26–28; vs. collaboration, 31–
33, 34; psychiatric symptoms and, 114;
therapeutic imperative and, 154; of
backache, 224, 226–28; understanding
vs. medication as, 279–80. *See also*
Prescriptions
Tricyclic agents, 148–49. *See also*
Antidepressants

Ulcer, 103, 217–18
Ulcerative colitis, 103
Understanding: naming and, 20–21, 26, 69;
biological vs. personal, 32–33, 37, 38–40;
collaboration and, 40–41; patients'
concern for, 279–80; personal
responsibility and, 329. *See also* Listening

University of Rochester School of
Medicine (New York), 3
Unknown etiology, 83, 88, 205–6
Uterine fibroids, 90

Vaillant, George E., 102
Vasconcellos, John, 110

Walter G. (case study), 56–57
Weakness, chronic, 61
Weight, *see* Overweight
Weight loss, 61
Women: chronic pelvic pain in, 18–23, 60,
90–92, 220–23, 311; training in health
care of, 22; abuse of, 314f. *See also*
Gender
Workup, and collaborative approach,
295–96
World Health Organization, 108

Yalom, Irvin D., 322
"Yeast connection," 93

Zung Self-Rating Anxiety Scale, 276
Zung Self-Rating Depression Scale, 276

Library of Congress Cataloging-in-Publication Data

Barbour, Allen B., 1918–1993.
Caring for patients : a critique of the medical model / Allen B.
Barbour.
p.   cm.
Includes bibliographical references and index.
ISBN 0-8047-2389-3 (cl.) : ISBN 0-8047-3153-5 (pbk.)
1. Medicine and psychology.   2. Medical care.   3. Physician and
patient.   4. Medicine—Philosophy.   I. Title.
[DNLM: 1. Patients—psychology.   2. Professional-Patient Relation.
3. Attitude to Health.   4. Models, Psychological.   W 85 B239c 1994]
R726.5.B346   1994
610.69'6—dc20
DNLM/DLC
for Library of Congress
94-27113   CIP

This book is printed on acid-free, recycled paper.

Originally published in 1995

Printed in the USA
CPSIA information can be obtained
at www.ICGtesting.com
JSHW021437221024
72172JS00003B/34

9 780804 731539